Clerkships

The Answer Book

SAINT-FRANCES GUIDE

Clinical Clerkships

The Answer Book

Jeff Wiese, MD, FACP
Associate Professor of Medicine
Chief of Medicine, Charity and University Hospital
Associate Chairman, Department of Medicine
Program Director, Internal Medicine Training Program
Tulane University Health Sciences Center
New Orleans, Louisiana

EDITORS

Stephen Bent, MD
Assistant Professor of Medicine
Associate Director, Clinical Research Fellowship
Division of General Internal Medicine
University of California, San Francisco
San Francisco, California
Attending Physician, San Francisco VA Medical Center
San Francisco, California

Sanjay Saint, MD, MPH
Associate Professor of Internal Medicine
Director, Patient Safety Enhancement Program
University of Michigan Medical School
Research Investigator, Ann Arbor VA Medical Center
Ann Arbor, Michigan

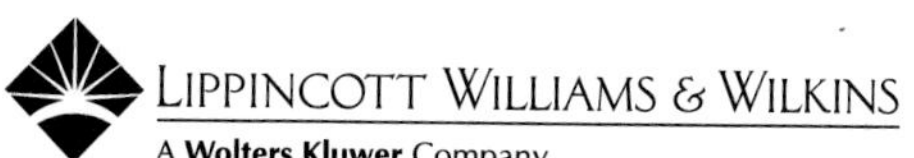
LIPPINCOTT WILLIAMS & WILKINS
A **Wolters Kluwer** Company
Philadelphia • Baltimore • New York • London
Buenos Aires • Hong Kong • Sydney • Tokyo

Acquisitions Editor: Donna Balado
Developmental Editor: Kristi Barrett
Managing Editor: Cheryl W. Stringfellow
Marketing Manager: Emilie Linkins
Production Editor: Kevin Johnson
Compositor: Maryland Composition Co., Inc.

351 West Camden Street
Baltimore, Maryland 21201-2436 USA

530 Walnut Street
Philadelphia, Pennsylvania, 19106-3621

Printed in the United States of America

Library of Congress Cataloging-in-Publication Data

Wiese, Jeff.
The answer book : the Saint-Frances guide to the clinical clerkships / Jeff Wiese, Stephen
Bent, Sanjay Saint.
p. ; cm.
Includes bibliographical references and index.
ISBN 0-7817-3754-0 (alk. paper)
1. Clinical clerkship—Handbooks, manuals, etc. 2. Clinical medicine—Handbooks, manuals, etc. 3. Diagnosis—Handbooks, manuals, etc. I. Bent, Stephen. II. Saint, Sanjay. III. Title. IV. Title: Saint-Frances guide to the clinical clerkships. II.
[DNLM: 1. Clinical Clerkship—Handbooks. 2. Clinical Medicine—Handbooks. 3. Diagnostic Techniques and Procedures—Handbooks. WB 39 W651a 2006]
R839.W57 2006
610′.71′1—dc22
2005019189

To purchase additional copies of this book, call our customer service department at (800) 638-3030 or fax orders to (301) 824-7390. For other book services, including chapter reprints and large quantity sales, ask for the Special Sales department.

For all other calls originating outside of the United States, please call (301) 714-2324.

Visit Lippincott Williams & Wilkins on the Internet: http://www.lww.com. Lippincott Williams & Wilkins customer service representatives are available from 8:30 am to 6:30 pm, EST, Monday through Friday, for telephone access.

Dedication

To my medical students and residents, past, present and future; they have taught me more than I have taught them. May they fulfill the role of the professional: to profess who they are in the practice of their art.

And to the staff of Charity Hospital, who since 1737, have not forgotten that the first principle of medicine is about service, and that providing the best possible care regardless of race, religion, or socioeconomic background is the first step to guaranteeing the dignity that every person deserves.

Jeff Wiese, MD

Contents

PART V APPROACHING THE CORE CLERKSHIPS

PART VI SELF-IMPROVEMENT STRATEGIES: MAXIMIZING YOUR POTENTIAL

APPENDICES

Contributors

Patrick Gaston
Tulane University
New Orleans, Louisiana
Original Illustrations

S. Andrew Josephson, MD
Neurovascular Fellow
Cognitive/Behavioral Fellow
Department of Neurology
University of California, San Francisco
San Francisco, California
Chapter 34: The Tier II Neurologic Examination

Allen Kachalia, MD, JD
Division of General Medicine
Brigham and Woman's Hospital
Boston, Massachusetts
Chapter 8: Financial and Legal Medicine

Jay Keyes, MD
Strong Memorial Hospital
Rochester, New York
Chapter 38: Surgery

Anda K. Kuo, MD
Assistant Clinical Professor
Director, Pediatric Leadership for the Undeserved (PLUS)
Department of Pediatrics
University of California, San Francisco
San Francisco, California
Chapter 40: Pediatrics (co-author)

Jeffrey A. Linder, MD, MPH
Instructor in Medicine
Harvard Medical School
Boston, Massachusetts
Chapter 23: The Tier I Head and Neck Examination
Chapter 29: The Tier II Head and Neck Examination

Malia McCarthy, MD
Assistant Clinical Professor
Department of Psychiatry and Behavioral Sciences
School of Medicine
University of California, Davis
Sacramento, California
Chapter 41: Psychiatry

Theodore D. Ruel, MD
Clinical Instructor
Department of Pediatrics
University of California, San Francisco
San Francisco, California
Chapter 40: Pediatrics (co-author)

Mona Saint, MD, MPH
Attending Physician
Department of Obstetrics and Gynecology
Saddleback Hospital
Laguna Hills, California
Chapter 39: Obstetrics and Gynecology

Preface: How *The Answer Book* Came to Be.

As a clerkship and residency program director, I practice medicine on the clinical wards with medical students and residents constantly at my side. A major portion of my time is spent giving advice to students as they make the transition from student to physician. This book is essentially a summation of the letters, emails and hallway advice given over the last ten years. I wrote the book because I thought it was unfair that some students were lucky in finding excellent mentors who gave them sound advice, while others were not. This is an advice book, and like all unsolicited advice, it may sound condescending at times. Please do not take it that way. You have worked hard to this point, and you deserve respect; no one should talk down to you, least of all me. Rather, see it as a series of emails or letters or brief phone calls from your *clinical coach*: someone who cares about nothing more than helping you become the best doctor you can be. Some of the advice will resonate with you, some will not. Embrace that which does, and discard the rest. The advice in this book is merely a summation of the methods, skills and qualities that I have found the greatest physicians to share. Congratulations on finishing the first phase of medical school; hopefully this book will provide you with the answers to your clerkship questions and help you in becoming a superb physician. I wish you the best.

Jeff Wiese, MD
New Orleans, Louisiana
January 2005

Acknowledgments

Jeff Wiese would like to acknowledge the personal support of those who have made this book possible: Janice Wiese, JT, Margaret and Grant Biehler, Stephanie and Paul Oseland, and Moni. And the educational support of Lawrence Tierney, Tom Evans, Kelly Skeff, Warren Browner and the faculty of The Drake University, The Johns Hopkins School of Medicine, The University of California San Francisco and The Tulane University Health Sciences Center. And finally the inspirational support of Jules Puschett, Dwayne Thomas, Ian Taylor, and E. Yorick Davis.

Stephen Bent would like to acknowledge the support of the Department of Medicine at the University of California, San Francisco, the General Internal Medicine Section at the San Francisco VA Medical Center, and the outstanding mentorship, guidance, and friendship of Andrew Avins, Deborah Grady, and Michael Shlipak. He also gives the deepest thanks to his family, Christine, Blake, and Chase, who provide unending support and love.

Sanjay Saint thanks two first-rate organizations–the Department of Veterans Affairs and the University of Michigan–for supporting his development as a faculty member, and acknowledges the superb and ongoing mentorship of Larry Tierney (aka "LT"), Larry McMahon, Rod Hayward, Steve Fihn, and Tim Hofer. He would also like to thank Veronica Saint, Sean Saint, and Kirin Saint for their love, devotion, and great senses of humor.

All of us thank Camilla Payne for her terrific and incredibly diligent work as our manuscript coordinator; the book would not have been possible without her help. We also acknowledge the assistance of all of the wonderful people at Lippincott Williams & Wilkins who helped in shepherding this book from conception to completion: Elizabeth Nieginski, Beth Goldner, Donna Balado, Emilie Linkins, and Cheryl Stringfellow.

PART I

Orientation to Clinical Medicine

1. The Purpose of *The Answer Book*

I INTRODUCTION

A. *The Answer Book* will help you make the transition from the classroom to the clinical wards more easily. This book will teach you to develop habits that will help you succeed not only as a medical student, but more importantly, as a physician. The habits you establish now will define the physician you will become.

B. One of the discriminating features of the clinical wards is that students who have the most knowledge do not always become the best physicians. Knowledge is necessary, but not sufficient. The ability to *apply* knowledge is what defines the best physicians. This book will teach you how to do that by giving you good methods. These methods will ensure that you do not succumb to common pitfalls, and that you establish good habits that will be the foundation of your lifelong success as a physician.

C. This book is not designed to give you the details of clinical medicine such as diagnostic criteria and management; for that you will need a medical reference book. See Chapter 45 for a list of high-yield books to get you started.

II CHALLENGE PRESENTED BY THE CLINICAL WARDS

There are two features of the clinical wards that make it different from the preclinical years.

A. Clinical medicine is not about how much you know. Instead, it is about:

1. **Methodically applying what you do know;**
2. **Recognizing when you do not know;** and
3. **Knowing how to find the knowledge you need.**

B. Clinical medicine is about caring for people, not diseases. Because each patient is complex, treating the same disease in two different patients can be quite different. On the same call night, you may have two patients with asthma: the first with a history of multiple intubations, and the second who has had only four mild attacks in her life. Although the pharmacology may be the same, the first patient will require greater vigilance during her hospital stay.

III Solution to the Clinical Challenge

A. **Recognize that human interactions are complex.** The quality of your medicine will be proportional to your ability to recognize and handle complex human interactions. **Expect complexity; use the strategies in this book to deal with it.**

B. **Resolve to develop methods of clinical practice.** Sound clinical methods prevent you from being deceived by complex cases. Clinical medicine requires a **methodical approach** of solving one problem at a time, beginning with the most difficult.

C. **Accept that true success is not attained quickly.**

   1. As a third- or fourth-year student, you are not expected to be a seasoned, competent physician. Your success hinges upon your ability to develop a **foundation of methods** for solving clinical problems. This book is your "clinical coach" and provides you with the methods necessary to manage the most common ward scenarios; acquiring new methods along the way will define your greatness.
   2. This book provides **strategies and methods for long-term success**. Quick-fix strategies may make you appear better in the short run, but ultimately they will put you at risk for falling into numerous pitfalls along the way. Quick-fix strategies also require energy because it takes a lot of energy to appear better than you really are. They will deprive you of the energy and focus you need to develop the methods that will help you. You will be only as good as the methods you use.

IV Supplementing Your Clinical Knowledge

A. This book is an **adjunct to the lessons you will learn from your supervisors**. It is unlikely that you will find one physician who has the time to give you the advice contained in this book. This book supplements what you learn from your attending physicians.

B. **Tacit knowledge may limit the ability of your superiors to teach you**. Tacit knowledge means knowing how to perform a task but not remembering how you learned it. Once a skill has become tacit, it is difficult to teach it to students. This is why experts in a topic can be the worst teachers and why some of your best attendings may find it hard to explain to you how they do the great things they do. This book provides insight into what has made your great role models great.

V USING *THE ANSWER BOOK*

A. This book is divided into six sections. Feel free to skip around; it is designed to be read one chapter at a time in any order, as your clinical situation requires.

B. Consult *The Answer Book* as the year progresses. Consider quickly rereading Chapters 1 to 20 after every 50 to 100 patients you see. This will reinforce your methods, making them routine. Remember Aristotle's words, "We are what we repeatedly do. Excellence then is not an act, but a habit."

2. Roles and Expectations

I Introduction

A. The first 2 years of medical school are like college. You attend lectures, read books, and take tests to prove competency. The expectations for the clinical clerkships are different. Not only must you master the knowledge necessary to diagnose and treat patients, you must also learn to assume the role of the physician. Although it seems like a distant goal, the process of deciding what type of physician you will become begins now.

B. On the road to becoming a physician are the roles of sub-intern, intern, and resident. The only way to achieve your goal is to master each role as you encounter it. You can get a head start on becoming a great intern, resident, or attending by carefully observing the team members who are in these roles and thinking about what you will emulate, and what you will discard, when it comes time for you to assume that role. As you observe your team members, remember these four principles:

1. **Medicine requires teamwork.** The entire team and its patients will suffer if team members do not fulfill their roles. Like a pyramid, the whole structure crumbles if one team member does not fulfill his role (Figure 2-1).
2. **Each team member has a role.** Each role has responsibilities that are consistent with the average person's ability at that stage of training. Although the intern's role of completing discharge paperwork is not as much fun as the resident's role of teaching the team, it is the intern's work that frees up the resident, who is then better able (based upon experience) to teach the team. This does not mean that the intern cannot also teach, but it does mean that if the resident is saddled with intern tasks, the team will suffer because resident teaching is lost. Your abilities may be greater than those of the average person at your level of training, which means you may be able to perform tasks above those of the typical student. Feel free to perform these tasks, but not at the expense of failing to perform the tasks within your role.
3. It is important that each team member master his role before moving up to the next role. A resident who has not mastered intern-level skills cannot teach future interns how to perform those skills and, in the absence of the intern, cannot step in to ensure that the intern's tasks are performed.
4. **Roles are ultimately established by the team.** This chapter is a guide to the roles of most team members. Always ask your

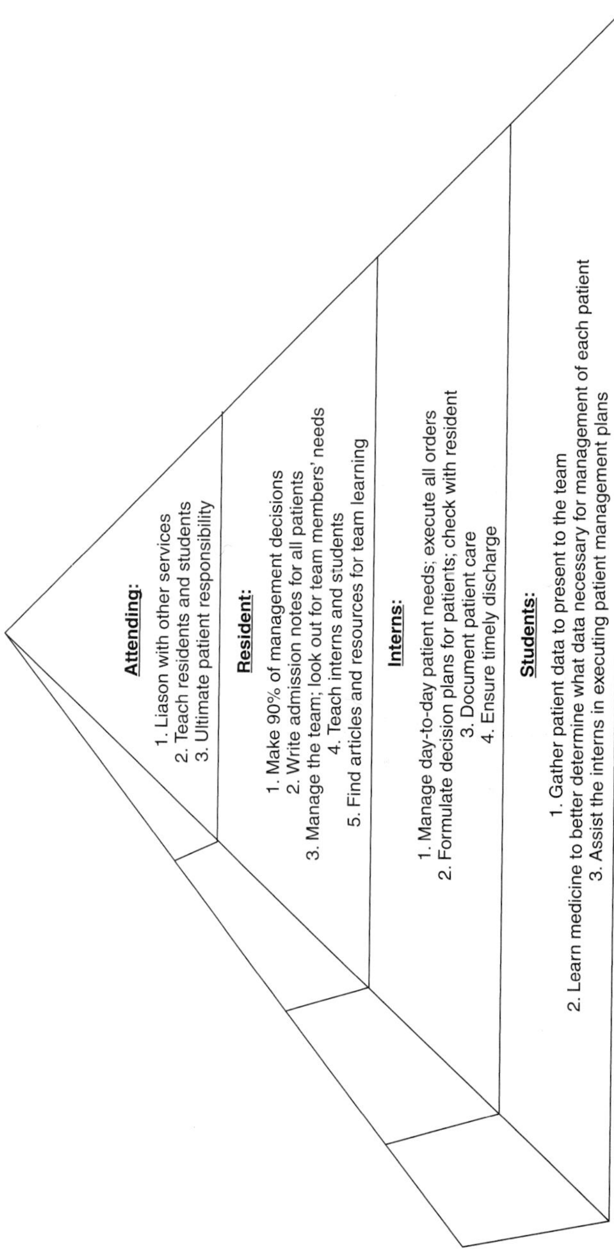
Attending:
1. Liason with other services
2. Teach residents and students
3. Ultimate patient responsibility
Resident:
1. Make 90% of management decisions
2. Write admission notes for all patients
3. Manage the team; look out for team members' needs
4. Teach interns and students
5. Find articles and resources for team learning
Interns:
1. Manage day-to-day patient needs; execute all orders
2. Formulate decision plans for patients; check with resident
3. Document patient care
4. Ensure timely discharge
Students:
1. Gather patient data to present to the team
2. Learn medicine to better determine what data necessary for management of each patient
3. Assist the interns in executing patient management plans

FIGURE 2-1. Osler's pyramid.

team leader to define your role, because it may vary from service to service.

II ROLES ON THE TEAM

The **team leader** establishes roles and defines expectations.

A. Identify the team leader. The attending physician has the highest rank but is rarely in charge of the day-to-day activities of the team. The **senior resident** usually is in charge of day-to-day team operations.

B. Insist on a 15-minute conference with the team leader early in the month. Most residents intend to do this but get too busy and forget. A simple question will do the trick: "Do you have a few minutes later today to talk about what you expect of me and what I can do to help the team?" This will give your resident the option of choosing a time that is not rushed.

1. Tell the team leader what you want to learn from the rotation. Everyone wants "to learn as much as possible" from the rotation. Take it to the next level: "I would like to better improve my physical exam skills, and I could use some help with rheumatology. Could you help me with these?"
2. Ask the team leader for his specific expectations of you. Write these down.

III SPECIFIC INFORMATION YOU MUST KNOW

A. **Schedule**

1. What time should I be ready to round? What would you like me to have prepared when rounds start (e.g., vital signs, physical exam data, etc.)?
2. When to leave. Be careful asking this question, because you risk sounding like a slacker. An easy way is to ask what the typical day looks like. Listen for the last task on the typical day; after this task is the normal exit time.

B. **Conferences**

1. Find out which conferences are mandatory and which are not. Try to attend all conferences, but if you are involved in active patient care (the OR, labor and delivery suite, etc.), leave your team only if the conference is mandatory. Clinical medicine is better learned on the wards than in the lecture hall.
2. Some residents may not know which conferences are mandatory. If you have to leave patient care for a mandatory conference, make sure you let your supervisor know that the conference is mandatory.
3. Assume that your residents will want you to return after your conference unless they tell you differently.

C. **Clerkship duties**
   1. Are students on call expected to stay overnight?
   2. What procedures am I expected to perform (e.g., draw blood, insert IV lines)?

IV Role of the Medical Student

A. **Know your patients.** You will have the most time of any team member to spend with your patient. You can be the *expert* when it comes to your patient's social and personal concerns if you assume the role of the liaison between the patient and the team. (See IV E for strategies to fulfill this role.)

HOT 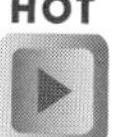 KEY

Do not assume primary responsibility for too many patients. You should begin with no more than one or two patients at a time, depending upon the complexity of the patients on your rotation. As you master the variety of skills, you can accept more patients (one to two per call day; three to four total on service).

B. **Learn as much as you can.**
   1. Read about your patients' conditions (see Chapter 45). This will keep your reading focused on important topics (i.e., those that you actually see). It will also link your reading to a live person; this has great power in enabling you to retain what you have read.
   2. Listen to medical discussions about other patients on the service. This will expand your ward experience.
   3. Try to attend all conferences and lectures.
   4. Hone your data gathering and clinical reasoning skills.

C. **Document your patient's care** (see Chapter 15).

D. **Always be prepared to present your patients succinctly and clearly** (see Chapters 3 and 16).

E. **Assume the role of the patient's primary physician.** The attending physician and the resident have the final say regarding the ultimate decisions relating to your patient, but you will learn the most about the role of being a physician if you take the attitude, "Although I am not the physician ultimately in charge, this patient is my responsibility." Here are a few strategies to do this:
   1. **See your patients at least twice a day.**
   2. **Assume responsibility for your patient's sign-out report.** At the conclusion of the day, each patient is handed off from the primary team to the night-float physician. The following morning, the night-float physician will give a sign-out report about what happened to each patient overnight to their primary doctors (i.e., you). Arrive early each morning to obtain a sign-out report from the night physician; ask your intern if you can be responsible for the sign-out report at the end of each day. Chapter 3 will show you how to do this.

3. **Do your own pre-rounds on your patients. Pre-rounds** includes everything you do in collecting patient data to prepare for work rounds. Chapter 3 will give you everything you need to know about succeeding with pre-rounds.
4. **Always develop your own assessment and plan (A&P) for your patients.** As you present it to your resident, listen carefully to how she modifies your plan; ask questions about the modifications. Making decisions is the hardest skill for a physician to master. Even though many of your decisions will be incorrect, you'll master this skill quicker by actively participating instead of passively waiting for the resident to tell you what to do.
5. Insist on doing everything related to your patient: the pre-rounds, presenting the patient, scrubbing in on the surgery, doing the procedures, giving the night-float sign-out report, and dictating the discharge summary.
6. Be present even for the things you cannot do by yourself (e.g., obtaining consents, family discussions).

HOT
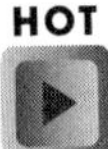
KEY

Try to participate in the care of your patients as much as possible, but if you are confused or unsure of what to do, tell your resident and ask him to teach you. This is not a sign of weakness; it is a sign of responsibility.

V Role of the Sub-Intern

A. The roles and responsibilities of the third-year student also apply to the 4th-year student sub-intern (sub-I; also called the acting intern [AI]). The change in roles is an **added emphasis on designing management plans** for patients. The sub-intern functions as an intern (see VI), with the following exceptions:
   1. The sub-intern must still have his orders co-signed by his supervising resident.
   2. Typically, the sub-intern does not have the same teaching responsibilities required of the intern.

B. The sub-intern typically works parallel to the intern (i.e., they have primary responsibility for different patients) and answers directly to the resident.

VI Role of the Intern

A. **The intern is responsible for executing day-to-day patient management.** The attending physician or resident may suggest a consultation, a test, or a discharge decision, but it is usually the intern who ensures that the plan is carried out. Great interns are efficient, organized, and skilled in prioritization.

B. **Documenting care.** Although the medical student may write a note on the same patient, the intern still must write a physician note of his own.

C. Teaching students the practical aspect of the physician's job. The best way to learn from an intern is to watch what he does, and then ask *why* he is doing it. You will note that the best interns go one step beyond: actively telling the students why they are doing each task and why they have chosen to sequence the tasks in a certain order (e.g., "Let's get the blood cultures now because if we wait an hour, the ER will have started antibiotics and that will taint our cultures.").

D. Formulating an assessment and management strategy. The best interns do not wait for the resident or attending physician to make management decisions. Instead, they formulate their own assessment and plan and then review this strategy with the team leader. **Independent decision making is the defining characteristic of successful advancement from one role on the team to the next.**

VII ROLE OF THE RESIDENT

A. The resident **organizes and runs the team.** The resident, more so than any other team member, is the key to a successful team. The best residents are great leaders. Functions of the resident include:

1. Informing all members of the team of their roles.
2. Establishing times for beginning and ending of rounds.
3. Delegating specific tasks to each team member (e.g., discharge paper work, follow-up on a radiology study, blood drawing, discharge summaries).

B. The resident makes **most final management decisions.** The resident is responsible for deciding which decisions need to be reviewed by the attending physician.

C. The resident **sets the agenda for attending rounds** (see Chapter 3).

1. The best residents organize their rounds by prioritizing severity of illness: the sickest patients are discussed first because these patients require immediate decisions. The discussion then proceeds to patients who require consultations, procedures, or radiographic studies (e.g., CT scans). This gives the resident the luxury of releasing an intern from rounds to get the ball rolling in ordering these tests or consults. Finally, patients who are ready for discharge are discussed. All other patients are then addressed.
2. The attending physician will modify treatment plans and teach (see below), but it is the resident who will manage the time of attending rounds so that all patients are discussed.

D. Evaluation and feedback

1. It is the resident's responsibility to give mid-month feedback to each member of the team.
2. Although the attending physician assigns the final grade for each student, it is the resident who provides comments about each team member's performance.

E. Teaching interns and students. Specific responsibilities include:
   1. Teaching methods of diagnosis and treatment.
   2. Supervising procedures.
   3. Formal teaching of students (e.g., "chalk talks").
   4. Providing the team with learning resources (e.g., suggested reading, articles, electrocardiograms).

F. Documenting care. The resident is responsible for ensuring that the chart documentation accurately represents the intended treatment plan. Residents usually write an admission note focused on the assessment and plan for each patient, in addition to the intern and student notes, but write progress notes only when a patient's condition dramatically changes (i.e., when a new assessment and plan is warranted).

VIII Role of the Attending Physician

A. Physician of record
   1. The attending physician is ultimately responsible for all decisions regarding her patients. Although residents and interns make most of the ward decisions, the attending physician is responsible for every decision.
   2. Any decision that might have significant consequences (e.g., discharging a patient, transferring a patient to another service, starting a risky medication) or any decision of which the team is unsure should definitely be discussed with the attending physician.

> **HOT KEY**
> It is crucial that the attending physician receive good communication from the team regarding the condition of the patients and management decisions.

B. Teaching. The attending physician teaches students and residents, either during attending rounds or at the bedside, and reviews and modifies the management plans of the residents or interns.

C. Evaluation and feedback. The attending physician assigns the final evaluation for each student, intern, and resident. The attending physician may not directly observe you performing the tasks that she is asked to evaluate; her impression of your performance will likely rely on the input from your residents or interns.

D. Interaction with other services. Occasionally there is a difference of opinion regarding which service (e.g., medicine vs. surgery) should assume primary responsibility for a patient. When conflict appears inevitable between two services, it is best to involve the attending physician early in the discussion.

3. Performing on Rounds

I INTRODUCTION

Most clinical services begin the day with pre-rounds and work rounds. If you use your experiences on these rounds well, you will have all you need to be good in attending rounds.

II PRE-ROUNDS

A. Pre-rounds include everything you do before you join your team for work rounds. The purpose of pre-rounds is to gather the necessary information to make management decisions about your patients.

B. Pre-rounds begin at different times on different services, and usually they take up to 1 hour.

C. Use the number of patients in your care, the severity of their illnesses, and the start time of work rounds to judge when you should begin pre-rounds. Give yourself 15 minutes to collect necessary information on each patient. Devote an extra 5 minutes for each of the following:

1. Patients who are very ill (i.e., have multisystem diseases).
2. Patients with multiple consultants attending to their care. You will want to review their recommendations from the previous day.
3. Patients whose daily physical examination involves time-consuming maneuvers (e.g., gait evaluation, detailed neurologic examination, dressing changes).
4. Patients who are to be discharged that day. Begin the paperwork before work-rounds start.

D. You do not need to gather all the data for your patients. It is unlikely that laboratory data or consultant recommendations will be available this early in the morning. **Your time is limited, so focus on the following:**

1. Obtain a **personal sign-out** report (see Chapter 2 IV E) from the covering night physician. He will tell you if any events occurred overnight.
2. Obtain **vital signs** for each patient.
3. Obtain an updated, focused **history** from the patient. The questions to ask are:
   a. **What has changed since yesterday?**
   b. **Have your symptoms improved?**
   c. **Do you have any new symptoms?**

4. Perform a **focused physical examination.** Focus on what has changed since yesterday. Do not examine organ systems that are not actively involved in patient management. If necessary, an expanded physical examination can be performed in the afternoon.
5. If possible, **ask the nurse about any overnight events.** Nurses are generally changing shifts during this time, so this may be difficult.
6. If your patient is on telemetry (electronic monitoring of the heart rate and rhythm), **check the telemetry section** in the chart to ensure no abnormal heart rhythms have occurred.
7. Determine whether there has been any change in the patient's laboratory values. The morning laboratory results may not be back by the time you do pre-rounds. If not, it is still worth checking old laboratory results that may have changed during the past 24 hours (e.g., blood cultures, urine cultures).

E. Do not worry about writing progress notes during your pre-round time unless your resident tells you to do so. The quality of the note will be compromised by lack of data; your assessment and plan (A&P) may change as you receive input during work rounds and attending rounds. Early afternoon is a good time to complete progress notes.

F. Be ready to start work rounds on time. Even if you have not obtained all the information on each of your patients, do not keep the team waiting. When you present these patients, tell your resident that you do not have all of the data; make a mental note to start earlier tomorrow.

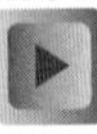

Do not worry about writing progress notes during pre-rounds. Save them until early in the afternoon, when you can incorporate your team's input in the patient's management plan.

III WORK ROUNDS

Work rounds include the entire team, except the attending physician, and are generally directed by the senior resident.

Most management decisions are made during **work rounds.**

A. **Presenting on work rounds.** Unlike the formal admission presentation, the work rounds presentation must be focused. Time is critical. **Consider what the team needs to know to make management decisions** (see Chapter 16 XIV).

HOT KEY

The most difficult skill to learn in medicine is the ability to make decisions. The only way to master this skill is to actively make decisions yourself and then check these decisions with your supervisors. **Do not worry about being wrong;** take the opportunity to learn as much as you can now, when you have the luxury of supervisors to correct your mistakes.

B. Keys to great work rounds presentation

1. **Know the data for each of your patients.** Know the results of what has happened overnight and the results of tests from the previous day.
2. **Stay organized.** Keep a patient card with all of the patient information in one place (Figure 3-1). In medical practice, it is usually the rate at which numbers change, not the absolute number, that is concerning. A sodium level of 128 mEq/L may not be concerning for the patient who has had the same value for the past 3 days; however, a sodium level of 130 mEq/L may be life-threatening if yesterday's sodium level was 145 mEq/L. Your data card must allow you to see these trends (i.e., it has past as well as present laboratory data and vital signs).
3. **Know your patient's medical regimen.** Write all medications on your patient card.
4. **Err on the side of saying too little** as opposed to saying too much. Your resident can ask for information you do not present.
5. **Stay focused.** Do not waste time with commentary on signs and symptoms. Present all data first; save your interpretation thoughts until you get to the A&P.

HOT 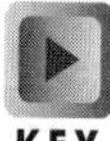 KEY

Pay attention to the discussion about the patients of other team members. You may be called on to help others in completing their work later in the day.

C. Asking questions on work rounds. Most residents want to answer your questions on work rounds. It is the pressure of finishing on time that prevents them from doing so.

1. **When you are considering asking a question, consider the needs of your team.** If there are several patients on the service, write down your questions and wait until the end of rounds to ask them.
2. **If you have a question that must be answered to advance your patient's care, however, ask immediately.**

D. Professionalism. You are a professional, and you know that. The problem is that the patient will not know that when he first meets you. First impression is everything; don't risk a wrong impression by doing things that create an impression of unprofessionalism.

Name				#

History

PMH:

Meds:
1.
2.
3.
4.
5.
6.
7.
8.
9.
10.
11.
12.
13.

All:_______ ETOH: ______/d Tob _____pk/yrs Drugs ____________

Physical Exam

Problems/Assessment

1)________	2)________	3)________	4)________	5)________
* * * * *				

Day 1	Day 2	Day 3
Day 4	Day 5	Day 6

Date								
BP								Echo: ____ EF%
Pulse								
T max								
RR								
Sat %								
Weight								Cath: ____ LAD ____ RCA ____ Circ
HCT								
WBC								
PLT								CT:
PT/INR								
PTT								
Na+								
K+								
Cl–								
HCO3–								
BUN								
Creat								
Gluc								
Trop								
AST								
ALT								
Alk. P								
T. bili								
UA								
Cultures								

FIGURE 3-1. Sample data card (front and back).

1. Do not eat, drink, or chew gum on work rounds.
2. Dress appropriately.
3. Do not slouch, lean against the wall, crouch on the floor, or sit in wheelchairs or on gurneys.

HOT 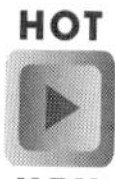 KEY

Talkative patients can greatly impede the efficiency of pre-rounds and work rounds. See your patients in the afternoon, as well as the morning. If they know they have another opportunity to talk with you, they are less likely to try to "get everything in" in one visit.

IV Special Circumstances in Pre-rounds and Work Rounds

A. **Surgery** (see Chapter 38). Usual start time: 5:00 AM.
1. **Check drains** in postoperative patients every morning. Record the amount of fluid and the character of the fluid (e.g., blood, serous fluid, pus) coming from each tube. Never remove tubes unless your resident tells you to do so.
2. **Present the input/output totals.** Record the amount of oral or IV fluid the patient received, including total parenteral nutrition and blood products, as well as volume lost from urine, stool, nasogastric tubes, and other tubes.
3. **Check bowel function.** The decision to feed a patient postoperatively depends on the function of the bowels. If bowel sounds are present, the patient is ready to be fed (i.e., peristalsis has returned and the bowels can accommodate the food). You must listen for at least 2 minutes to reliably say bowel sounds are *not* present.
4. **Check wounds.** Do not undress wounds covered by extensive bandages. These wounds will be evaluated during work rounds, and the process of undressing and dressing them takes up precious pre-rounds time. Simple bandages can be removed, and these wounds should be checked.
5. **Check the adequacy of pain control.**
6. **Writing notes.** Work rounds on surgical services may run right up to the first operating room case. You may be asked to write a brief note while on work rounds. In this case, keep the note focused on what is said. Work with your intern and other students to make sure that charts are available to the team as you do work rounds.

B. **Pediatrics** (see Chapter 40). Usual start time: 7:00 AM.
1. It is not always necessary to wake children for pre-rounds. **Talk with the parents** if they are present and awake.
2. Most drugs in pediatrics are administered based on body weight (kg). **Make any dose calculations during pre-rounds.**

C. **Obstetrics and gynecology** (see Chapter 39). Usual start time: 6:00 AM.
  1. As with surgery, **check wounds and tubes.**
  2. Check fundus size, and record any bleeding or fetal monitor events.

D. **Internal medicine** (see Chapter 37). Usual start time: 7:00 AM.

E. **Neurology.** Usual start time: 7:00 AM.

F. **Emergency medicine.** There are no pre-rounds.

G. **Psychiatry** (see Chapter 41). Usually there are no pre-rounds.

V Attending Rounds

A. Attending rounds are an important feature of medicine, pediatrics, and psychiatry. In attending rounds, the decisions made during work rounds are checked and evaluated. There may be no attending rounds for surgery or obstetrics and gynecology, because most of the attending contact is in the operating room. Your goals for attending rounds are to:
  1. Be prepared to present the information about your patient and the A&P, as modified during work rounds (Chapter 16).
  2. Further learn about the diseases your patients have, based on your attending physician's teaching.
  3. Assess the quality, including any weaknesses, of your clinical reasoning.

B. The key to getting the most from attending rounds is to ask the right questions. Read about your patient's disease before attending rounds. This enables you to ask about any issues you do not understand and identify what are the most important elements of the disease (see Chapter 44). It also allows you to learn what you cannot learn from textbooks: the methods and clinical reasoning necessary for managing your patient's disease.

HOT
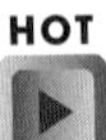
KEY

Asking your attending physician the right question is vital. For example, asking, "What is *your approach* to a patient with chest pain?" is a better question than asking about the electrocardiogram changes found in myocardial infarction. The latter can easily be looked up in a textbook.

D. If the team succeeds on attending rounds, so do you. Three pitfalls are commonly encountered on attending rounds.
  1. **Never upstage interns** by presenting data of which they are not aware. If data become available to you between work rounds and attending rounds (e.g., a nurse pages you with a laboratory result of which the interns are not aware), always precede your presentation of this information with a disclaimer that you just discovered it. This avoids embarrassing the interns.

2. Although you should design your own management plans, **attribute all clinical decisions to your team.** Never take credit for a good patient intervention.
3. Other medical students are a part of the team, and you must **respect their sovereignty over their patients.** If the attending physician asks another student a question about one of her patients, be courteous and let her answer. Answer the question only after she has had a fair chance. It is very tempting to try to make a good impression on your attending physician, but the best impression you can make is by making *others* look good. Remember, most of the attending's evaluation of you will come from input from your resident and interns.

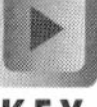
HOT KEY

Most attending physicians, regardless of how "out of touch" they may appear, can usually spot the student who tries to shine at the expense of others.

VI Sign-out Reports

A. Do not let the care of your patients stop at the end of your work day. A good progress note helps ensure that the cross-covering physician understands the plans for a patient, and this note is **essential to ensuring your patient receives the best possible care if an unexpected event occurs.**

B. There are many methods of signing out, depending on your service (e.g., printed computer sheet, 3 × 5 note card). **Ask your intern how she signs out.**

C. Do not burden the cross-cover physician with too much information. She has access to the progress note in the patient's chart. **Components of a good sign-out include** (Figure 3-2)**:**

1. Patient's name, identification number, and location.
2. A one-line description ("56-year-old man with congestive heart failure") and any active treatment regimens of which the cross-covering physician should be aware ("He is going to the operating room tonight for a pacemaker replacement.").
3. Anything you want the cross-covering physician to check or do. ("Check the potassium level at 10 AM. Give 40 mEq KCl if the potassium level is less than 3.3 mEq/L."). As a rule, if you ask the night-float to check something, tell him what you want him to do with the results.
4. **How to manage the three most common calls**
   a. **Replace the IV?** If the IV comes out and the nurse cannot replace it, do you want it replaced during the night or can it wait until morning? If you want it replaced, this usually means that a central line will be placed. If the patient needs a continuous infusion (antibiotics, chemotherapy), a new IV is neces-

Ignatius Riley, 899504921		Room 535
56 yo man admitted for heart failure. He is being diuresed and ruled out for MI.		
Check urine output at 9 pm. Give 500 cc bolos if <1L. Check potassium at 9 pm. Give 40 mEq if <3.3.		
Full code	+ IV	+ Culture
Holden Caulfield, 988114322		Room 635
24 yo man admitted for a broken hand and delusions of phony people haunting him. He is on suicide precautions.		
Full code	+ IV	+ Culture

FIGURE 3-2. Sample sign-out card.

sary; if the IV is for maintenance fluid or intermittent doses only, it can probably wait until morning.

b. **Culture for fever?** If the patient spikes a fever, do you want blood cultures to be ordered? You may expect a fever spike with some diagnoses (e.g., pneumonia, endocarditis, tumor fever). Tell the night-float if a culture is not indicated; this spares the patient unnecessary discomfort of repeat cultures.

c. **Code status?** If your patient has expressed a desire not to be resuscitated or intubated, and this has been confirmed by a "do not resuscitate" (DNR) or "do not intubate" (DNI) order from the attending physician, tell the night-float. When the code pager sounds, there may not be enough time to carefully review the chart to decide if full resuscitation efforts should be initiated or not.

5. It is extremely poor form to sign-out urgent laboratory results or radiographic studies that are pending. Results of urgent tests should be checked and acted upon before you leave the hospital.
6. Do not ask the night-float to check on routine studies unless you expect him to act on the results (e.g., "Check the exercise stress test." There is no immediate action to take on this result; the patient will need additional tests that you can schedule tomorrow.).

HOT

KEY

If you ask the night-float to check a test result for you, make sure you write the order for the test before leaving the hospital.

4. Ward Structure and Working with Nurses and Ancillary Staff

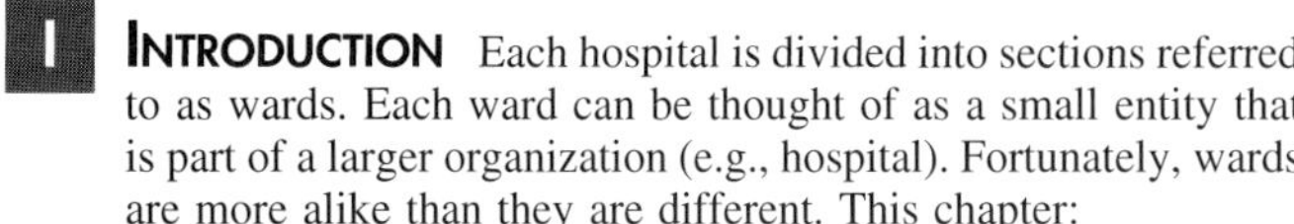

I INTRODUCTION

Each hospital is divided into sections referred to as wards. Each ward can be thought of as a small entity that is part of a larger organization (e.g., hospital). Fortunately, wards are more alike than they are different. This chapter:

A. Introduces you to the features that are similar for all wards and offers a strategy for discovering the idiosyncrasies of different wards.

B. Gives you the fundamentals of working with non-physician staff. The practice of medicine is a team activity, and although the physician runs the team, the contributions of the non-physician staff are equally vital to the care of your patients.

HOT

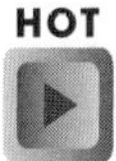

KEY

Respect all hospital staff; you will need their help.

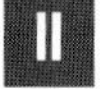

II ESTABLISHING A GOOD WORKING RELATIONSHIP WITH STAFF

A. Introduce yourself to each member of the ward team at the appropriate time. The introduction should be brief and sincere. For example, "Hello, my name is Jeff Wiese, and I am the medical student working on the medical service this month. Dr. Bent is my resident. Let me know if there is anything that I can do to help."

B. You may also want to tell each staff member that you would like to be the first medical staff contacted with any news about your patients.

III KEY NON-PHYSICIAN STAFF

A. Ward secretary (ward clerk)

1. Duties. The ward secretary is in charge of the administrative issues of the ward. Some of his duties include:

a. Making clinic appointments.

b. Calling messengers to pick up laboratory specimens.

c. Notifying residents about incoming admissions.

d. Entering orders into the computer system.

2. **Using the talents of the ward secretary.** Ask for assistance only when necessary.
   a. Tell the ward secretary if you have ordered a laboratory, diagnostic, or dietary order that is particularly important. However, be judicious. If the order is not vital, the best way to communicate with the ward secretary is via the orders on the chart.
   b. Always personally inform the ward secretary if one of your patients is being discharged. This allows him to prioritize the discharge order so your patient is discharged early, reducing work for the nursing staff.

B. **Registered nurses (RNs).** RNs can accomplish a tremendous amount of work in a short time. Do not waste their time on unnecessary tasks.

1. **Duties**
   a. Administering pharmacy orders.
   b. Maintaining IV and nasogastric access.
   c. Notifying interns about a change in the patient's condition.
   d. Performing daily physical examinations, including obtaining vital signs.
   e. Performing all aspects of daily patient care.
2. **Establishing a relationship.** There are too many RNs for you to introduce yourself to all of them on the first day. However, you should introduce yourself to each nurse that is caring for your patients. Good ward manners include:
   a. Cleaning up after yourself (e.g., putting charts back where you found them, disposing of bandages).
   b. Not using the ward phone for personal pages except when absolutely necessary.
   c. Not surfing the Internet on ward computers.
   d. Not having food and drinks on the ward.
3. **Using the talents of the RN**
   a. **Patient contact.** The RN is the only person who has more contact with your patient than you do. He knows what treatments are working and what new symptoms have developed. If you are planning to start a new therapy whose success is uncertain, ask the RN how well he thinks it will work for this particular patient.

HOT
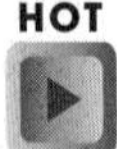
KEY

Check with the RN at least once a day on the progress of your patient.

   b. **Nursing intuition.** After years of caring for patients, RNs often know when a patient's condition may change for the worse, even before there are objective signs. If an RN is concerned about a patient, you should be too.

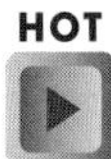

HOT KEY

Listen carefully to what an experienced RN tells you.

c. **Where to find what you need.** RNs know where all supplies are kept. If you want to know where to find a central line kit, for example, first make an attempt to find it yourself, and then ask the RN. Request a good time to ask the question (e.g., "When you have a minute, can I ask you a question?") If an RN is very busy, this gives her the opportunity to defer the request to a more convenient time ("Yes, in just a minute."). It also shows respect for how busy she is.

d. **Fulfill your role.** Offer to help if you have extra time to do nursing duties (e.g., start an IV line). However, never do something you are uncomfortable doing, even if the nurse asks you to do so; if this happens, ask your resident for help.

C. **Nurse Supervisors and Charge Nurses.** The charge nurse is in charge of the non-physician staff for an entire ward. The nurse supervisor is in charge of the non-physician staff for the entire hospital. If you have an opportunity, introduce yourself to these influential and important people.

D. **Other nurses.** Licensed practical nurses (LPNs) are licensed to do noninvasive tasks such as obtaining vital signs and hygienic care of patients. In some states, LPNs may administer medications and start IVs. LPNs may supervise nursing aides and nursing assistants.

IV OTHER NON-PHYSICIAN STAFF

A. **Respiratory therapists** are technicians who provide supplemental oxygen via various delivery systems. They also administer nebulized drugs and perform postural drainage. In the intensive care unit (ICU), they determine ventilator settings. **Any changes in ventilator settings must be discussed with the respiratory therapist.**

B. **Dietitians** care for patients who are severely malnourished and require special diets and for those who are receiving enteral feeding (via a feeding tube) or parenteral feeding (via an IV catheter).

C. **Physician assistants (PAs) and nurse practitioners (NPs)** perform many of the tasks of a physician, such as performing physical examinations and writing diagnostic and medical orders under physician supervision. Most PAs and NPs have their own patients and verify treatment plans with their supervising physician.

D. **Social workers** handle the non-medical patient issues. Social workers are extremely knowledgeable about support groups, forms of financial support, arranging home visits, and preparing the family for taking patients home. **Social workers are essential in discharging patients.**

E. **Pharmacists** can be helpful with patients with impaired drug clearance (renal or hepatic disease) or with patients who are taking multiple medications (drug–drug interactions).

F. **Technicians** perform simple tests with expertise. Examples include phlebotomists, ultrasound technicians, and radiology technicians. They can be a valuable educational resource if their skill is something you will ultimately use (e.g., phlebotomy).

G. **Therapists**

1. **Occupational therapists** help patients learn or relearn skills necessary to live independently.
2. **Physical therapists** help patients regain and maintain strength and mobility after disability or injury.
3. **Speech therapists** help patients develop or recover communication skills. They also work with patients with swallowing disorders, oral motor problems, hearing loss, and cognitive disorders.

H. **Janitors** are often completely ignored and allowed to go about the business of cleaning up after others. They deserve respect.

V Maintaining Efficient Patient Flow Through the Hospital

A. Almost all hospitals are near capacity each day; to accommodate additional patients, each patient's hospital stay (the time from admission to discharge) must be as efficient as possible. You want your patients to stay as long as necessary, but not longer. Non-physician staff are vital to this efficiency.

B. **Key steps in flow through the hospital**

1. Flow through the hospital begins with early patient discharge from the wards. It may take up to 6 hours between the time a discharge order is written and the time the bed is ready to accommodate a new patient. The IVs must be removed, the prescriptions filled, transportation called, and the bed cleaned.

HOT
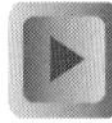
KEY

Even if you later change your mind about discharge, it is easier to stop a discharge process than it is to get it started.

2. Once ward patients have been discharged, patients from the ICU can be transferred to the ward. This frees ICU beds for new admissions.
3. Patients admitted from clinics and the emergency department can also then be admitted to the ward beds.

C. How you can help accelerate flow through the hospital

1. Begin thinking about discharge planning on the first day a patient is admitted. On the first day, ask these three questions:
   a. **Where is the patient going after hospital discharge** (e.g., nursing home, home with family, home with home care)?
   b. If the patient is going home, **what home therapy is necessary** (e.g., home oxygen)?
   c. **Are there any tests the patient needs before leaving the hospital?** (Some nursing homes require a tuberculosis skin test and chest radiograph.)
2. If there is any question about where the patient will go on discharge and whether there are special discharge needs (see above), **contact the social worker immediately.**
3. Communicate with the ward staff. If you suspect a patient may go home the following morning, write an order in the chart: "Anticipate discharge tomorrow morning." Complete discharge paperwork the night before discharge, so that the pharmacy can fill the outpatient medications during off-peak times.
4. On the morning of discharge, let the nurse and ward secretary know early, even if you have to check the decision with your attending physician or wait for a result of a morning laboratory test. An early discharge obviates all of the required nursing rounds and notes; this nursing time can then be allocated to other patients that remain.

VI Resolving Conflict on the Wards

A. Expect that people will occasionally be unpleasant to you. The wards are stressful, and sometimes you may be the subject of another person's frustrations. As a medical student, you can do very little compared to the interns and residents (e.g., you cannot write orders, do solo procedures, etc.). Therefore, you may not receive the respect you deserve. Do not take it personally.

B. Despite what might happen, be sincere and pleasant to everyone. Above all, do not hold grudges. A grudge will eat you from within, robbing you of the emotional energy you need to help your patients.

C. If you feel very frustrated, leave the ward for a few minutes and then return. If you need a graceful exit, tell the nurse you have to "check on a radiograph." Leave and then return when the emotion of the situation has diffused.

D. If the problem with one of the ward staff members persists, have your intern or resident intervene on your behalf. Ancillary staff know that you will be there for only a month; residents will be there again and again for 3 or more years. They are much more likely to be amenable to resolving conflicts with the resident.

5. Common Ward Pitfalls

I INTRODUCTION

INTRODUCTION There are two major types of pitfalls in the clinical years: those that have a negative effect on your evaluations and those that undermine your effectiveness as a physician.

II WORKING WITH RESIDENTS AND ATTENDING PHYSICIANS

A. Challenging authority.

1. It is unlikely that you will like all your supervising residents and physicians. Nevertheless, it is to your advantage to remain respectful. They are the team leaders, and a lack of harmony on the team will adversely affect patient care and your learning experience. Focus on finding the positive and helpful traits of even the most difficult attending physicians and residents. Even the worst physicians can teach you lessons about things you do not want to emulate when you are in their role.
2. Do not be afraid to take a stand or challenge ideas, but focus on challenging the *idea* or the *decision*, not the physician's authority. There is an art to doing this in a nonthreatening way. Instead of, "I don't agree with that decision," try, "On my last rotation they taught us ________." If the team leader sees merit in your idea, this approach will allow him to change his mind without sacrificing his ego. He will be much more likely to modify the decision slightly and adopt it as his own. The team leader will value you more for introducing a new idea without emphasizing his errors.

B. Talking behind closed doors. Unfortunately, students are often put in the middle of residents who are temporarily at odds with each other. Avoid the temptation to take sides. If asked your opinion of another resident, stay neutral, "Well, like all residents, I guess he has his good and bad points," or "As a student, I don't get to see him in the contexts you do." This will prevent you from being labeled as the backstabber when the conflict ends.

C. Undercutting your interns and residents. This may occur in two situations.

1. **Attending rounds.** Between work rounds and attending rounds, you may learn something new about your patient but not have the opportunity to tell your intern or resident about it. If you have discovered new information and present it during attending rounds, state that the information is new so not to embarrass your resident for not knowing the information. For example, you might say, "The laboratory just informed me that the hematocrit is 20%."

2. **Disagreement in findings.** Always present what you found on *your* examination. Do not embarrass your resident by pointing out discrepancies between your examinations.

HOT
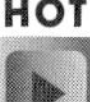

KEY

Try to make team members look good. As the team prospers, so will you. A team player is always rewarded at evaluation time.

D. **Garnering favor.** Medical school rotations are not the appropriate time to develop intimate friendships with residents. The power gradient prevents the true mutual respect requisite for friendship. It is fine to have common interests and friendly discussions (e.g., sports, art), but becoming close personal friends with a resident during a rotation may interfere with the teaching, learning, and evaluation that should occur. Defer personal relationships until after the rotation has ended.

E. **Not knowing what is expected of you.** Although it is your resident's responsibility to clearly communicate what is expected of you (see Chapter 3), not all residents do this. If your expectations are not communicated to you, use the strategy suggested in Chapter 2 II B. This is the time to ask about your days off. If there are days you have to have off, request them at this time, and offer to work any other days except those days. Try not to take weekdays off, because these are when teaching and conferences are most likely to occur.

F. **Not seeking feedback.** The month passes quickly, and residents may forget to give you feedback. If you have not received feedback after 2 weeks, approach your resident and say, "Do you have a few minutes later today to talk about what I can do to continue to improve?" This gives her the luxury of choosing the time so that the discussion is not rushed or tainted by a resident who is in a bad mood. The tone of your approach is also important. Instead of asking "How am I doing?", which implies "What is my grade?", focus on how you can improve. With this approach you will appear genuinely interested in learning and improving and you will receive higher quality feedback while simultaneously gaining the resident's respect.

III WORKING ON ROTATIONS

The hospital wards are not for us, they are for our patients. Reminding yourself of this daily will keep you from succumbing to the following pitfalls. Table 5-1 is copied from an intern locker-room wall. It's good advice.

A. **You will not like all rotations; do not pretend that you do.** Be honest when your resident asks you in what field of medicine you want to specialize. She will not like you less if your interests do not coincide with hers, and this may allow her to tailor your clerkship experience to your interests (e.g., if you are interested in surgery, a

TABLE 5-1. Eleven Commandments for Medical Students and Interns.

1. Play as a team.	Work hard to help your team; demand that your team works hard to help you. Work closely with staff. Treat everyone with respect.
2. Be honest.	Never lie to your patients or to your team. Honesty is requisite for truth. Truth is requisite for science. Science is requisite for your patients' health.
3. Communicate.	Keep everyone, including the night-float and your resident, informed of new events and problems you anticipate.
4. Participate in pre-rounds.	Show up early enough to see and examine your patients before work rounds. The more you can offer on work rounds, the more you advance your patients' care.
5. Write good notes.	A good note tells everyone exactly what you have found and what you plan to do. Write notes after you have discussed your patient with the team.
6. Show up.	You are paid for your work in the form of education. Every time you miss a conference, you are taking a pay cut.
7. Develop good methods and be thorough.	Ask residents to teach you *methods* for the clinical problems you encounter. Once you have mastered a method, apply it consistently.
8. Read.	It does not matter how much medical material you read, only that you develop the habit of reading something every day.
9. Keep your wits about you.	You only have so much energy; do not waste it on needless squabbles.
10. Keep something for yourself.	Preserve at least one activity in your life, such as working out, dining out, or reading a novel. This will keep you sane. You have little to offer your patients if you are sick.
11. Do not lose perspective.	Wards and rounds are not about you, they are about your patients.

medicine resident may devote more time to discussing coagulation disorders or preferentially assign you patients with abdominal pain).

B. Do not dismiss a rotation that does not interest you. This is your last opportunity for formal instruction in this field. If you choose a career in surgery, you are unlikely to have additional formal instruction in gynecology, although it is likely you will have surgical patients with gynecologic problems. Visualize yourself in your chosen career, and imagine scenarios in which the material on your current rotation will be useful.

C. Do not disrespect other specialties. Residents may make fun of or discredit other specialties. Do not engage in this behavior; it is a sign of insecurity, ignorance, and weakness. A surgeon may discredit an internist (forgetting it is the internist who keeps the patient alive after the surgery), and an internist may discredit a surgeon (forgetting that it is the surgeon who removes the cancer once it is diagnosed). The practice of medicine is a team effort, and physicians who discredit other physicians show their ignorance of this important concept.

D. Communicate with your team. The adage "it is easier to ask for forgiveness than permission" leads to disaster on the wards. If you must leave the ward for an extended time during your shift, let the team know where you are going and make it clear that you will come back if needed. Leave the resident your pager number. If you do not have a pager, get one.

E. Learn as much as you can.

1. Although there will be times when the service is so busy that you will receive little formal teaching, you are still learning great lessons merely by taking care of patients. The more patients you have, the more you learn.
2. Do not decline to help with "scut" work (i.e., patient-related work that must be completed to care for the patient, such as ordering tests, drawing blood, wheeling a patient to radiology). Remember, service to the patients is the primary focus. Make it a practice to say to your residents, "Tell me what I can do to help out. If this gives you a little extra time to teach, I would like to be around for that." In doing so, you are trading what you can offer (ability to do scut) for what the resident can offer (teaching).

F. Do not give up too soon. You are going to make mistakes, and many of these mistakes occur at the worst possible times. It is important to remember that one mistake does not ruin the entire month. Mistakes made in good faith are quickly forgotten.

HOT

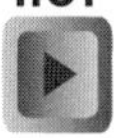

KEY

If you make a mistake, learn from it and then let it go.

G. **Be professional.**

1. **Respect hierarchy.** The chairperson runs the department. Never talk while she talks. Indeed, do *nothing* but stand at attention, even if you have already heard what she has to say. The same applies to your attendings and senior residents. Even if you do not respect the person, give due respect to the position and to the work it took to get there.
2. **Do not eat or drink on the wards.** The medical condition of patients is not a casual matter. Fulfilling the patient's expectation of the professional physician goes a long way in establishing his trust in you. Besides, food in a health care environment (e.g., the wards) is an OSHA violation.
3. **Do not talk about your patients** when there is even a remote possibility that someone may overhear your conversation.
4. **Never make fun of your patients.** Even if the resident encourages comments about how fat or debilitated a patient is, resist the temptation to join in the same behavior. Your patients may hear you, and senior physicians who witness your behavior will think less of you. They will immediately recognize this cynicism as the defense mechanism that it is: one that depersonalizes the patient so that the physician does not have to truly be involved in the patient's plight. Ridicule is inconsistent with the empathy and sincere concern that is an essential part of best patient care.
5. **Be on time.** This is a sign of respect for the team and for the patients. It also shows that you are in control of yourself and your schedule.

H. **Do not perform tasks that you do not know how to do.** If your resident asks you to do a procedure that you feel uncomfortable doing ("Jim, put a central line in Mr. Jones"), do not pretend to know how and try to figure it out later. This shows lack of judgment, not great bravery. Besides, the chance of successfully accomplishing a medical procedure that you do not understand is remote. You need not refuse to perform the task, however. Say, "I don't know how to do that safely alone. I'll get the catheter tray and materials ready to go if you'll walk me through it."

I. **Assume the role of the patient's primary physician** (see Chapter 2).

J. **Learn to make decisions.** Muster the courage to make decisions and be responsible for the consequences. This is the hardest lesson for physicians to learn. Now is the time to practice making confident decisions, while you have the luxury of supervising physicians to evaluate and correct your mistakes.

K. **Learn to be confident.** It is hard to be confident in discussing a patient's disease when you realize that most of the team knows more about the disease than you do. But although you are not the expert on the patient's *disease*, you *are* the expert when it comes to knowing the patient as a person. Know your patients well, and confidence will come to you. The appearance of confidence will also promote your team's confidence in what you have to say. Stand straight and look them in the eye. Do not be ashamed or afraid of not knowing something about a disease. This is why you are here.

L. Learn not to succumb to stage fright. Yes, you are on stage. Recognize that this is part of the experience. If you feel especially nervous during presentations on rounds, ask your resident for help and extra practice.

IV WORKING WITH OTHER STUDENTS

A. Undercutting one of your colleagues does not make you appear smarter; residents see through this (they've been there). At every turn, try to make your fellow students look good. This will gain your residents' respect.

B. Do not compare yourself with other students. It's easy to do so, especially when schools pit one student against another for the honors grade. Even so, try to keep your focus on the physician you are becoming; your ultimate competition is within you, not with another student.

V UNPARDONABLE OFFENSES

All mistakes by student physicians are forgiven except three:

A. Showing self-interest at the expense of the patient or the team.

B. Not being on time. Consistently arriving late or leaving early (or not showing up at all) is unacceptable.

C. Being dishonest. Everyone wants to be in control, but, occasionally, even the best interns forget to check a laboratory result. If you did not check a laboratory result, say so. Decisions are made based on your information. Your lie can have catastrophic consequences. You may receive justifiable chastisement for not checking that result, but that is mild compared to a bad patient outcome.

6. Bedside Skills and Dealing with Difficult Patients

I INTRODUCTION

The most challenging aspect of the clinical clerkship is adapting to the variety of patient demands. A few fundamental principles will help you alleviate even the most stressful situations.

II BEDSIDE SKILLS

A. **Establishing rapport** is critical, because it enables you to be **effective in making your therapeutic plans work.** Even if you are not in the mood to be compassionate or do not have time to listen to a patient's stories, establishing a bond is still important because it establishes trust. Once your patient trusts you, he will be open in sharing information about his symptoms and issues relating to compliance with his therapy. Without trust, you will be at a significant disadvantage; you will never know the whole story. Whatever it takes to establish rapport is worth the time.

1. When you are taking a history, patients will initially tell you only part of the whole story. If they sense your disapproval, they will never reveal the whole story.
2. Ultimately, patients must leave the hospital and live their own lives. Inspiring a patient to change his life (e.g., start a new diet, stop smoking) is impossible unless you inspire a genuine sense of concern for his welfare. Feeling concern is not enough; the patient has to see it in you for it to matter.

B. **Techniques that promote rapport**

1. **Be sincere.** Patients can sense obligatory compassion or sorrow. Insincere compassion is worse than no compassion at all; insincerity implies manipulation, and this will drive your patient farther from you.
2. **Be respectful**, even if it does not seem warranted. No one feels like being nice when she is sick. Expect patients (or their families) to sometimes talk or act in ways that are rude or insulting. When it happens, try to understand their position and respond respectfully. It is easy to be nice to people who are nice in return; it takes a professional to be nice in the setting of hostility. If necessary, excuse yourself and come back later.
3. **Avoid judging your patients.** As with insincere compassion, patients sense when they are being judged. Once they know they are being judged, they will shut off information from you,

for they can no longer trust you. As a physician, you have set high standards for your own health. It will be easy to look down on a patient who eats too much, smokes, drinks, engages in unsafe sex, or uses drugs. These are behaviors that you would abhor in yourself. Unless you consciously recognize your feelings toward these behaviors, you will be at risk for projecting these feelings to your patient in the form of judgment. The problem with judgment is that once you judge, you will emotionally feel responsible for enacting punishment. You cannot explicitly punish your patients, and thus an internal conflict will arise, manifested in many subconscious punishments (e.g., not seeing the patient as often as other patients, doubting what the patient is telling you), all of which result in sub-optimal care.

4. **Fulfill all promises.** Even small promises (e.g., "I'll tell that to the nurse") that you do not keep erode your rapport with the patient.
5. **Assume the role of a physician.** Patients expect attentive, friendly, professionally dressed, competent physicians. Remember that perception is reality; when it comes to patient interactions, it will not matter if you are professional on the inside if the patient sees you as unprofessional on the outside. Remember too that patients expect professionalism just as much at 2 AM as they do at 10 AM. Even when tired, try your best to act and look professional.
6. **Find common ground.** Ask about patients' lives outside of their illnesses. Even small talk, such as, "In what part of the city did you grow up?" or "What kind of work do you do?" conveys that you care more about the patient than you do about her disease.
7. **Let the patient do the talking.** The best way to show that you care is to listen. **Patients will not care about what you know until they know that you care.**
8. **See your patients more than once a day.** The patient will expect the first visit of the day because it is required. Additional visits are a bonus; he will know that you are not required to come back, but that you *choose* to return. It shows genuine concern, and it greatly builds rapport.
9. **Although it may not always be possible, ask to round and present at the bedside.** This allows patients to see how much time and thought you have put into their care.
10. **Try to make patients laugh or smile.** Even in moments of pain, a few seconds of laughter reminds the patient of what it was like to feel good, and what it will be like to feel good again. It's therapeutic.
11. **Interact with the family.**
12. **Empower your patients.** Nothing is more disabling than being hospitalized. Patients are away from home and at the mercy of

the disease; they no longer control what they eat, whom they see, when they have visitors (physicians come when it is convenient for them, not for the patients), and perhaps even when they bathe, urinate, or defecate. Giving back even the smallest amount of control goes a long way toward reempowering your patient. Allow patients to make decisions about the smallest of choices. "Would you like the door open or closed?" "Would you like the TV on or off?" "Would you like the light left on or turned off?"

HOT 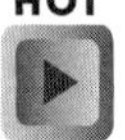 KEY

"Attending Syndrome." Patients may occasionally withhold information until they believe they are talking to the physician in charge. When you ask questions of patients, you may receive partial responses. However, when your attending physician asks the same questions, she receives complete answers. Patient rapport reduces the frequency of this syndrome.

C. **Make precious time.** Patients crave more time with their physicians, but your time is limited. To avoid sacrificing time with patients in lieu of getting ward work accomplished (or vice versa), you will have to optimize your efficiency in doing non-patient tasks. The other trick is to make time with patients seem longer than it is. Here are a few techniques:
   1. **Tell patients exactly how much time you have to spend, and then spend 20% more.** "I only have 5 minutes to talk." Then spend 6 minutes. The extra minute will be treasured.
   2. **See your patients more than once a day.** Seeing patients twice improves rapport (see above), but it also saves time. The patient who expects to see you only once a day will be under great pressure to cram all of his complaints and concerns into that one session. The pressure leads to a flustered, disorganized report of his symptoms; the disorganization leads to poor communication, which in turn leads to the patient frequently repeating himself in an effort to be understood. If he comes to expect additional visits, this pressure is relieved, and each visit will be more focused. You'll save time, and the patient will be more satisfied with each visit.
   3. **Sit down.** The gesture of sitting down sends the message that you plan to remain with the patient for a while. The patient will perceive the time you spend with him as longer than it really is.
   4. **Listen; do not talk.** Patients talk excessively because they think they are not being understood.
      a. Never interrupt. If you interrupt, the patient will feel as if he is not making his case clearly, and he will begin again from the start.
      b. For most patients, acknowledging the patient with "uh-hum," or "I see" shows that you are listening. For the excessively

loquacious patient, however, a different strategy is in order. Look directly at the patient and maintain complete silence. Do not utter a sound, not even the "uh-hum," or "I see." Even the most talkative patients will soon be cognizant of the unilateral conversation and will stop.

   c. When it is your turn to talk, summarize what the patient said and *immediately* ask your next question. This will keep the conversation moving forward. Do not ask if your summary is correct; the patient will correct you if it is not. Asking this question will return you to the beginning of the conversation.

5. **Focus and redirect** patients. Use the following techniques to keep the conversation focused and moving forward.
   a. Acquire data chronologically. Do not accept any history until you have established the time point at which it began. Do not accept the next piece of history until you have the preceding chronologic event. If information is not in chronologic order, say, "That's important, but let's go back a bit so I can keep this straight. The pain began 6 months ago; what happened 5 months ago?"
   b. Set conversational goals. This is especially useful for day-to-day visits. Identify what you need to know up front. "I need to know how your abdominal pain is today." If the patient begins to talk about knee and foot pain, redirect. "That is important, and I want to hear about it in a minute. Let's finish up with the abdominal pain." Continue redirecting until you have the information you need, then return to his other complaints.
   c. If you have to redirect the patient, validate as you go. Nothing kills a conversation like the feeling of being cut off. The patient may have many issues to discuss, and if he feels pressure to tell you about all of them, his reporting of them is likely to be flustered and disorganized. Validate that you are interested in hearing about each of them, and then redirect: "These are all very important points, and I want to come back to them and discuss them in detail. However, before we get to them, will you tell me again what happened after you left the hospital back in August?"
   d. Crystallize by rewinding. Sometimes you can help crystallize your patient's story by repeating it back to him; this reduces disorganized thought and keeps the history focused. "Your story is very complex. Do you mind if I piece it together?" Then start at the very beginning, quickly noting each part of the history in sequence, up to the part where the history became tangential. "OK, so that brings us to your discharge from the hospital. Tell me what happened then."
6. **Identify your talkative patients,** and see them last. Patients under pressure to tell you everything will feel more pressure if

they sense you are in a hurry to go somewhere else. Seeing them last relieves some of your time pressure and thus some of his pressure. This also gives you the luxury of a definitive stop time: "I have to start rounds at 8 AM, but I have until then to talk about how you are doing."

7. **Learn to read between the lines.** It may be difficult for patients to verbally express their fears or concerns, but they will continue to try until they feel you understand. Because emotions are hard to express verbally, a patient may never reach a point where he feels he has satisfactorily communicated his fears to you; the words will continue to flow to futility. Use verbal and nonverbal cues to determine what frightens him or what emotions are at play. If you can identify, validate, and address emotional concerns, the patient will feel relief and your time with him will be more efficient. "Let me stop you for a second, Mr. Aliota. If this were me, I'd be exceedingly scared. Do you feel scared?"
8. **If you are faced with a loquacious family, ask to do the history and physical examination alone with the patient.** Families often digress, and patients must compete to tell their side of the story. Briefly interact with the family, then say, "Could you excuse us for about 5 minutes while I do an examination?" If you have time, bring the family back and extend the history.
9. **Manage your own time well** (see Chapter 43).

III Difficult Situations

Problematic patient situations are bound to arise. This section explains how to defuse the most common situations.

A. **Patient disrespect**. "Hey honey, how do they get someone so good looking to work here?" The dilemma here is whether to be polite and maintain patient rapport or stand up for yourself and risk losing patient rapport. In reality, there is no patient rapport to maintain. Rapport is based on mutual respect, and you are not being respected as a physician. Be unemotional and firm. "I have been assigned to assist your doctor, and I want to help you in that role. I cannot fulfill that role and be your 'honey.' Let's start over and you can tell me what brought you here."

B. **Threatening patients.** Immediately leave the room if you feel threatened by a patient.
   1. If there is a question of safety, leave the door open or call for a chaperone. If necessary, call security to be with you or just outside the room.
   2. Always sit so that you are closer to the door than the patient. Do not block the entrance, however, because this may make the patient feel trapped. If he tries to escape, he will be escaping through you.

C. **Comatose patients.** Talk to comatose patients as if they are conscious. They may hear you, and there is also merit in hearing yourself verbalize what you plan to do.

D. Fearful or distrusting patients. Many patients distrust or fear the healthcare system, creating a dynamic that is frustrating and disruptive. Identify the fear, acknowledge it, and address it. Reasons may include:

1. Prior difficulty in gaining access to the healthcare system. This is especially a problem in emergency departments or clinics with long wait times. Separate yourself from the system; show the patient you are the exception. "I know the system can be frustrating, and I wish I could do more about it. The good news is that I'm with you now, and I think I can help you with your symptoms."
2. Fear that physicians will not take the complaint seriously. Say, "I haven't seen the CT scan yet, so I do not know if this abdominal pain is life-threatening or not. Even if it is not, I can see this is disrupting your life, and I want to make that better."
3. Fear their pain will be undertreated unless it is dramatized. Say, "I want you to know that whatever the cause of the pain, life-threatening or not, we will take care of it."
4. Fear they will be discharged from the hospital too soon. Say, "I don't want to keep you in the hospital too long; it puts you at risk of contracting someone else's disease. However, I am not going to let you go home until we are confident that you will do well." Do not promise that you will let him decide when he will be discharged, because this is a promise that you may not be able to keep.

IV Working with Patients Who Are Delirious

Delirium is a fluctuating level of consciousness. The therapeutic strategy should change based on the stage of the delirium.

A. Nonlucid periods. Ensure patient safety. If necessary, use fall precautions and restraints. Talk to the patients as if they are not confused.

B. Lucid periods. During times of lucidity, remind the patients who they are, where they are, and the date and time. Remind them that they are ill and that they have nonlucid periods as part of their illness. Reassure them that you are here when they are not lucid and that treating the illness will make them completely lucid again. This will reduce their fear.

V Working with Patients Who Have Dementia

A. Typically, patients with dementia are aware of who and where they are (as opposed to delirium), but cognitive function is impaired.

B. Short-term memory loss can lead to:

1. **Inaccurate historical data.** To avoid this problem, take these steps:

   a. Involve the patient's family in discussions about their symptoms and treatment. Family input is additional source of information and may prompt the patient to remember other information.
   b. Be diligent in getting old records to supplement your history. Ask the patient about old diagnoses to prompt his memory.
   c. Ask specific questions, but exercise caution. Many patients with dementia will confabulate, that is, make up answers to fill in the gaps where memory has failed them. Use the family and the medical record to confirm the accuracy of the patient's answers.
2. **Failure to remember treatment instructions.** To avoid this problem, take these steps:
   a. Repeat treatment instructions frequently.
   b. Ask patients to bring all of their medications on all visits.
   c. **Write out treatment instructions.**
   d. Simplify treatment regimens as much as possible.
      (1) Coordinate medications so that they are given only once or twice a day and correspond with a standard feature of the patient's life (e.g., meals, bedtime).
      (2) Sacrifice complicated regimens that may have marginally better efficacy in lieu of simpler regimens that still work.
   e. Use week-long pill boxes to dispense medications. A family member can load the pills at the beginning of the week, and can determine if a patient has taken his medications by looking in the pill box.

HOT
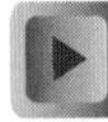
KEY

For the demented patient, do not propose treatments that require highly developed cognitive abilities.

3. **Sundowning** is a loss of orientation (person, place, time) and increased confusion as visual stimuli are removed (e.g., it gets dark when the sun goes down). Patients may exhibit great fear and anxiety in response to the confusion.
   a. Treat acute anxiety with benzodiazepines or haloperidol.
   b. Maximize the patient's sensory input.
      (1) Keep the lights on (at least a night-light).
      (2) Encourage the patient's family to bring favorite objects from home to the hospital.
      (3) Keep a calendar and clock clearly visible in the patient's room.

VI WORKING WITH PATIENTS WITH PERSONALITY DISORDERS

All patients have a personality; some you will like, some you will not. Some patients, however, actually have a personality that consistently disrupts their social function in life. This is the definition of a personality disorder (Axis II disorders). These disorders may interfere with the physician–patient relationship. You will have to modify your standard bedside manner for these individuals. Table 6-1 has a listing of the three clusters of personality disorders; Table 6-2 has a strategy for dealing with each type of patient.

VII Noncooperative Patients and Those Signing out Against Medical Advice

Some patients do not desire hospital care. This is frustrating, but you must respect their wishes.

A. Make sure that patients have the information needed to make good decisions.

B. Considerations of which you are not aware (family responsibilities, job security) may play a role in the patient's decision making. Acknowledge this by saying, "I know you have a life outside the hospital and a lot to do at home. Is there anything we can do to help you with this?" Resolving these issues will sometimes keep the patient in the hospital.

C. Do not be emotional. It is the patient's life, not yours. It is better to respect the patient's wishes to preserve the physician–patient relationship; if she leaves against medical advice and then has problems at home, she will be more likely to return.

D. If you believe that the patient should stay in the hospital, but she still asks to leave, you should ask her to sign out against medical advice (AMA). Ask the ward clerk for the necessary forms. Ensure that you document that you have:

1. Informed the patient about the risks of leaving.
2. Attempted to establish a method to follow up for additional care (ask the ward clerk to schedule an outpatient appointment for the patient).
3. Told the patient that she is welcome to return for care at any time.
4. Confirmed that the patient has the capacity to make an informed decision (patient is alert, lucid, and can understand the potential drawbacks of her decision).
5. Write prescriptions for the patient just as you would for any patient that is being discharged.

VIII Legal Issues

A. Psychiatric and medical holds (legal statutes 5150 and 5250). In these two situations, the patient cannot leave the hospital, even if he wishes. Establishing and maintaining a hold order is a limitation of a patient's liberty and should be used with the utmost precaution. The physician should be prepared to testify as to why the hold was

TABLE 6-1. Recognizing Axis II Personality Disorders.

	Character of the Personality
Cluster A	
Schizoid	• Unemotional, lonely, and indifferent to comments of others.
Schizotypal	• Anxiety in social situations. Magical thinking is used to explain eccentric behavior; digressive, overelaborate speech.
Paranoid	• Unwarranted suspicion and mistrust of others; suspicion evokes negative feelings from others, thus perpetuating the paranoia. Illness heightens the paranoia; litigious and hypervigilant.
Cluster B	
Narcissistic	• Grandiose self-importance, but extremely sensitive to criticism. • Require constant attention, and may abuse others for attention.
Histrionic	• Attention-seeking and excessive emotionality. Constantly seeking praise and reassurance.
Borderline	• Instability of self-image. Impulsive and self-damaging behavior.
Antisocial	• Cannot control impulses; engages in immediate gratification. Violates rights of others; lack of remorse. May be superficially charming but manipulative and rule-breaking.
Cluster C	
Avoidant	• Timid and shy; afraid of rejection; self-critical.
Obsessive-compulsive	• Preoccupied with the letter of the law, often missing the larger picture; perfectionist to the point of interfering with task completion; abhors changes in routine.
Dependent	• Allow others to direct their lives; lack self-confidence. Disease may aggravate fear of being abandoned.
Passive-aggressive	• Allow others to direct their lives; lack self-confidence. • Expresses anger by passively refusing to perform instructions. • Noncompliant; develop new symptoms just before discharge.

TABLE 6-2. Recognizing Axis II Personality Disorders.

Cluster	Patient Characteristics	Management Strategy
Cluster A	Patients are **lonely and isolated.** They compensate by **projection** (attributing unacceptable thoughts and feeling on others), **fantasy** (magical thinking), and **paranoia.** The patients' primary concern is to be well enough to return to their isolated world.	**a.** Remain aloof. For magical thinkers, the image of "doctor as wizard" may have its own therapeutic power. **b.** Do not try to establish an emotional relationship; patients are likely to rebel against it. **c.** State treatment plans clearly and in a matter-of-fact manner. **d.** Give instructions; admonishments may aggravate the paranoia. **e.** Do not "push" patients too hard, because they are likely to discharge themselves against medical advice (AMA).
Cluster B	Patients respond by using **dissociation** (forgetting unpleasant feelings and events), **denial, splitting** (dividing relationships and self-perception into all good or all bad), or **acting out** (aggression, violence, sex).	**a.** Set firm limits. **b.** Beware of seduction. Patients may use seductive tactics to gain what they desire. **c.** Beware of splitting of the hospital staff. Patients may try to divide the team, pitting one member against the others. **Round on these patients with the entire team present (i.e., no pre-rounds).**
Cluster C	Patients are **shy, compliant, and dependent.** They may at first appear to be perfect patients; however, separation anxiety may be a problem.	**a.** Set limits as to how often a physician or nurse will visit each day. **b.** Establish early the criteria for discharge and the date for discharge. **c.** Provide reassurance about continued care in the clinic.

absolutely necessary to prevent imminent danger to the patient or others.

1. **Psychiatric hold (5150).** Criteria are imminent danger to self (suicide) or others (homicide) or being so psychiatrically disabled as to be incompetent in making decisions for himself. Most psychiatric holds are enforceable for only 24 to 48 hours. Subsequent hold orders usually require physicians to petition the court to obtain a legal hold.
2. **Medical hold (5250).** Criteria are the same as for psychiatric holds; however danger to self is rarely evoked because patients have the right to refuse medical care if they are competent to do so. More commonly, a medical hold is based on the possibility of danger to others, such as with infectious tuberculosis. Like psychiatric holds, medical holds require a court order after 24 to 48 hours.

B. **Patient incompetence.** Patients may not have the capacity to make decisions about their care. Chapter 41 discusses the requirements for declaring a patient incompetent. A psychiatric consultation is often useful in determining competence.

C. **Durable power of attorney** (see Chapter 8). This is a legal transfer of decision making in which a patient has designated another person to make medical decisions for him if he lacks the capacity to do so.

IX Restraining Patients

A. **Indications for restraints.** Restraints should be considered for the following reasons only:

1. Patients are a danger to themselves.
2. Patients are sufficiently confused that they may dislodge an endotracheal tube, a urinary catheter, or IV lines. Patients who are incompetent or delirious may require restraints to ensure the best medical care.
3. Patients who are a danger to others.

B. **Types of restraints**

1. **Chemical restraints** are pharmacologic agents such as benzodiazepines, neuroleptics, or narcotics, that are used to sedate patients. They increase the risk of aspiration and hypotension; they must be used with caution.
2. **Physical restraints** refer to tie-down devices, including soft nylon and leather restraints.

C. **Guidelines for using restraints**

1. Use the least restrictive device necessary.
2. Make sure the restraint is properly tied to the bed *and* to the patient.
3. Never restrain the feet without also restraining the hands (the patient will fall out of bed).

4. Review the indication for restraining a particular patient at least daily; remove them as soon as possible. A new restraint order must be written each day.
5. Be careful with patients who vigorously fight against the restraints. This isometric muscle contraction results in liberation of heat (hyperthermia) and muscle break down (rhabdomyolysis).

HOT  KEY

Anxiety may be a sign of significant physical abnormalities (e.g., new infection, myocardial infarction, perforated organ), especially in the elderly, demented, or delirious patient who cannot communicate details about the pain. **Do not treat anxiety without seeing the patient. Do not chemically restrain a patient until you have ruled out organic causes of anxiety.**

7. Being on Call

I INTRODUCTION

As a medical student, you may or may not be asked to take overnight call with your team. If you are taking overnight call, this chapter gives you some fundamental principles that will make it easier. If not, then this chapter gives you some early insight that will be useful in learning from your intern's and resident's experiences; you'll be better prepared when your time comes.

II FUNDAMENTAL PRINCIPLES

The key to great performance while on call is threefold:

A. **Conserve your energy.**

B. **Maintain your appearance and composure** to meet your patients' expectations and needs. Unfortunately, patients do not understand the amount of work that goes into your call night; they will expect the same from you at 4 AM as they do at 10 AM. Furthermore, people will react to you based on your appearance and how you first interact with them. If you look professional and composed, you are much more likely to get respect and professional treatment from nurses, ancillary staff, and other physicians. This will decrease your stress level dramatically.

C. **Head into call with a great attitude.** See call nights as a great opportunity. In your medical training, **it is important that you are exposed to a diverse range of both diagnosed and undiagnosed diseases.** Being on call puts you on the front lines, thereby enabling you to see undiagnosed patients.

III ESSENTIALS OF BEING ON CALL

A. **Anticipate the busiest part of the day** and work hard during this time. Rest or relax during the down times. If you expend too much energy during a slow period, you will struggle through the busy periods. If you expend too little energy during the busy periods, these parts of the day will extend into the rest periods.

1. **Surgical specialties** are usually busiest in the morning and early afternoon. Most admissions to a surgical service come from elective admissions or transfers from other services. The down time is in the late evening. Expend energy earlier in the day and rest in the late evening or night.
2. **Obstetrics/gynecology** is busy in the morning because of elective surgeries, induced pregnancies, and cesarean sections. The rest

of the day varies, depending on when newborns decide to enter the world. Expend energy early; rest in the late evening.

3. **Medicine, neurology, and pediatrics** usually are busiest in the late afternoon and evening, when late clinic admissions arrive and patients begin to present to the emergency department. Sick patients struggle through the work day, hoping their illness will subside, or they survive during the day while other people are around. However, the fear of being sick at night without help prompts the rush to the emergency department at the end of the day, resulting in maximum admissions in the late hours. Conserve energy early; plan on expending energy during the evening and night.
4. **Psychiatry** has a more varied schedule. Count on admissions throughout the day. Late evening and night is light. Expend energy during the day, because you will likely be able to rest at night.

B. **When on call, adjust your daily routine to conserve energy.** Many ward activities must be completed with great precision and thoroughness on noncall days but are not as critical on call days.

1. **Progress notes.** Label your progress notes "On-Call Progress Notes." The purpose of the progress note is to communicate your clinical reasoning to the cross-covering physicians so that they can maintain continuity of patient care. When on call, you are the cross-covering physician, so there is little need for a detailed progress note. Instead of giving a complete assessment and plan (A&P) for each problem, note only the current intervention. At the end of your note, write, "I am on call and present for the next 24 hours. Please page me if there are questions (555–1234)."
2. **Patient visits.** Make patient visits brief. Say, "I only have a few minutes this morning, but don't worry. I'm here for 24 hours, so I will come back and see you later today." If you say this, you *must* go back and see your patients later that day. Never sacrifice patient trust for efficiency.

C. **Rest when you can.**

1. Take **naps** during down times. Even a 30-minute nap can go a long way in sustaining energy for late-night hours. Do not nap for more than 1 hour at a time. Anything more than this will keep you from falling asleep at night if the opportunity arises.
2. If you have down time after 9 PM, go to sleep and sleep as long as you can.
3. Do not abandon your team when you rest, and never nap during busy times. Tell your intern, "I'm going to rest for 30 minutes so that I will be ready to work hard tonight. If you need anything, page me." Any initial weakness on your part will quickly be forgotten when you come through strong later that night.

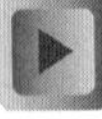
HOT KEY

As a rule, when you can sit, sit. When you can lie down, lie down. When you can sleep, sleep. Even lying down awake saves vital energy.

4. **Get enough sleep the night before call.**
5. **Eat well.** Do not skip meals in anticipation of eating better meals at a later time. If you wait too long, the cafeteria will close, and you will be left with the high-fat, high-sugar snacks from vending machines that offer little sustainable energy. If the call day is especially variable, pack your own lunch so that you eat well when you do have time.
6. **If you use caffeine, use *it*; do not let it use *you*.** Caffeine can give you a much-needed boost during crunch times but will leave you tired after an hour or two. As a rule, have no caffeine 3 hours before expected down time. It is worth being sleepy during the last three hours of the up time so that you can easily fall asleep during the down time. After 12:00 midnight, do not drink caffeine unless you plan to stay up for the duration of the call. Nothing is worse than not being able to sleep when the opportunity finally arrives.

D. **Complete time-consumptive tasks while on call.** This will make your postcall day shorter, and noncall days easier.
   1. **See your patients** a second or third time during the call day. If the call day is light, this is the time to have time-intensive conversations such as family meetings, do-not-resuscitate (DNR) discussions, and disposition planning.
   2. **Dictate discharge summaries.** Complete prescriptions and discharge forms for patients who may be going home in the next 2 days. Write discharge orders and put them in your pocket or in the back of the chart; it is easier to stop an anticipated discharge than it is to start it once the day has begun.
   3. **Write orders for consults and tests.**
   4. **Perform necessary procedures.** Do not put off that inevitable paracentesis for the postcall day.

E. **Bring medical material to read.** Do not count on reading on postcall days and do not count on reading on your days off. On average, a "q 4" call rotation means 4 days off, 7 call days, 7 postcall days, and 10 other work days. Ten days is not enough time to accomplish the reading you need to do. Bring books that have concise chapters that you can read during down times while on call (e.g., books in the *Saint-Frances Guide* series).

F. **Look good.** Patients have an image of what they want their physicians to be. No patient imagines a sloppy, beaten-down, postcall doctor in "pajamas" as his physician. They know that the "real" physicians (the attendings) never wear "pajamas" (scrubs). If you want to play the role of the patient's primary physician, play it completely. Looking the part goes a long way in convincing your patient of your professionalism.

G. **Do not become overwhelmed.** A lot of energy goes into worrying. If your team has five admissions in an hour, this does not mean it will have five admissions every subsequent hour. If necessary, prioritize tasks and do all that you can in the time allowed. If the call becomes excessively busy, just remind yourself that no matter what happens, they cannot stop the clock. The call night will end soon.

H. **If you stay overnight on call, make sure you have a place to sleep.** It is an Accreditation Council for Graduate Medical Education/Liaison Committee on Graduate Medical Education (ACGME/LCGME) rule that you must be provided a place to sleep if you are asked to stay overnight. Empty patient beds and hospital couches do not count. If a bed has not been provided for you, talk with the clerkship director. Be direct. "I need a place to sleep when I stay overnight with my team. Can you help me out?"

I. **If you go home when you are on call, find out when you should leave.** If activity is picking up, stay with your team until you are dismissed.

J. **Going home**

   1. Think about where you park your car as you come to work on call. For a Wednesday call day, it may appear to be safe to park in a "No parking on Thursday: Street Cleaning" space; it will not be all right the following day when you pay that $35 penalty on your way home after call. Also, parking spaces that seem physically safe during the day may not be safe at night when you go home.
   2. It is always worth the 30 minutes to wait for security to take you to your car if you are uncertain whether it is safe. If you do walk alone, don't make yourself out to be the doctor going home. Leave the doctor's bag at home; put your stethoscope in your pocket. Have your keys in hand as you approach your car.

IV A GOOD CALL BAG

The best possible scenario is to have a locker at work. If you do, stock it early. If you do not, pack a call bag the night before you are on call. It should contain the following items:

A. **An alarm clock.** This will allow you to take 30-minute naps. A pager that has an alarm feature will suffice.

B. **Shower supplies.** Pack liquid soap (it is less messy), shampoo, a toothbrush, and a towel.

C. **An inexpensive Walkman.** Call bags are stolen frequently. Listen to your $30 Walkman at work and your MP3 player at home. Wear no jewelry on call days; expensive jewelry is for noncall days if you choose. If you choose to carry a PDA, be careful on call. When you get busy, it will be easy to set it down; once it's down, it's all but stolen. Laptops are absolutely unnecessary on call.

D. **A change of clothes.** At the very least, bring clean underclothes and socks.

E. **Material to read** (see above).

V POSTCALL

A. **Take a shower.** Get up 30 minutes early and take a shower. Part of the misery of being postcall is the sweaty, hot feeling that is associated with clogged pores. "A shower is worth an hour (of sleep, that is)."

B. **Look professional.** In fact, try to look the same on postcall days as you do on noncall days. The first step in preventing call from defeating you is to refuse to let it defeat you. If you look as if you have just been on call for 24 hours, people will respond to you as if you have been on call. You react to the way they respond, and soon you feel very much postcall. Have pride in your appearance postcall; pride is a great source of positive energy.

C. **Complete pre-rounds early.** Remember, morning rounds is a "game of inches" (like getting to the freeway at 7:45 instead of 8:00, when traffic increases). Your team's patient orders will compete against the orders of other teams for the priority in which they are carried out. Being postcall gives you an advantage: you have the opportunity to have your orders co-signed and taken off the chart before the other teams arrive at the hospital.

8. Financial and Legal Medicine

I **INTRODUCTION** Quality of care *should be* independent of a patient's ability to pay. However, when it comes to designing therapeutic plans, you must understand how healthcare is reimbursed to protect your patient from unnecessary charges. More importantly, understanding financial constraints is the key to preventing the most common cause of noncompliance with outpatient prescriptions: the inability to afford the medication.

II **FINANCIAL STATUS OF PATIENTS** If the patient has no medical insurance, he can still potentially be eligible for benefits. Involve the social worker on the first day of admission. Healthcare is often paid by a **third-party payer,** defined as any party other than the patient or the hospital that is paying for the healthcare. There are several types of third-party payment.

A. **Private insurance.** The degree of benefits and limitation of care depend on the specific insurance company. Prescriptions may or may not be covered. Even when covered, expensive medications still usually require preapproval by the insurance company.

B. **Health maintenance organizations (HMOs)** hire their own physicians, staff, clinics, and sometimes hospitals. Because HMOs control the physicians, staff, and facilities, they contain the cost of healthcare. The HMO contains cost by requiring physicians to use preset protocols to optimize financial efficiency.

   1. If you are working in an HMO system, you may need to obtain approval before ordering expensive tests or procedures. Ordering an MRI without prior approval may leave your patient holding the bill.
   2. Approval of some medical decisions (tests, therapeutic regimens, etc.) may be required before ordering them. Although this seems unfair, patients join HMOs voluntarily, and in doing so they have agreed to trade physician flexibility for lower health care costs.
   3. When an HMO patient is admitted to a non-HMO hospital, the HMO will want him transferred to an HMO-member facility as soon as it is safe to do so. For each day the patient remains at a non-HMO facility, the HMO must pay the other facility.

C. **Preferred provider organizations (PPOs)** are similar to HMOs but do not have hospital facilities and staff. PPOs contract with physicians who receive payment in agreement for providing discounted services. PPOs, like HMOs, want member patients cared for by member physicians, because this enables them to control expenses.

D. Medicare is a federally funded program mainly for patients 65 years of age and older. It provides good overall coverage for most home services and clinic and hospital benefits. However, it will not cover expenses without justification, and the rationale for treatment must be documented.

1. There is a limit to benefits. After the amount per year has been exceeded, the patient may not be reimbursed for medical care.
2. Medicare does insure some patients with disabling chronic diseases that are likely to have a limited life span (e.g., dialysis-dependent patients).
3. The Medicare bill passed in 2004 will phase in coverage of outpatient prescription medications. Depending on how the legislation progresses, your Medicare patient may still be on her own in paying for prescriptions. Exercise caution with prescribing expensive medications.

E. Medicaid (Medi-Cal in California) is a federally funded program that provides each state with money to care for the poor and uninsured. To qualify for Medicaid, a patient must have less than $500 in assets and no insurance. In most states there is no outpatient prescription coverage. Many states (e.g., Tennessee and Louisiana) have established a PPO-like network in which each Medicaid recipient is assigned to a primary provider who must authorize subspecialty referrals.

F. Worker's compensation is an agreement between an employer and an employee that the employer will pay for the medical care of any on-the-job injury. In turn the employee agrees not to sue the employer for accidents sustained while on the job. Any job-related injury must be documented in the physician note. Be careful with your documentation; reimbursement of care depends on the quality of documentation.

G. Supplemental Security Income (SSI) requires proof of mental or physical disability and provides the patient with early social security-type payments.

H. Veterans services. Veterans Administration (VA) hospitals provide primary care, specialized care, and related medical and social support services to veterans of the U.S. military. In addition, VA hospitals offer multiple clinical programs and initiatives. Not all care is 100% free to every veteran, however. The amount of coverage depends on service-connected disability, time served in the military, and the setting of military service (e.g., domestic vs. overseas; wartime vs. peacetime).

HOT
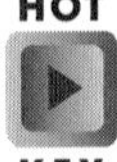
KEY

Capitated care refers to the agreements between an insurance company and a physician in which the physician receives a fixed amount of money to provide care for each of his or her patients for the entire year, regardless of the actual amount of money that the patient spends on healthcare.

III Durable Power of Attorney (DPOA).

Competent persons may legally transfer decision making about their healthcare to another person. Involuntary DPOAs can be established only when a patient has been declared incompetent by a judge of the courts. There are three types of DPOA: financial (concerning financial decisions for the patient), medical (concerning medical decisions for the patient), or comprehensive (both types of decisions).

IV Legal Restraints

(see Chapter 6)

V Legal Liability

Lawsuits are a major concern of all physicians. Although they may not win the suit, patients may sue their physicians for virtually any reason. The possibility of being sued should not keep you from practicing medicine; you simply must learn to practice smartly. Even though students are rarely sued, it is important to know what prompts lawsuits so that you can develop sound methods to prevent lawsuits as part of your future career.

A. The high-risk settings

1. **Inappropriate discharge.** The risk of a lawsuit increases any time a patient is discharged from the hospital. The very act of discharge implies that the physician has no longer chosen to care for the patient (as the patient's lawyer will argue). After discharge, the physician is not in a position to witness the consequences of a suggested therapy and cannot act to correct the treatment plan; this increases the probability of a poor outcome. Exercise great caution when the time for discharge arrives (the suggestions below will help mitigate risk).
2. **Dissatisfied patients or family.** Patients are less likely to initiate a lawsuit if they feel that their physician has done her best to help them. In any venue, if the patient or the patient's family is upset, be cautious. Even if their anger is completely unrelated to the medical care, remember that it is emotion and not facts that drives most lawsuits. If the family is upset, spend as much time as necessary to reduce their frustration. If the patient or family is still upset after this time, involve your attending physician immediately.

B. Methods for reducing legal risk

1. **"Do no harm."** When there is no good evidence that an intervention will work, do not use it. Novel, untested therapy, even if it might prove effective, will be difficult to defend if a bad result occurs. Let the standard of care as defined by your attending physicians and the medical literature guide your decisions.
2. **Spend time with your patients.** Even if you do the wrong thing (e.g., prescribe the wrong medicine or the wrong dose), your

error will usually be forgiven if the patient and her family see that you are doing your absolute best and that you are honest in admitting your mistakes. The only way to show your effort is to spend time at the bedside explaining what you are doing and why you are doing it.

3. **Clinically reason through your treatment plans.** Paradoxically, empiric treatment out of fear of lawsuits may increase the risk of a lawsuit. Unless you have a solid reason for your actions, you will be unable to justify them later. **Document your clinical reasoning** in the medical record (see Chapter 13).
4. **Never alter the medical record.** Never scribble out an entry in the medical record; it looks as though you are trying to hide something. Likewise, never remove an entry. As a rule, never change a note once it has been written. If you have a correction to make, mark one line through it (so people can see what is beneath the line) and date and initial the correction.
5. **Never criticize other students or physicians in the presence of a family member or patient.** This creates an environment of blame and mistrust, from which lawsuits flourish. Remember that the patient may be angry at the mere fact of having a disease, and it will be easy to place this anger on another physician. If a patient asks you if another physician made the right decision, simply state, "Well, hindsight is 20/20. I think we have the luxury of more information than he did at the time. What I *do* know now is that we need to do ________ (etc.)." If you have a legitimate concern about a physician, let your attending physician handle it.
6. **Do not engage in chart wars.** Do not place blame on other physicians or dispute their decisions in the medical record. If one physician has a disagreement with another physician or consulting service, it should be discussed person-to-person. A patient-care decision may be contested in the medical record, but the physician who suggested it should not be personally defamed.
7. **Take responsibility for finding follow-up care arrangements for the patient.** You know the hospital system better than your patient, and therefore you will be much more effective in ensuring follow-up care (e.g., clinic appointments). Do not release your patients until they have a follow-up clinic appointment arranged (the ward clerks are a valuable service here). Also, make sure the patient has discharge instructions that are legible and detailed and that he understands them. Take the time to go over the instructions and ask him to repeat them back to you in his own words. Document that discharge instructions have been given.

C. **Requirements for medical malpractice and medical negligence.** Malpractice is a medical mistake that has resulted in sustained physical injury or mental anguish. Both components are necessary for a successful suit. Negligence, on the other hand, is failure to provide the standard of care (e.g., the patient was refused therapy, the physician did not visit the patient in the hospital each day), resulting in physical or emotional injury. There will be little you can do to prevent malpractice suits, because you are bound to make mistakes. Medical negligence, however, is completely under your control. Spend time with your patients and let them know you are there for them, even when they leave the hospital.

VI Medical-Legal Acronyms Worth Remembering

A. Healthcare Information Privacy Protection Act (HIPPA). This act stipulates that:

1. Healthcare providers should make a "reasonable effort" to prevent others from hearing discussions about patients.
2. Patient data recorded in the medical record should be secure. There should be only one medical chart or record, and any data recorded electronically must be secure.

B. Emergency Medical Treatment and Active Labor Act (EMTALA). This act stipulates that patients who present to one hospital cannot be refused emergent treatment based upon their inability to pay. It also stipulates that before a patient is transferred from one healthcare facility or service to another, there must be a direct physician-to-physician communication. As a rule, the transferring physician assumes liability for the patient's safety until the patient is under the care of the accepting physician.

C. Joint Commission on Accreditation of Healthcare Organizations (JCAHO). This organization sets the minimum standards of healthcare for each hospital. A JCAHO visit is important because loss of accreditation means the hospital and its physicians are not eligible to receive Medicare and Medicaid reimbursement. If JCAHO visits your hospital, wear your name tag and know how to save a patient if there is a fire. If you are asked any other questions, take the surveyor to the nearest charge nurse.

D. Resident Review Committee (RRC). Each specialty has its own RRC that is an extension of the ACGME (see below). The RRC will use the ACGME general regulations and the specialty's board regulations to set the standard for residency training for that specialty, including work hours, curriculum, and competencies.

E. Liaison Committee on Graduate Medical Education (LCGME). This organization, which sets standards for medical schools, has a similar mission as the RRC.

F. Accreditation Council of Graduate Medical Education (ACGME). This organization oversees all residency training programs. Its focus is primarily on work hours, core competencies, curriculum, resident supervision, and evaluation and feedback.

9. Death and Dying

I INTRODUCTION

There will be times when patients come to you not for diagnosis or cure but rather because they sense that they are dying. They may be seeking guidance in how to have a peaceful and meaningful death, free from fear, pain, and angst, although they may not be able to communicate this. They are not necessarily asking for euthanasia; they are looking for an ambassador to guide them through life's last voyage. For the patient, this will be his first experience with death; the physician, on the other hand, will go through over a hundred deaths as a part of his career. Who better to be this ambassador than the physician?

II UNDERSTANDING DEATH

A. **Death is not necessarily a sign of failure on the part of the physician.** Unfortunately, mistakes are a part of practicing medicine, and although death may be caused by a medical error, most deaths are not. A death does not necessarily mean the physician failed the patient; to the contrary, for some patients a peaceful death may be a successful outcome.

B. **Help patients focus on peace, not pain.**

1. Most patients do not know what to expect from death and the fear that results from this uncertainty prevents them from truly sharing life's last moments with their family and close friends.
2. The physician experiences death hundreds of times in his career. He knows what to expect. He has seen peaceful deaths and painful deaths, and this experience, if conveyed to the patient, allows him to relieve the patient's fear and uncertainty. A peaceful death begins with knowing when to stop using measures to prolong life when the quality of life has long since stopped (e.g., dialysis and mechanical ventilation to prolong the life of a patient with end-stage lung cancer).

C. **Talk to physicians on your team about death at an appropriate time.** When you first encounter a death of one of your patients, you may feel a range of emotions: fear, responsibility, anger, disappointment. It may even spark thoughts about your own mortality. It is worth talking about these emotions, because only by engaging in the experience will you garner the experience of having lived through the death experience. This will be important for subsequent patients who rely upon your experience to guide them. Despite the temptation to address these emotions immediately, however, it is important to respect the emotions of your team, who may be feeling a similar sense of loss or anger. Immediately after the patient's death may not be the time to discuss it. Wait a day or two, and then address it with your team.

D. **Do not deprive yourself of contact with death.** Someday your patients will depend on you to help them have a peaceful death. If you avoid contact now, you will not gain the experience you'll need later.

III DISCUSSING CODE STATUS: DO NOT RESUSCITATE/DO NOT INTUBATE ORDERS

A "full code" order designates that full resuscitation measures should be employed in the event a cardiac or respiratory arrest occurs. A patient may designate that he does not want to be resuscitated or intubated (or both) should an arrest occur. It is important to discuss code status with your patient early. It will be an uncomfortable conversation at first, because it seems as if you are giving up on your patient. The art is in relieving this discomfort and assuaging their concerns about abandonment. Tell your patient that you will do everything for him, but that you also want to represent his wishes during a time when he will be unable to tell you what to do. Keep the following in mind as you watch your intern or resident have this conversation with patients.

A. **Choose the proper time.** Emotional, fearful settings may not allow the patient to think through his options. If possible, choose a time when you can sit with the patient without being in a rush and when the emotion of the acute illness has resolved. After the patient has arrived at his hospital room or the day after admission is usually a good time to begin the discussion.

B. **Address the topic directly.** "Mr. Capulet, I want to talk to you about what you would want a doctor to do in the event that your heart stopped beating or you stopped breathing." At this point, he may reflexively say "Do everything," or "Save me." This may be his true wish, but it may also be a sign that he is unprepared for the topic. Do not change the subject; reassure the patient and explain why you want to discuss it.

C. **Reassure the patient that you are not going to abandon him.** "I know this seems frightening, and I want to assure you that we are going to do everything we can to help you. Nothing we decide now will change that."

D. **Give a rationale for the discussion**. "The reason I bring this up is that I want to do what you want. If your heart stops, you are not going to be able to tell me what to do. I will do whatever you want me to do, but I feel I should tell you what is involved so that you can make an informed decision."

E. **Give the patient the freedom to make this decision and to change his mind.** "You do not have to make this decision now; take some time to think about it. Talk about it with your family. Also, once you make the decision, you can change your mind at any time. Regardless of what you decide, I am still your doctor and I will do anything I can to help you."

F. Whatever the patient decides, **leave the discussion open.** "OK, that is what we will do. If you want to talk more about this, I am here."

IV Hospice

A. **Definition.** Hospice is a designated program for patients who have a life expectancy of less than 6 months. Patients are given emotional and spiritual support, as well as adequate pain relief. Patients should have a DNR order on the chart. The commotion surrounding an attempt at full resuscitation in a hospice facility is traumatic for the other patients who are near death themselves.

B. **Setting of hospice care.** Hospice care can be delivered in two ways.
   1. **Home hospice** involves visits by support staff to provide pain medication and other medications. This generally requires that a family member live with the patient, because the support staff is not constantly with the patient.
   2. **Institutional hospice** is geared toward providing emotional, spiritual, and physical comfort in the last few months of life.

V Facilitating Death

A. **Allay the patient's fear of death.** Discuss what patients may expect, based on your experience with other patients with this disease. Do not discuss grim details. Instead, discuss each intervention as it occurs and each new symptom as it arises. Establishing yourself as the patient's guide will help reduce her anxiety.

B. **Look for signs of patient guilt** (e.g., "I should have stopped smoking" in a patient dying of lung cancer). These thoughts are nonproductive and only detract from the positive emotional energy he can direct toward his family during the last few moments of life. If patients express such thoughts, you might respond, "Well, maybe, maybe not. Either way, it is not worth thinking those thoughts now. Let's focus on when your kids are going to visit."

C. **Reflect on the good things in the patients' lives.** The goal is to help patients get the most out of the last days of their lives. Focus their thoughts, not on what they should have done, but on the good things that they did do. Ask them about past work experiences, exciting stories, or their happiest moments.

D. **Provide pain control as necessary.** Good pain control reduces fear and allows the patient to focus on his final affairs.

VI RUNNING A CODE

A. What to do if you are the first one to arrive

1. **Stay calm.** Use body actions that subdue the emotions. For example, just before you *walk* into the patient's room, take a deep breath and let it out slowly. Speak deliberatively and in a normal tone; do not yell or think randomly out loud. If the code has not been called, call a nurse or pick up the telephone and call the operator. Speak calmly, "Please call a code blue in room 355."
2. **Begin basic life support: cardiopulmonary resuscitation (CPR).** Remember the first step in CPR is to assess the airway and breathing. Until help arrives, CPR is the only step you can take alone.

B. How to run a code (when your time comes). You will not be asked to run a code as a medical student, but it is worth knowing what goes into a well-run code so that you can begin to prepare for the day that you are in that position. Well-run codes have this in common: the code leader prevents panic by establishing herself as the team leader and remaining calm herself. This allows every team member to do his or her best.

1. It is key that **one person assumes control and directs the team.** This person should announce that she is running the code. This person should be emotionally composed to ensure rational decision-making and leadership in directing the team. Emotion will not heighten authority or ability; to the contrary, it will panic the team. To maintain full control and rational thought, the team leader should not be distracted in performing other tasks; *all* tasks should be assigned to other team members.
2. **Each person has an assigned task** appropriate to her ability. The code leader should assign tasks directly using names; for example, "Emma, please place the IV." If you are asked to do a task that you do not know how to do or feel uncomfortable doing, tell the code leader, "I don't know how to do that. I can do something else."

VII FUTILE THERAPY

A futile intervention offers no benefits, only harm.

A. You are not obligated to institute any therapy that you consider to be futile, even if the patient or family demands it.

HOT

KEY

The first directive of a physician is "Do No Harm."

B. If in doubt, consult your hospital's ethics committee.

VIII Death Protocol

A. Pronouncing death. A physician must pronounce the patient dead. The time of death, suspected cause of death (if known), and that the family and coroner (if indicated) have been contacted should be noted. The pronouncement note should include:

1. The patient has no pulse and no respirations by palpation and auscultation.
2. The patient does not respond to noxious stimuli (sternal rub, corneal brush).
3. The patient has been observed for at least 1 minute with no change in the above observations.
4. The patient has not recently been hypothermic or immediately subject to anesthesia (these conditions can simulate death).

B. Notifying the coroner

1. The coroner should be notified in the **following circumstances. If in doubt, call the coroner.**
   - **a.** Unexpected death.
   - **b.** Death in criminal circumstances (e.g., death from a gunshot or knife wound).
   - **c.** Death less than 24 hours after admission.
   - **d.** Death after having surgery or a procedure.
   - **e.** Death from aspiration or sepsis.
   - **f.** Death from neglect or abuse.
   - **g.** Death from drug overdose.
2. Even if some of these criteria are present, it is likely that the coroner will release the body, which means that no autopsy will be performed. In this case, ask the family for an autopsy (see VIII D).

HOT

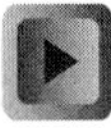

KEY

Always try to have an autopsy performed. This is a valuable tool in learning about physical manifestations of disease.

C. Completing the death certificate. Each state has its own specific type of death certificate. All require the time of death and the cause. Be as specific as possible in identifying the cause of death; vague diagnoses that are the result of the true etiology (e.g., respiratory failure instead of pneumonia) should not be listed.

D. Requesting an autopsy. This task is very important for your training as a physician. Requesting and obtaining an autopsy does not put you or your team at increased legal risk. Diagnoses discoverable only by autopsy are unlikely to be held against physicians.

1. **Recognize the awkwardness of the situation.** Show empathy; “Mrs. Darcy, I know this is a difficult time, but I have a very important question to ask you.”

2. **Be direct.** Get to the point; "We would like to ask your permission to do an autopsy on your husband."
3. **Tell why the autopsy is important.** "It is only by seeing how disease kills people that we are able to learn to conquer it. Your husband could teach us valuable lessons that might be able to save other patient's lives."
4. **Rectify misconceptions.** "The autopsy will not change the appearance of your husband. You will still be able to have an open casket funeral if that is what you would like. If you are really concerned about the autopsy, we can do the autopsy on only the heart (i.e., the organ of interest in the patient's death)."
5. **Respect the family's wishes** regardless of what they decide.

PART II

The Fundamental Skills of Clinical Medicine

10. Clinical Reasoning

I FUNDAMENTALS Clinical reasoning is the process of determining which disease is causing the patient's symptoms. While on the wards you will note that some physicians are superior to others in their diagnostic abilities. All physicians use the same laboratory and radiographic tests; thus **the quality of a physician's diagnostic ability is proportional to the quality of her clinical reasoning.** This chapter teaches you the three pillars of clinical reasoning: 1) using the history to establish a differential diagnosis and assess the confidence you have in each specific diagnosis being considered (pretest probability), 2) knowing the diagnostic power of examination maneuvers and laboratory tests, and 3) knowing what to do with the posttest probability for each diagnosis you are considering in choosing to treat or not. Table 10-1 is a summary of the seven-step clinical reasoning process.

A. **Pillar I: Long list to smart list and pretest probability.** Chapter 11 gives you techniques for obtaining a medical history. After hearing the patient's history, the first step is to create a "long list" of diagnoses that could explain the patient's chief complaint. For example, Table 10-2 has a sample "long list" of diagnoses that could explain a 25-year-old man's abdominal pain. After constructing the long list, the next step is to construct a "smart list," that is, the four or five diagnoses that fit the pattern of the patient's presentation. **This smart list is known as the differential diagnosis.** The next step is to begin mentally ranking each of the diagnoses on the smart list based on their probability of being the correct diagnosis. **The pretest probability for a disease is the chance that the patient has that disease based solely on the historical information** (i.e., before laboratory tests are ordered). If you were to actually assign a numerical value to the pretest probability of each diagnosis (e.g., 40% appendicitis, 20% gastroenteritis, etc.), the sum of all of these

TABLE 10-1. Clinical Reasoning Using the Seven-Step Approach.

Procedure	Steps
History	1. Take a history (see Chapter 11). 2. Create a list of possible diagnoses (four or five). 3. Ask questions about each of these diagnoses. 4. Mentally assign a pretest probability to each diagnosis.
Physical examination	5. Perform a physical examination (see Chapter 12). Focus the examination on the diagnoses you are considering. Change the probabilities of each diagnosis based on the examination results. Reorder the diagnoses.
Laboratory tests and other studies	6. Order laboratory and other studies. Focus these tests on the diagnoses you are considering. Change the probability of each of the diagnoses based on the laboratory test and study results. Reorder the diagnoses.
Assessment and plan	7. Make an assessment and plan based on the remaining diagnoses.

numbers would add up to 100%. This is based on Occam's razor, which states that only one diagnosis should explain a patient's symptoms. That is to say, if we were to discover one diagnosis as the cause, with 100% certainty, the probability of all other diagnoses will have to go to 0%. This is important because the reverse is also true: by making some diagnoses' probabilities 0% (i.e., ruling them out), the probabilities of the remaining diagnoses increases. This enables deductive reasoning. The important point is that the history establishes the differential diagnosis and the probability that each diagnosis being considered is correct; these probabilities will change as the examination is performed and laboratory tests are ordered (next pillar).

B. **Pillar II: Predictive power of a test.** Each physical examination maneuver, laboratory test, or radiographic study will either increase (if the test is positive) or decrease (if the test is negative) the probability of a diagnosis being considered. **Powerful tests greatly increase or decrease a diagnosis' probability.** We measure the power of a diagnostic test by looking at its likelihood ratio, which is a statistic

TABLE 10-2. A 25-Year-Old Man with 3 Days of Abdominal Pain and Nausea.

Long List (diagnoses that fit the patient's chief complaint)	Smart List (diagnoses that fit the pattern of the patient's presentation)	*Ranked* Smart List (probability of each diagnosis based on the prevalence of disease in all 25-year-old men)	Smart List II (after further questions, physical examination, and laboratory testing)
Stomach			
Gastroenteritis →	Gastroenteritis →	Gastroenteritis (40%) →	Gastroenteritis (50%)
Peptic ulcer			
Duodenum			
Duodenal ulcer			
Liver/bile duct			
Cholangitis →	Cholangitis →	Cholangitis (5%)	
Cholecystitis			
Hepatitis →	Hepatitis →	Hepatitis (20%)	
Pancreas			
Pancreatitis →	Pancreatitis →	Pancreatitis (5%)	
Spleen			
Splenomegaly			
Bowels			
Bowel obstruction			
Appendicitis →	Appendicitis →	Appendicitis (25%) →	Appendicitis (35%)
Diverticulitis →	Diverticulitis →	Diverticulitis (5%) →	Diverticulitis (15%)
Bacterial colitis			

composed of the test's sensitivity and specificity for a particular disease (see below).

C. **Pillar III: Integrating posttest probability and treatment thresholds.** After all of the tests are done, the ranking of the diagnoses in the initial differential diagnosis will be different from before; some diagnoses will be more likely than they were before and some will be less likely. The goal is to get one diagnosis to 100% probability. Achieving 100% certainty is rarely reached, however, and it is likely that you will be left to decide whether to start treatment for a disease that is highly probable (say, 80%) but is not yet 100% certain. In most circumstances the physician cannot wait until he has 100% assurance that a diagnosis is correct; to do so would deny many patients who need treatment the benefits of the treatment until it is too late. For example, if you routinely wait until you are 100% sure that the patient has appendicitis before doing surgery, some patients will experience rupture of their appendix and die. **The level of confidence at which you decide to administer therapy** (e.g., 60% certain vs. 80% certain) **is called the <u>treatment threshold.</u>** If your level of confidence is above this threshold, even if you are not 100% sure, treatment should be administered. **The treatment threshold is determined by looking at the costs and benefits of the therapy being considered** (see discussion of treatment thresholds below).

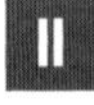

II Putting the Three Pillars Together: Clinical Reasoning

A. **Step 1: Determining the pretest probability of disease.**

1. Determining an accurate differential diagnosis and pretest probability for each diagnosis is challenging, but it is this accuracy that defines the master clinician. There are three components to great accuracy:
    a. **Knowing the prevalence of disease** in the patient being treated based on age, gender, geographic location, and ethnicity. This is why the first line of every patient presentation (see Chapter 16) begins with a demographic description of the patient: "A **54-year-old Caucasian woman** who presents with chest pain."
    b. **Knowing disease patterns.** After a chief complaint is identified, the physician begins making a mental list of diseases that can cause that complaint (the long list). Knowing the pattern of how each of these diseases typically presents allows the physician to select those diagnoses whose typical patterns closely match the character and time course of the patient's complaint. The closer the match, the higher the pretest probability for that disease.

c. **Experience** in treating patients will allow you to improve your accuracy in estimating pretest probability by having seen the diagnoses in previous patients. Be warned, however. Practice does not make perfect; perfect practice makes perfect. Only by learning from your mistakes will you improve your clinical reasoning. Section V gives you a method for identifying the precise error in your clinical reasoning when mistakes occur.

2. Example. Let's say a 25-year-old man presents with 2 days of abdominal pain and vomiting. The physician will mentally go to his "file cabinet" of diseases that cause nausea and vomiting and create a **"long list"**—every diagnosis it **could** be (Table 10-2; Column 1). The physician will then elicit the time course and character of the complaint and, by using pattern recognition, will select those diagnoses that appear to fit the pattern of the patient's complaint. This is the **"smart list":** the diagnoses it is **likely to be** (Table 10-2; Column 2). In this example, the patient's pain began with anorexia and nausea, followed by gradual periumbilical pain that then moved to the right lower quadrant. After hearing this, the physician then mentally ranks the diagnoses on this smart list based on the prevalence of each disease in a population of 25-year-old Caucasian men. Appendicitis is much more prevalent than diverticulitis in 25-year-old men, so at least initially it is of higher probability. **Great physicians will then begin targeting their questions at the diagnoses being considered on their smart list.** The smart list is what keeps their history focused and efficient. Table 10-2 does not have all of these questions, but you can imagine a few you might ask: "Do you drink alcohol (pancreatitis)?" "Have you had unprotected sex (hepatitis)?" The list is then mentally reordered based on the answers to these questions (Table 10-2; Column 3). Once the questioning is done, the smart list is advanced to the physical examination for more refinement. (NOTE: The numbers in this example are used only to make the concept more tangible. In real life, instead of hearing a physician say "I have a 60% pretest probability that appendicitis is the right answer," you are more likely to hear, "I have a strong hunch that this patient has appendicitis.")

B. **Step 2: Obtain diagnostic tests.**

1. **After the differential diagnosis is established,** physical examination maneuvers are performed and laboratory and other diagnostic tests are ordered. The goal of each is to increase (if the test is positive) or decrease (if the test is negative) the probability of the disease being considered. This is why it is vital that the history precede the physical examination and the ordering of tests. This allows the physician to target the physical examination and laboratory testing toward what really counts: the diagnoses being considered. It also allows her to exclude or confirm diagnoses as the examination and laboratory testing proceeds.

2. Let's say the patient in our example had a fever, rigidity on palpation of the abdomen, no scleral icterus, and a normal liver size. The fever increases the probability of an infectious etiology such as appendicitis, hepatitis, diverticulitis, and cholangitis. The normal liver size and the lack of jaundice significantly reduce the probability of hepatitis and cholangitis. In this example, the laboratory tests ordered to evaluate the diagnoses on the smart list revealed normal liver enzymes, normal amylase, and normal serum bilirubin, but an elevated white blood cell count. The normal amylase significantly reduces the probability of pancreatitis, and the normal liver enzymes and bilirubin significantly reduce the probability of hepatitis or cholangitis. The elevated white blood cell count increases the probability of an infection (e.g., appendicitis, diverticulitis, cholangitis).

C. **Step 3: Determine the posttest probability of disease and decide whether to treat or not.**

1. After the results of the diagnostic tests are obtained, the probability of each disease changes; positive results have increased the probability of a specific diagnosis, and negative results have decreased it. The probability of the disease being the correct diagnosis after testing is known as the **posttest probability.** Column 4 of Table 10-2 shows how the probabilities of our initial diagnosis have changed based on the laboratory results. If the posttest probability of disease is extremely low, the diagnosis can be excluded. Note how hepatitis, pancreatitis, and cholangitis fell off the list; the negative examination and laboratory test findings reduced their posttest probability to essentially 0%. The probability they previously owned has been transferred to those diagnoses still in the race: the probability of appendicitis, gastroenteritis, and diverticulitis all increase. This is a useful clinical strategy; **some diagnoses can be made more probable by excluding other diagnoses on the differential diagnosis.**
2. As noted above, in most circumstances the physician does not have the luxury of waiting until she is 100% sure of the diagnosis to institute treatment. The question then is "How sure do you have to be to institute therapy?" The answer is that it depends on the potential costs and benefits of the therapy for the patient being considered. **The combination of the potential costs and benefits of treatment defines the treatment threshold.** If the benefits are high and the costs are low (e.g., treating suspected pneumonia with antibiotics), the probability of disease needed to start antibiotics for a suspected pneumonia is low (e.g., 30%). If the potential costs are high and the benefits are low (e.g., chemotherapy), we have to be absolutely certain the diagnosis is

correct (e.g., the diagnosis must be confirmed by tissue biopsy). In simple terms, when the probability of disease exceeds its treatment threshold, treatment should be given, even if you are not 100% certain the patient has the disease. This also explains why you may see your attending physician treating two diseases simultaneously (e.g., pneumonia and asthma), even though statistically (by Occam's razor) the patient has only one disease explaining his symptoms. If the probability of both diseases has crossed their respective treatment thresholds, both diseases should receive treatment.

HOT 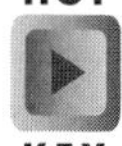 KEY

There are two ways to make a diagnosis more probable:
1. Confirming the diagnosis by finding a test result that is positive for that disease.
2. Excluding other diagnoses on the differential diagnosis by finding test results that are negative for those diseases.

III ESTIMATING THE DIAGNOSTIC POWER OF THE TEST

Up to this point, the whole process may sound nebulous. After all, how do we know that the pretest probability for hepatitis (estimated to be 30%) was reduced to zero with normal liver enzymes? The key is in knowing the diagnostic power of liver enzymes in confirming or excluding hepatitis. The sensitivity and specificity of a test is the measure of that test's diagnostic power.

A. Sensitivity is the ability of a test to detect a disease when it is truly present. Sensitivity is the percentage of all patients *with* a disease who have a *true* positive test result [**true** test positive/**all** patients with disease a/(a + c)] (Figure 10-1). Highly sensitive tests are almost always positive when a patient truly has the disease. Airport metal detectors are examples of very sensitive tests; if there is any metal on you at all, the test will register a positive result (beep). Therefore, when highly sensitive tests are negative, we can be fairly confident that the patient does not have that disease (the disease has been "ruled out"). Elevated liver enzymes are always present with hepatitis (the liver is inflamed, releasing the enzymes); therefore, if the liver enzymes are normal, hepatitis is virtually excluded.

B. Specificity is the ability of a test to correctly identify a disease as being absent when it is truly absent. Specificity is the percentage of all patients *who do not have the disease* who are correctly identified by the test as having a *true* negative test result [d/(b + d)]. Cinderella's slipper is an example of a highly specific test: the slipper will not fit (negative test result) all people who are not Cinderella (those without the disease). It will have a positive result only when the disease is present (e.g., Cinderella is present). Therefore, when

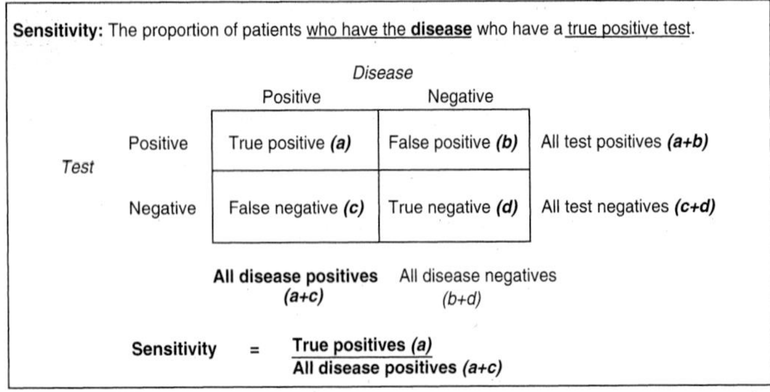

Sensitivity: The proportion of patients <u>who have the **disease**</u> who have a <u>true positive test</u>.

		Disease: Positive	Disease: Negative	
Test	Positive	True positive ***(a)***	False positive ***(b)***	All test positives ***(a+b)***
	Negative	False negative ***(c)***	True negative ***(d)***	All test negatives ***(c+d)***
		All disease positives *(a+c)*	All disease negatives *(b+d)*	

Sensitivity = True positives *(a)* / All disease positives *(a+c)*

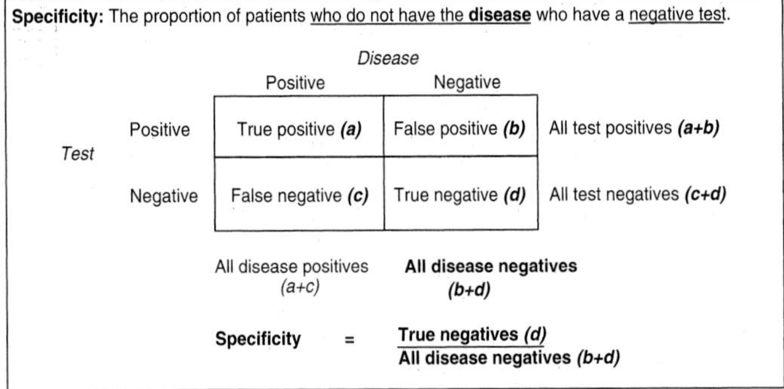

Specificity: The proportion of patients <u>who do not have the **disease**</u> who have a <u>negative test</u>.

		Disease: Positive	Disease: Negative	
Test	Positive	True positive ***(a)***	False positive ***(b)***	All test positives ***(a+b)***
	Negative	False negative ***(c)***	True negative ***(d)***	All test negatives ***(c+d)***
		All disease positives *(a+c)*	**All disease negatives *(b+d)***	

Specificity = True negatives *(d)* / All disease negatives *(b+d)*

FIGURE 10-1. Calculating sensitivity and specificity. **A,** Sensitivity answers the question, "How good is this test at detecting patients <u>with</u> disease?" A sensitive test is very good at ruling a disease out. **SNOUT, sen**sitivity rules disease **out. B,** Specificity answers the question: "How good is this test at detecting patients <u>without</u> disease?" A specific test is very good at ruling a disease in. **SPIN, sp**ecificity rules disease **in.**

highly specific tests are positive, they are very useful for "ruling in" a disease. In the example above, a CT scan demonstrating a swollen, inflamed appendix is very specific for appendicitis, because no other diagnosis can cause this finding.

HOT KEY

To remember the formula for sensitivity and specificity, remember "What is <u>**true**</u> over <u>**all**</u>?"

Sensitivity = <u>**True** positives</u> / **All** patients *with* disease

Sensitivity = <u>**True** negatives</u> / **All** patients *without* disease

Also remember the "SNOUT" and "SPIN" mnemonics:
SeNsitive tests rule **OUT** disease.
SPecific tests rule **IN** disease.

C. **Combining sensitivity and specificity.** The problem with using either sensitivity or specificity alone in assessing the value of a test is that very sensitive tests tend not to be highly specific and very specific tests tend not to be highly sensitive. Note that in the above examples, airport metal detectors are not specific for guns (they often go off when no gun is present) and Cinderella's slipper is not sensitive in detecting a suitable partner for Prince Charming (this test will miss many great people who would have fit Prince Charming just fine). When we order a test, we are interested in both confirming a diagnosis if it is present *and* excluding the diagnosis if it is not. To accurately estimate a test's diagnostic power, then, we need to know the *combination* of a test's sensitivity and specificity. Likelihood ratios are just that combination. Figure 10-2 illustrates how sensitivity and specificity are used in calculating positive and negative likelihood ratios.

D. **The Positive Likelihood Ratio** is used when a test result is positive. Positive likelihood ratios are always greater than 1, which means when you multiply the likelihood ratio by the pretest probability, the posttest probability will always increase (i.e., the diagnosis becomes more likely than before the test was ordered). (NOTE: If you were to actually make the multiplication, you would multiply by pretest

When a test result is positive, use the Positive Likelihood Ratio. The result will always be a number >1 (i.e., it makes the disease *more* probable)

$$+LR = \frac{\text{Sensitivity}}{1 - \text{Specificity}}$$

When a test result is negative, use the Negative Likelihood Ratio.The result will always be a number <1 (i.e., it makes the disease *less* probable)

$$-LR = \frac{1 - \text{Sensitivity}}{\text{Specificity}}$$

(In both formulae, sensitivity is always on top; only the "1 − " changes position.)

FIGURE 10-2. Positive and negative likelihood ratios.

odds, not pretest *probability*) [Figure 10-3]. How much it increases is reflected in the positive likelihood ratio: the bigger the number, the better the test.

E. **The Negative Likelihood Ratio** is used when a test result is negative. Negative likelihood ratios are always less than 1, which means when you multiply the negative likelihood ratio by the pretest probability, the posttest probability will always decrease (i.e., the diagnosis becomes less likely than before the test was ordered). How much it decreases is reflected in the negative likelihood ratio: the smaller the number, the better the test.

F. In simple terms, **the best test is the one that has a very high positive likelihood ratio and a very low negative likelihood ratio.**

G. An important word of caution. Because likelihood ratios are built on the test's sensitivity and specificity for identifying a particular disease, **the test's likelihood ratios will change for different diseases.** For example, an ECG may have good likelihood ratios for myocardial infarction (+LR = 14; −LR 0.3), but lousy likelihood ratios for pneumonia (+LR 1.1; −LR 0.99).

H. Practically, it is impossible to remember the likelihood ratios for every test for every disease. Most physicians come to appreciate a test's strength for a certain disease as a part of their clinical experience. There are two occasions in which knowing a test's likelihood ratios is important, however, and looking up the test's sensitivity and specificity in the medical literature can solve both.

1. You may find yourself wondering which of two tests (e.g., ultrasound vs. CT) is the best for diagnosing a particular disease (e.g., appendicitis). The medical literature will provide sensitivity/specificity data (and perhaps likelihood ratios already calculated for you) on each test.
2. Most importantly, if you make an error in your clinical reasoning, the test's likelihood ratio will tell you if your error was due to overestimating or underestimating the power of the diagnostic test you used (see Section V).

I. Table 10-3 has some general guidelines for interpreting likelihood ratios.

HOT KEY

Order a test only if you think it has the potential to change what you will do for a patient (e.g., it will increase the probability of a disease above its treatment threshold or help rule out the disease). Tests that have little power (e.g., likelihood ratios close to 1) have little use in clinical medicine.

TABLE 10-3. General Rules for Interpreting Positive and Negative Likelihood Ratios.

Positive	Negative
A likelihood ratio of 2 increases the probability about 15%.	A likelihood ratio of 0.5 decreases the probability about 15%.
A likelihood ratio of 5 increases the probability about 30%.	A likelihood ratio of 0.2 decreases the probability about 30%.
A likelihood ratio of 10 increases the probability about 45%.	A likelihood ratio of 0.1 decreases the probability about 45%.

IV THE ANATOMY OF A MISTAKE: IDENTIFYING WHERE YOU WENT WRONG

A. When you make the wrong diagnosis it is due to one of eight errors in the clinical reasoning process (Table 10-4).

B. When you make a mistake in a diagnosis, it is worth mentally walking through the clinical reasoning process (Figure 10-3). The math in this figure is only to make the process more tangible. Note, however, that there are only two components to the equation. If you find yourself very confident in a diagnosis that was not the correct diagnosis, you either overestimated the pretest probability of the diagnosis or you overestimated the power of the diagnostic test. Review the literature, and if the test's diagnostic power is similar to what you thought it was, go back and look carefully at the history you obtained from the patient. Somewhere in there is some data that you gave too much credence in making your diagnosis. Once you appreciate this, you can then ask the questions of your attending that you cannot get from books: "I clearly gave too high a pretest probability to pulmonary embolism (the incorrect diagnosis). What about this patient's clinical presentation made you think congestive heart failure (correct diagnosis) was more likely?" In this way you can tap into the attending's experience and truly learn from your mistake.

V ADVANCED CLINICAL REASONING.

A. Dealing with protean diagnoses. Some diagnoses are universally consistent in their presentation. Cellulitis, for example, almost al-

TABLE 10-4. Types of Medical Mistakes.

DIAGNOSTIC ERRORS

Type A Error: You Supported the Wrong Diagnosis.

Error 1: You overestimated the pretest probability of a wrong diagnosis. *Example:* You were overconfident in the diagnosis of tuberculosis because the patient had once spent time in a jail.

Error 2: You overestimated the power of a diagnostic test whose results were positive (i.e., you overestimated its positive likelihood ratio), thereby suggesting the *wrong* diagnosis. *Example:* You thought it was definitely a urinary tract infection because there was 0–5 WBC in the urine.

Error 3: You underestimated the power of a diagnostic test whose results were negative (i.e., a negative likelihood ratio). *Example:* You persisted in believing the patient had a myocardial infarction (instead of pericarditis), even after the troponins were negative.

Type B Error: You Did Not Support the Correct Diagnosis.

Error 4: You underestimated the pretest probability of the correct diagnosis. *Example:* In a patient with dyspnea, you failed to note the patient's history of an around-the-world airplane flight as a risk factor for pulmonary embolism.

Error 5: You underestimated the power of a diagnostic test whose results were positive for the *correct* diagnosis. *Example:* you discounted the T wave inversion on the ECG as a sign of myocardial ischemia.

Error 6: You overestimated the power of a diagnostic test whose results were negative (i.e., a negative likelihood ratio) for the *correct* diagnosis. *Example:* You excluded sepsis because the first blood culture was negative.

TREATMENT ERRORS

Error 7: You correctly estimated the posttest probability of the disease, but you withheld treatment from a patient who needed it because you **set the treatment threshold too high.** This occurs as a result of **overestimating the potential risks of the therapy or underestimating the potential benefits** (i.e., you established a reasonable probability of appendicitis, but you did not take the patient to the operating room because you overestimated the potential complications of the surgery or you underestimated the potential benefits of the surgery).

Error 8: You correctly estimated the posttest probability of the disease, but **you gave treatment prematurely because you set the treatment threshold too low.** This occurs when a physician clearly sees the benefit of potential treatment, but does not see the potential harm. *Example:* You established a reasonable probability of myocardial infarction so you gave the patient thrombolytics (blood thinners), resulting in a fatal gastrointestinal hemorrhage. You failed to note the history of a bleeding stomach ulcer 1 month earlier. Although the decision to treat (treatment threshold) may have been appropriate for most patients, the potential risks were much higher in this patient; to justify therapy, the probability of myocardial infarction would have to be almost certain.

Step 1	Step 2	Step 3	Step 4	Step 5
Establish a pre-test probability for a disease	**Convert to pre-test odds***	**Multiply by the likelihood ratio. Use the positive LR if the test was positive; the negative LR if it was negative**	**Convert back to probabilities****	**This is your post-test probability**
60% appendicitis	60% yes / 40% no	CT of abdomen is positive. The +LR for appendicitis is 10		
60%	$\frac{60}{40}$	$\times 10 \quad \frac{600}{40} \quad =$	$\frac{600}{(600+40)}$	94%

FIGURE 10-3. Quantitative decision making. * Note: Likelihood ratios are expressed in the mathematical form of "odds." To multiply a pretest probability by a likelihood ratio, you first have to convert the probability to the form of "odds." This is simply the probability/(1-probability). ** Note: The result of the pretest odds multiplied by the likelihood ratio is the posttest odds. To convert this back to a posttest probability, divide the top number in step 3 by the sum of the top and bottom numbers [i.e., top/(top + bottom)].

ways presents with a red, warm area of skin. Other diagnoses are protean, meaning they can present in many different clinical patterns (e.g., pulmonary embolism). Because protean diagnoses lack a consistent pattern, they are hard to recognize using pattern recognition alone. With experience, you will learn to differentiate the consistent from the protean diagnoses. When a protean diagnosis does appear on your differential, try to exclude the other diagnoses on your differential diagnosis before addressing the protean diagnosis. Remember, all pretest probabilities must total 100%. Thus, as other diagnoses become less likely (e.g., as the probability of pneumonia decreases from 50% to 0%), the other diagnoses become more likely (i.e., 50% must be added to the other diagnoses). For example, consider a patient who presents with sudden shortness of breath. You go after the "easy" diagnoses by ordering an ECG, complete blood count, and CXR; all of which were normal. These findings decrease the likelihood of pneumonia, pneumothorax, myocardial infarction, congestive heart failure, and anemia, thereby increasing the probability of pulmonary embolism.

B. Multiple complaints. On occasion, a patient may present with multiple complaints, and it will be tempting to suspect that the patient is succumbing to a multitude of diseases. The reality is that in the absence of an immune-compromising condition, it is very unlikely that the patient's acute problems are due to more than one primary disease. The best strategy is to address each complaint as if it were the only complaint by making a differential diagnosis for each. Once the differential diagnosis for each complaint is assembled:

1. See if the complaints can be linked together as pathophysiologic consequences of the one disease process. For example, leg swelling, renal failure, and shortness of breath may all be due to a new cardiomyopathy that is impairing blood flow to the kidney and creating a backup of blood volume in the lungs and legs, causing shortness of breath and edema.
2. Create a Venn diagram by overlapping the differential diagnosis for each problem; see if there is one disease that each differential diagnosis shares.

C. If, after collecting the history, physical examination, and laboratory data, you feel overwhelmed with the number of problems the patient has, step back and look at your admission note (see Chapter 13). Go through the admission note front to back and circle the solvency issues. **Solvency issues** are those problems (symptoms, physical findings, or laboratory abnormalities) that must be solved before the patient goes home. Not all problems will be solvency issues (e.g., the patient may have a history of asthma or gout; if these are not active, they are not solvency issues). In the margin of the admission note, write the solvency issues. Focus your clinical reasoning on these issues.

D. No answers. If after extensive history-taking, examining, and testing there is still no answer for your patient's diagnosis, do not fall victim to the temptation to extend testing for fantastical and rare diseases. If there is no answer after doing all of things that make common sense, take out a fresh piece of paper and go back to the patient as if it was the first day you had admitted him. Begin the history from scratch, repeating all of the examination maneuvers and laboratory testing that made sense the first time around. The answer may very well reveal itself to you. If you still cannot figure out what is wrong, then knock yourself out with fantastical testing.

11. Taking a History

It is important that you read Chapter 10 (Clinical Reasoning) before reading this chapter.

I **THE IMPORTANCE OF THE HISTORY** The history is the most important element of the patient's evaluation, because it enables you to build a strong differential diagnosis (see Chapter 10). If done correctly, it will also enable you to accurately assess the probability of each diagnosis on your list. The differential diagnosis sets the stage for the rest of the patient's evaluation (Chapter 10); therefore small errors here will result in exponential errors when the evaluation is complete. A strong differential diagnosis will also enable you to efficiently choose the physical examination maneuvers and laboratory tests that will be useful in increasing or decreasing the probability of each diagnosis being considered. In addition, the history also offers two important benefits:

A. **The history establishes physician–patient rapport.** Patients trust physicians who take time to listen to their stories. Patients are more likely to give you complete, accurate information if they believe they can trust you. Even if portions of the history seem like a waste of time, carefully listening will facilitate the release of valuable information from the patient.

B. **The history keeps the diagnostic workup focused on the patient, not the disease.** It is easy to get lost in chasing laboratory abnormalities during the course of a patient's evaluation. It's equally easy to lose sight of the patient as you descend complicated algorithms. A good history will keep you focused on what is most troublesome to the patient. Curing the disease is priority No. 2; addressing the patient's primary concern is priority No. 1.

II **THE THREE STEPS IN A GREAT HISTORY OF PRESENT ILLNESS** The order of these three steps is very important, because each step depends on information obtained in previous steps.

III **STEP 1: IDENTIFY THE CHIEF COMPLAINT** The chief complaint is the reason the patient came to see you. The chief complaint can be subjective because some words have different meanings for different people (e.g., "falling out" = "passing out" =

"losing time"). You can minimize this subjectivity by using the following guidelines:

A. Ask the patient to describe the chief complaint as accurately and concisely as possible ("shortness of breath with exercise," not "shortness of breath").

B. When a chief complaint has multiple interpretations, ask the patient specific questions for further clarification. For example, for a patient who complains of dizziness, you might ask, "Do you mean the room is spinning, or do you mean you feel lightheaded, as if you had stood up too quickly?"

IV Step 2: Characterize the Chief Complaint

A. The goal of the history is to establish a list of diagnoses that could explain the patient's symptoms and to establish a probability of being correct for each diagnosis. One of the three techniques for establishing each diagnosis' probability of being correct is **pattern recognition (see Chapter 10).** Accurately establishing the pattern of the symptoms will ensure an accurate differential diagnosis. There are two key components to pattern recognition: the character and the time course of the chief complaint.

1. **Step 2a: Describe the chief complaint/symptoms using the "FAR COLDER" mnemonic:**

Frequency of occurrence
Associated symptoms
Radiation of the symptom
Character of the symptom
Onset of the symptom
Location of the symptom
Duration of the symptom
Exacerbating/**R**elieving factors

2. **Step 2b: Establish a time course of the chief complaint.** Each patient presentation is a story, and establishing this story **as you take the history** will greatly assist you in recognizing the time course of the chief complaint. It will also be of great help later when you present the patient's history to your attending physician (see Chapter 16).
   a. Begin by asking when the symptom first appeared. Then ask the patient to describe what has happened up to the time of admission.
   b. The patient is likely to skip around, but do not let him. Try to coach him into presenting the story in its **exact chronologic order.** This will allow you to fully see the temporal pattern. The sample dialog in Figure 11-1 illustrates how this can be

Physician: "When did the chest pain begin?"

Patient: "Four months ago, but yesterday I noted shortness of breath and nausea."

Physician: "Ok, good. You know it will help me to keep this straight if I can keep it in all in order. Let's go back to four months ago. Did anything change between four months ago and now?"

Patient: "Well, two months ago I noticed the pain was occurring twice a week."

Physician: "Ok good. But before I hear more, did anything change between two months ago and now?"

FIGURE 11-1. Establishing a chronologic time course during questioning.

done without offending the patient or closing the conversation. The key is to keep going back to the most distant piece of history and clearly establishing what changed between each point of time as the symptoms progressed. Do not move forward in the history until the link between each time point is clear (e.g., 4 months ago to 2 months ago to 1 week ago).

c. See Chapters 13 and 16 for how a concisely obtained history translates into a cogent and concise admission note and oral presentation.

3. Step 3: Questions directed at the list of possible diagnoses.

a. After establishing the time course and character of the chief complaint, take a minute and think about what diagnoses might fit the patient's presentation. **This is the differential diagnosis that will guide the rest of your history** (and indeed, the rest of the patient evaluation as a whole). For a 54-year-old man with 3 days of chest pain, you might choose the following diagnoses: myocardial infarction, pneumonia, pulmonary embolism, costochondritis, or gastric reflux (heartburn).

HOT
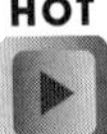
KEY

As you are taking the history, it is useful to write the list of diagnoses you are considering in the margin of the page. This will remind you to focus your subsequent questions on these diagnoses.

b. Use the remainder of the history to ask questions that help to increase or decrease each diagnosis' probability on your differential diagnosis. For example, to evaluate the possibility of myocardial infarction, ask about past coronary disease, smoking history, family history of heart disease, etc. For heartburn, you might ask if the pain is worse after eating or worse when lying flat. Do this for each diagnosis on your list.

HOT 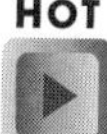 **KEY**

The second part of the history can be very brief if the diagnosis explaining the chief complaint is obvious after hearing the time course and character of the chief complaint. If the diagnosis is uncertain, expand the questions targeted at the diagnoses on the differential diagnosis.

V PAST MEDICAL HISTORY

PAST MEDICAL HISTORY The past medical history chronicles all past medical and surgical history. Although important, it is less so than the history of present illness.

A. **Allergies.** First ask about allergies to medications. Also ask about allergies to iodine/shellfish (e.g., potential reaction to contrast media), latex, and foods. If there is an allergy, ask the patient to describe the symptoms of the allergic reaction (e.g., rash, facial swelling, etc.).

B. **Medications.** Next, ask about the patient's medications. If possible, ask to see them. Record the dose and frequency at which the patient is *actually* taking each medication, not merely the dose and frequency written on the label. Ask the patient why she takes each medication. This question will reveal insight into her understanding of her disease, and it may reveal diagnoses that she has failed to mention. For example, the question, "I see you are taking metformin; what is that for?" yields the answer "I have diabetes." It is also important to ask about over-the-counter medications and any alternative medications (e.g., herbs).

C. **Past diagnoses**

1. List each diagnosis, including when the diagnosis was made and any residual complications (e.g., stroke, 1998: residual left hemiparesis).
2. For adults, ask about childhood illnesses only if they affect adult health (e.g., rheumatic heart disease; childhood asthma). Childhood illnesses are always important in taking a history for pediatric patients.
3. Patients may not remember the details of all of their past diagnoses. The past medical record is a valuable resource to prompt the patient's memory (see Chapter 14).

D. **Health-related habits.** It is important to ask about social and sexual habits that may predispose to disease. Asking these questions may feel uncomfortable at first. To relieve the tension (for both you and your patient), follow this technique:

1. Begin with the most innocuous habit or sexual practice, then progress to more contentious topics. For example, start with tobacco, then alcohol, then sexual behavior, then illicit drugs.
2. Preface uncomfortable questions with extremes of possible answers so that the patient's answers will fall in a comfortable range. For example, "Some of my patients have never had sex, others have had sex with over a thousand people. Where do you fall in this spectrum?" or "Some of my patients have never used heroin or other drugs; some spend $1,000 a day on their heroin. Where do you fall in this spectrum?" Make sure the extremes are sufficiently broad so that the patient's answer falls somewhere between the two.
3. **Important topics**
   a. **Alcohol.** Quantify in amount per day (e.g., one-fifth of vodka/day for 20 years). A fifth is 750 ml (one large bottle), or a fifth of a gallon. Two pints roughly equal one fifth. One case of beer (24 cans) equals a fifth of alcohol.
   b. **Tobacco.** Quantify in pack-years: number of packs × number of years smoking (e.g., two packs/day for 20 years is 40 pack-years). Also ask about chewing tobacco.
   c. **Other street drugs** (e.g., marijuana, cocaine, amphetamines, heroin). Note the type of drug used, how often it is used, and the method in which the drug used (e.g., smoked, inhaled, intravenously injected).
   d. **Sexual activity.** Ask about sexual preference, number of partners, condom use, anal sex, and any history of sexually transmitted disease.

E. **Occupational history and other social history.** Learn the patient's occupation, marital status, and domestic and financial situation. If the patient does not currently work, ask about types of previous employment. Some diseases may result from occupations years earlier (e.g., asbestosis).

F. **Family history of medical disease.** Focus the family history on heritable diseases that may put the patient at greater risk for that disease (e.g., colon cancer, breast cancer, early myocardial infarction). Except in rare cases, family history of non–first-degree relatives is unlikely to be important.

G. **Other aspects of the past medical history that may be useful.** Other issues useful in some patients include transfusion history, immunization history, dietary habits, screening tests (e.g., PPD, Pap smear, mammogram, cholesterol level), and obstetrics/gynecology information (e.g., number of pregnancies, number of live births, number of abortions, menstrual history, contraceptive method). Whether you ask these questions or not depends on the patient's chief complaint and the service on which you are working.

VI Review of Systems

A. At this point, it is likely that you will have all of the history you need. To ensure that you have not missed anything, however, make a quick run-through with the review of systems questions (Figure 11-2). This list of symptoms is long, and this review is often tiresome for the patient.

B. Remember that its purpose is to serve as a "clean up" and not the focus of the history. Be brief with your questions. Do not dwell on elaborating on the answers unless they sound concerning.

General: fever, chills, weight loss or gain, weakness, fatigue

Skin: rashes, loss/gain in hair, change in moles/lesions

Eyes: changes in vision, scotoma

Head: headache, dizziness, vertigo

Ears: ringing, hearing loss

Nose and sinuses: drainage, nosebleed

Mouth and throat: sore throat, bleeding gums, loose teeth

Neck: lumps, pain

Breasts: discharge, tenderness, lumps

Lungs: cough, shortness of breath

Heart: chest pain, orthopnea, paroxysmal nocturnal dyspnea

Gastrointestinal: change in bowel habits, constipation, diarrhea, melena, hematochezia, vomiting, nausea, abdominal pain

Genitourinary: dysuria, change in stream, discharge, impotence, lesions

Gynecologic: abnormal menses (pain, amount, duration), pain with intercourse, incontinence

Vascular: claudication, edema

Musculoskeletal: aches, joint swelling

Neurologic: dizziness, paresthesias, weakness

Hematologic: bleeding, bruising, clotting

Psychiatric: nervousness, phobias, anxiety

FIGURE 11-2. The review of systems run-through.

THE IMPORTANCE OF BEING TERSE Ask as many questions as necessary, but not more. Each question comes at a cost to the reliability of subsequent questions' answers. Extensive questioning will fatigue the patient, and, once fatigued, he may reply with short agreeable answers just to complete the history as soon as possible. Remember too, that by the time you get to the patient, he has already answered similar questions from several other healthcare providers.

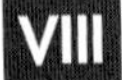

OLD MEDICAL RECORDS Old medical records, discharge summaries, and transfer summaries are a valuable adjunct to the patient's report in completing the history. Always put uppermost emphasis on the patient's first-hand report over archived data, however. Chapter 14 will give you advice in efficiently navigating through old medical records.

12. The Physical Examination and Laboratory Testing

I THE ROLE OF THE PHYSICAL EXAMINATION

A. The patient's history will have established your differential diagnosis and your relative confidence in each diagnosis you are considering (Chapters 10 and 11). The role of the physical examination is to refine this differential diagnosis by changing the probability of each diagnosis on the list. Some will be made more probable, some will be made less.

B. Each physical examination maneuver is a "test." Like other tests (e.g., CBC, ECG, or CXR), its sole purpose is to evaluate the diagnoses you are considering.

C. Each maneuver has a positive and negative likelihood ratio (Chapter 10), and this increases or decreases the probability of a particular disease.

1. Some maneuvers are so powerful (large positive likelihood ratios or small negative likelihood ratios) that the diagnosis can be established or excluded by the maneuver alone. For example, the presence of cervical motion tenderness virtually confirms the presence of pelvic inflammatory disease (very large positive likelihood ratio); further testing may not be necessary. The absence of crackles virtually excludes left-sided heart failure (very low negative likelihood ratio); again, further testing may not be necessary.
2. Other maneuvers are less powerful but may still be useful in increasing the probability of a diagnosis to a point at which laboratory or radiographic tests make sense. For example, the probability of colon cancer in a 42-year-old man with anemia may be initially too low to justify spending money on a colonoscopy. Although a positive stool guaiac card on rectal examination does not confirm the diagnosis of colon cancer, it will increase the probability of colon cancer sufficiently such that spending money on the colonoscopy now makes sense.
3. In this way, **the physical examination does not compete with laboratory testing but rather *guides* it.** Indiscriminate ordering of tests is wasteful, inefficient (hospital length of stay is increased waiting for test results), and may endanger the patient. **The physical examination is useful in choosing which tests are appropriate and the order in which they are performed,** thereby reducing this waste, inefficiency, and endangerment.

4. Finally, there are maneuvers that are of little diagnostic usefulness because their positive and negative likelihood ratios are close to 1. Chapters 24 to 38 will highlight the physical examination maneuvers that are diagnostically useful.

II Using Laboratory Tests

A. When should I order tests? Testing thresholds.

1. In Chapter 10, you learned that if the cost of the treatment is small and the benefit is large (e.g., antibiotics for suspected pneumonia), you need only minimal suspicion of pneumonia to begin therapy. Conversely, if the cost of the treatment is large, and the benefit is small (e.g., chemotherapy for cancer), you need to be very confident in the diagnosis to begin treatment.
2. The same principle applies to testing. If the risk or cost of the test is low, and the benefits of making the diagnosis are high (CXR for pneumonia), you need only minimal suspicion of the disease to order the test. Conversely, if the risks or costs of the test are high and the benefits are low, you must have a high clinical suspicion (e.g., a liver biopsy for liver cancer) for ordering the test.
3. Before ordering a test, consider the financial cost, the discomfort to the patient, and the potential complications of the test. It is also important to consider the implications of a false-positive test result. A false-positive test result will prompt further testing, resulting in additional cost and may introduce further harm to the patient (e.g., a false positive ventilation/perfusion scan results in a pulmonary angiogram, which may cause dye-induced anaphylaxis).

B. A testing strategy

1. **First, use your differential diagnosis to guide your testing strategy.** Test only for those diagnoses you are considering in your differential diagnosis.
2. Second, **think about what you will do with the results of the test.** If you are very confident in the diagnosis, there is little need to test, because a negative test result is unlikely to change your mind about the diagnosis. If a diagnosis is very unlikely, there is similarly little need to test, because a positive test result is unlikely to prompt you to treat the disease. In sum, **if the test result is likely to change your management of the patient, it is a good test to order.**
3. **Use the physical examination to exclude diagnoses that can be easily excluded.** The physical examination is free and does not pose a danger to the patient. Do not order tests to confirm diagnoses that have already been confirmed by the physical examination. Confirmatory tests run the risk of false-negative re-

sults that will confuse you and delay appropriate treatment of the diagnosis you already knew to be correct.

4. **Cascade testing.** Instead of ordering all diagnostic tests at one time, order them in phases using the following guidelines.
   - **a.** If there are multiple diagnoses on your differential diagnosis, focus your laboratory testing on excluding the easiest diagnoses first (see Chapter 10 V A).
   - **b.** If inexpensive and noninvasive tests will suffice in excluding a diagnosis, order these first. For example, a chest CT may be unnecessary if the CXR is normal.
   - **c.** If you are looking to exclude a disease, order the most sensitive test first (e.g., order an ANA before a ds-DNA to exclude lupus.) If you must confirm a disease, order the most specific test first (e.g., order a troponin I before you order a CK-MB).

HOT  KEY

To keep the physical examination focused and concise, concentrate on maneuvers that evaluate the diagnoses being considered.

13. The Admission Note

I Introduction

The admission note (write-up) documents the results of the history, physical examination, and laboratory studies. It is essential to patient care because it enables other physicians (e.g., consult services) and team members (e.g., social workers, nurses) to access the patient's information quickly without repeating the entire evaluation. For this reason, it is important that you document your findings accurately and neatly.

A. The admission note is organized so that the information contained in the note exactly parallels the order in which it was obtained.

B. In doing so, it also exactly parallels the clinical reasoning process (e.g., history, physical examination, laboratory tests, assessment and plan [A&P]).

C. The A&P contained in the admission note outlines the patient's anticipated course through hospitalization. Subsequent progress notes modify this course, but it is the admission note that identifies the solvency issues, establishes the goals of the hospitalization, and sets the trajectory for the hospital course.

HOT KEY

Solvency issues are issues that must be resolved before a patient may return home. Not every abnormality is a solvency issue. Focus your plan on issues that need to be addressed before discharge.

II Components of the Admission Note

A. Chief complaint (first line)
B. History of the present illness
C. Review of systems
D. Past medical history
E. Physical examination
F. Laboratory tests and study results
G. A&P

III Chief Complaint and History of the Present Illness

A. First line. Begin with the patient's age, gender, ethnicity (if significant to your differential diagnosis), and chief complaint. Do not include past medical history in the first line, because it introduces the risk of focusing on the past medical history rather than on the chief complaint.

B. Paragraph 1. Characterize the chief complaint and provide a time course. See the FAR COLDER mnemonic in Chapter 11. Instead of just listing the information, take the time to synthesize it into a story. This will greatly improve its readability, which will in turn greatly increase the chance that people who read it will understand what you know about the patient.

C. Paragraph 2. Provide answers to the questions you asked when you took the history to evaluate the diagnoses being considered.

1. Do not list the diagnoses you considered; just provide answers to the questions you asked.
2. Although paragraph 2 will focus on information related to your differential diagnosis, do not try to "spin" the history by selectively including some information that makes one diagnosis appear more probable than another. The reader of your note should have unbiased historical information.

HOT
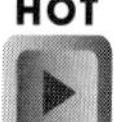
KEY

The assessment portion of the A&P is where you get a chance to "editorialize."

IV Past Medical History

A. Allergies. List the allergy and the reaction (e.g., penicillin = rash). (see Chapter 11 V A).

B. Medications. Record the dose and frequency with which the patient is actually taking the drug. Include over-the-counter drugs (e.g., aspirin, ibuprofen, herbal supplements) (see Chapter 11 V B).

C. Past diagnoses. List each diagnosis, including when the diagnosis was made, and any residual complications resulting from the diagnosis (e.g., stroke, 1998: residual left hemiparesis). You may omit further details about past diagnoses unless it relates to the diagnoses being considered (see Chapter 11 V C).

D. Health-related habits (see Chapter 11 V D)

1. Alcohol
2. Tobacco
3. Intravenous drug use
4. Sexual activity

E. Occupational and social history. Record the patient's place of birth, marital status, occupation, and domestic and financial situation (see Chapter 11 V E).

F. Family history. Especially note family history that might put the patient at greater risk for that disease (e.g., colon cancer, breast cancer, early heart attack). Except in rare cases, family history of non–first-degree relatives is unlikely to be important (see Chapter 11 V F).

G. Other aspects of the past medical history that may be useful (see Chapter 11 V G).

V REVIEW OF SYSTEMS (see Chapter 11 VI)

A. Note only abnormal findings. Refer to the list of systems and associated symptoms in Figure 11-2.

B. Do not duplicate recording abnormalities that have been noted in the history of present illness.

C. If there are no additional abnormalities elicited by the review of systems, note: "ROS normal except as noted above."

VI PHYSICAL EXAMINATION

A. Always record vital signs as numbers, not notations such as "stable" or "normal."

1. Remember that other physicians will compare these initial values with subsequent values.
2. Values that are abnormal in certain patients may be normal in others. For example, some patients whose blood pressure is chronically elevated may suffer hypotensive consequences if their blood pressure suddenly declines to a normal level.

B. Organize the physical examination by organ system (see Figure 13-1).

1. Note all abnormal findings.
2. Note the absence of an abnormality (e.g., "no egophony") if it helps evaluate the diagnoses being considered on your differential diagnosis (e.g., absence of egophony decreases the probability of pneumonia).
3. **Use your differential diagnosis to determine what you record in the physical examination section.**

HOT

KEY

Avoid using jargon (terms only physicians in your specialty would know) and nonstandard abbreviations. If your readers cannot understand your notes, you have failed to communicate to other physicians (and all team members).

VII LABORATORY TESTS AND OTHER STUDIES

A. Note all results of laboratory tests. Even if the results are normal, documenting the results provides a baseline for comparison of subsequent laboratory values. Use shorthand notation to record laboratory results in the admission note as well as on the patient's chart (Figure 13-2).

HPI:

The patient is a 54-year-old day-care worker who presents with three days of a progressively worsening headache and a pruritic rash over all extremities. The headache began three days ago when she awoke from sleep. It initially abated for two hours, but then returned while she was at work. Since that time it has been persistent without periods of relief. She notes an acute worsening of the headache this morning, and also noted the presence of photophobia. The maximal area of pain is in the posterior neck. It is associated with nausea but there has been no vomiting. The pain is characterized as a "vice-like" pain that is exacerbated by flexing the neck. It does not change when lying flat. Nothing improves the headache, including acetaminophen and codeine. The rash is characterized as "itchy" with involvement of the arms and legs initially, then progressing over the past two days to involve the trunk and back. It has been associated with fever.

She has a history of migraine headaches, though she notes that this pain is different from her typical migraine headaches. She has had no trauma to her head and she describes no recent falls. She has had no sinus congestion. There is no history of cancer in her family, and she notes no recent weight loss, breast swelling or blood in the stool. She was exposed to a child who was diagnosed with meningitis within the day-care center. She has had no recent travel or insect bites.

Review of Systems: All nine review of systems were reviewed. This was negative except as noted above.

Past Medical History:

Hypertension
Peptic Ulcer Disease (1999)
Seizure Disorder; the last seizure was 2002.
Status-post Hysterectomy (2002)
Status-post Appenedectomy (1997)

Allergies: Sulfa drugs (rash)

Medications:

Omeprazole 10 mg q d
Dilantin 300 mg q d
Aspirin 325 mg q d
Metoprolol 50 mg BID
Acetaminophen prn

FIGURE 13-1. Sample admission note. *(continues)*

Past Social History:
She lives with her husband in an apartment in New Orleans. She is still sexually active and practices unprotected sex with her husband only.
She has a 10 pk/year smoking history.
She does not drink alcohol or use intravenous drugs.

Family History:
There is no family history of malignancy. Family history is otherwise non-contributory to her present complaint.

Physical Examination:
BP 110/54; HR 112; RR 16; Temp 39.8°C; 98% Saturation (RA)
- Pupils were normal with 4mm→2mm constriction bilaterally without afferent papillary defects. The sclera were non-icteric. There were no signs of head trauma; no ecchymosis, no scalp or spinal tenderness. There was no sinus tenderness. The external auditory canals and the tympanic membranes were normal. The mouth and pharynx were normal. There was nucal rigidity; Kernig's sign was present. There was no lymphadenopathy.
- The lungs were clear to auscultation; there were no signs of consolidation or obstruction.
- S1 and S2 were normal; the PMI was non-displaced and normal size. There were no murmurs. The JVP was < 5 cm.
- The abdomen was soft and non-tender. The liver size was 9 cm. The spleen was not palpable. Bowel sounds were present.
- The genitourinary examination was normal. The rectal exam was normal.
- The neurologic examination was normal; there were no focal deficits in strength and all reflexes and sensation were normal.
-There was a non-blanching macular rash on the extremities and trunk. There was no edema or joint tenderness.

Laboratory and Studies:

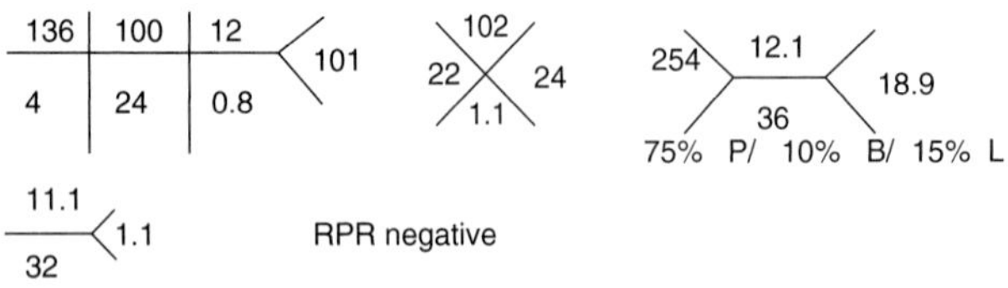

136	100	12	101
4	24	0.8	

102 (top); 22 (left); 24 (right); 1.1 (bottom)

254 (left); 12.1 (top); 36 (bottom); 18.9 (right)
75% P/ 10% B/ 15% L

11.1 / 32 ⟨ 1.1

RPR negative

FIGURE 13-1. (*continued*) JVP, jugular venous pressure; LVH, left ventricular hypertrophy; MCV, mean corpuscular volume.

EKG: Rate-112, normal rhythm; No ST-T wave abnormalities. No Q waves. Normal intervals. No hypertropthy.

CXR: Normal.
Head CT with contrast: No masses or enhancement. No midline shift or hemorrhage.

Blood cultures: Pending
Urine cultures: Pending
Lumbar puncture: 100 WBC; 80% polys/20% lymphs. No RBC. Gram-negative diplococci. Glucose 20; Protein 52. VDRL negative.

Assessment and Plan:

1. Headache-
I believe this is due to meningitis from *Neisseria meningitidis.* The time course, the exposure history as part of her day-care employment, and the findings on lumbar puncture support this diagnosis. Other diagnoses considered include sinusitis, migraine headache, intra-cerebral bleeding and a metastatic tumor. The lack of sinus tenderness and congestion, the character of the pain atypical for her migraine, and the lack of red cells on lumbar puncture make these diagnoses unlikely. She has no evidence of breast or colon cancer on examination, though her screening is not up-to-date. The negative head CT makes the diagnosis of metastatic tumor less likely.

Our plan is to give ceftriaxone 2 gm IV every 12 hours. Close personal contacts will be contacted to receive prophylaxtic antibiotics. We will await final culture results from the blood, urine and CSF fluid.

One of the potential complications of *Neisseria meningiococcus* infection is adrenal infarction. She does not appear to have signs and symptoms of this syndrome, though we will be vigilant for hypotension and hyponatremia. Hydrocortisone 100 mg IV will be administered if these signs become apparent.

2. Skin Rash-
I believe this is due to the *Neisseria meningitidis* as noted above. Other diagnoses we considered were disseminated intravascular coagulation due to sepsis, TTP, secondary syphilis, Rocky Mountain Spotted Fever, and a drug reaction. The normal coagulation studies, the normal renal function and the findings on the lumbar puncture make these diagnoses less likely. She

FIGURE 13-1. *(continued)*

has not been exposed to insect vectors, her RPR was negative and she has not begun any new medications. We will treat with ceftriaxone as noted above.

3. Seizure Disorder-
We will continue her standing dose of 300mg of dilantin each evening.

4. History of Peptic Ulcer Disease-
We will discontinue her aspirin and continue the omeprazole. Acetaminophen will be given for pain relief.

5. Health Care Maintenance-
She will receive a pneumococcal vaccination. We will arrange for a colonoscopy and a mammogram as an outpatient. A breast examination will be performed prior to discharge.

FIGURE 13-1. *(continued)*

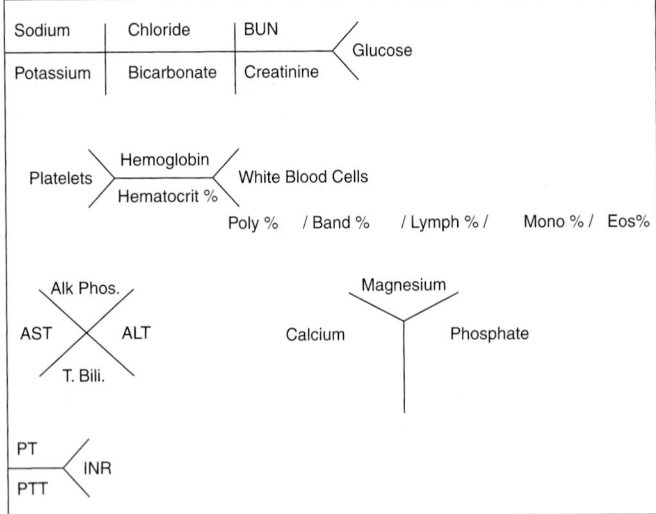

FIGURE 13-2. Shorthand notation for recording laboratory results.

B. Note all results of other studies. Common studies include ECG; CXR and other imaging studies, such as CT, MRI, and bone films; echocardiography; and ultrasonography.

C. Note results of previous studies if they:

1. Are relevant to the diagnoses you are considering on your differential diagnosis. For example, it would be useful to note a past echocardiogram result if congestive heart failure is being considered on your differential diagnosis.
2. Might preclude performing a test again (e.g., having the results of a recent cardiac stress test might preclude its repetition).
3. Provide insight into the rate of how current laboratory results may have changed. Remember, the significance of any single laboratory text result is not in its current value, but how it has changed over time.
4. Note the dates the results were obtained to distinguish them from the admission laboratory results.

VIII Assessment and Plan

A. Do not provide a summary of the case; this merely reiterates what the reader can find in the first portion of the admission note.

B. Organize the A&P by ***problem***. The A&P should focus on the main problem (e.g., "Problem No. 1: shortness of breath"), which is usually the patient's chief complaint. If the diagnosis is known (e.g., the patient presented for chemotherapy for an established diagnosis of leukemia), use the *diagnosis* instead of the symptom as the title of "Problem 1" (e.g., "Problem No. 1: leukemia"). Other problems should be addressed as subsequent problems (e.g., "Problem No. 2," etc.), but most of the A&P should be devoted to Problem No. 1.

C. Structure of the A&P for each problem.

1. List the problem (e.g., Problem No. 1: shortness of breath).
2. State your hypothesis (e.g., "We believe this is due to congestive heart failure...").
3. Support your hypothesis with data (e.g., "The associated edema, crackles, S_3, and cephalization on the CXR support this diagnosis").
4. List other diagnoses you considered and any data that support or refute these diagnoses. (e.g., "We also considered pneumonia, pulmonary embolism, and pneumothorax. The absence of fever, cough, and the CXR findings argue against these diagnoses.")
5. State the plan.
   - **a.** Use action verbs to describe clearly what is being done. For example, state, "We will treat with antibiotics," not "We will consider using antibiotics."
   - **b.** Be as specific as possible. State, "We will treat with ampicillin 500 mg PO bid," not "We will treat with antibiotics." This

allows the reader to make specific changes in the management plan if necessary.

c. If there is a contingency plan, make it clear what contingencies will change the management (e.g., "If the spiral CT is positive for pulmonary embolism, we will start enoxaparin").

IX SAMPLE ADMISSION NOTE (Figure 13-1)

14. Finding Your Way Around the Chart

I INTRODUCTION

A. The practice of medicine is a team effort; physicians, nurses, therapists, social workers, and other team members must coordinate their services. The medical chart is the common point of communication and coordination between these team members.

B. It is important that no items be removed from the chart, including progress notes, laboratory or radiology reports, or ECG findings. In addition, the chart may not be removed from the ward. If removed, other team members will be without this information and communication between team members will disintegrate. See Chapter 20 for how to put patient information on data cards so that you have this information even when you are not near the chart.

II INSURANCE AND ADMINISTRATION

The front section of the chart contains the patient's demographic, insurance, and administrative paperwork, which you need only rarely. Included are living wills, advanced directives, next-of-kin contact information, and durable power of attorney information.

III GRAPHICS

This section shows the hour-to-hour changes in vital signs. Vital signs are plotted versus time, which allows you to see trends as well as sudden variations from the baseline condition (Figure 14-1).

IV ORDERS

Progress notes tell what clinicians planned to do, but orders tell what *actually* happened. Chapter 19 discusses writing orders.

V ADMISSION NOTES/PROGRESS NOTES

Chapter 13 describes admission notes, and Chapter 15 describes progress notes. Both types of note may be combined in one section, or there may be two sections. If the admission note is separate, it is usually also the place to find consultant's notes. If not, you'll find the consultant notes with the progress notes.

VI NURSES' NOTES

The nurses' notes document the patient's hour-to-hour progress, especially with respect to subjective

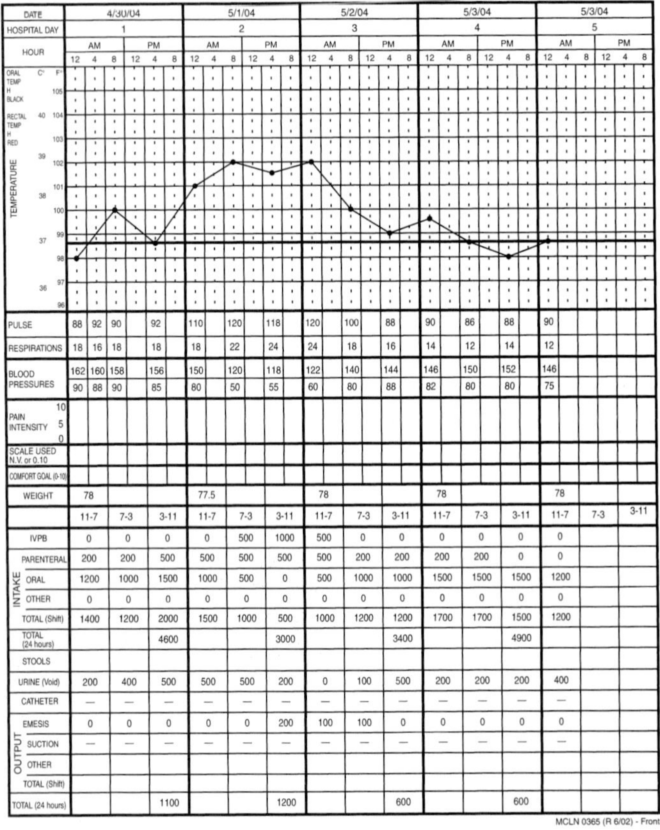

Louisiana State University Health Sciences Center
Medical Center of Louisiana at New Orleans

GRAPHIC AND I & O RECORD

DATE	4/30/04	5/1/04	5/2/04	5/3/04	5/3/04
HOSPITAL DAY	1	2	3	4	5

ORAL TEMP C° F° H BLACK · RECTAL TEMP H RED · TEMPERATURE 40 104, 105, 103, 39 102, 101, 38 100, 99, 37 98, 97, 36 96

4/30/04 (Hospital Day 1)

HOUR	AM 12	AM 4	AM 8	PM 12	PM 4	PM 8
PULSE	88	92	90		92	
RESPIRATIONS	18	16	18		18	
BLOOD PRESSURES	162/90	160/88	158/90		156/85	

5/1/04 (Hospital Day 2)

HOUR	AM 12	AM 4	AM 8	PM 12	PM 4	PM 8
PULSE	110		120		118	
RESPIRATIONS	18		22		24	
BLOOD PRESSURES	150/80		120/50		118/55	

5/2/04 (Hospital Day 3)

HOUR	AM 12	AM 4	AM 8	PM 12	PM 4	PM 8
PULSE	120		100		88	
RESPIRATIONS	24		18		16	
BLOOD PRESSURES	122/60		140/80		144/88	

5/3/04 (Hospital Day 4)

HOUR	AM 12	AM 4	AM 8	PM 12	PM 4	PM 8
PULSE	90		86		88	
RESPIRATIONS	14		12		14	
BLOOD PRESSURES	146/82		150/80		152/80	

5/3/04 (Hospital Day 5)

HOUR	AM 12	AM 4	AM 8	PM 12	PM 4	PM 8
PULSE	90					
RESPIRATIONS	12					
BLOOD PRESSURES	146/75					

PAIN INTENSITY 10 5 0 · SCALE USED N.V. or 0.10 · COMFORT GOAL (0-10)

	4/30/04			5/1/04			5/2/04			5/3/04			5/3/04		
WEIGHT	78			77.5			78			78			78		
	11-7	7-3	3-11	11-7	7-3	3-11	11-7	7-3	3-11	11-7	7-3	3-11	11-7	7-3	3-11
INTAKE IVPB	0	0	0	0	500	1000	500	0	0	0	0	0	0		
PARENTERAL	200	200	500	500	500	500	500	200	200	200	200	0	0		
ORAL	1200	1000	1500	1000	500	0	500	1000	1000	1500	1500	1500	1200		
OTHER	0	0	0	0	0	0	0	0	0	0	0	0	0		
TOTAL (Shift)	1400	1200	2000	1500	1000	500	1000	1200	1200	1700	1700	1500	1200		
TOTAL (24 hours)			4600			3000			3400			4900			
STOOLS															
OUTPUT URINE (Void)	200	400	500	500	500	200	0	100	500	200	200	200	400		
CATHETER	—	—	—	—	—	—	—	—	—	—	—	—	—		
EMESIS	0	0	0	0	0	200	100	100	0	0	0	0	0		
SUCTION	—	—	—	—	—	—	—	—	—	—	—	—	—		
OTHER															
TOTAL (Shift)															
TOTAL (24 hours)			1100			1200			600			600			

MCLN 0365 (R 6/02) - Front

FIGURE 14-1. Sample graphics sheet.

progress, patient mobility, compliance, and social factors (e.g., who visited the patient). It is a good place to see how the patient is subjectively responding to therapy and his functional status (e.g., Is the patient responding to his medications, is pain control adequate, is he ambulating?).

LABORATORY TESTS AND OTHER STUDIES

There is usually a time lag between when laboratory results are actually available and when they are placed on the chart, so this section is of little practical use with regard to day-to-day patient care. However, it may be useful for examining long-term trends in laboratory values.

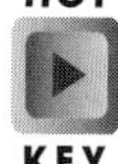

HOT KEY

To obtain the most recent laboratory results, check the computer or call the laboratory. If you need to obtain the most recent results of radiographic tests, call the radiologist directly.

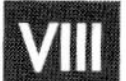

RADIOGRAPHIC REPORTS

Like laboratory results, radiographic reports are usually placed on the chart several days after they are practically useful. If you need the results of a recent study, call the radiologist. Alternatively, you can call the radiologist's dictation system, which will play the results of the test back for you. Ask your resident for this number.

ELECTROCARDIOGRAMS (ECGS)

With ECGs, it is very important to interpret each ECG in the context of past ECGs to look for changes over time. A normal-appearing ECG may actually be abnormal if it is a change from a previously abnormal ECG. Do not remove ECGs from the chart and do not mark on the ECG, even if the ST-segment depression is so remarkable that you feel you must circle it. Each ECG "lives in perpetuity" as a comparison to subsequent ECGs; graffiti makes comparisons difficult.

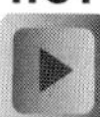

HOT KEY

If you want to bring the ECG on attending rounds, make a copy of the original. Keep the original ECG in the chart.

MEDICINE ADMINISTRATION RECORD

The medicine administration record (MAR) is a list of medications currently being administered, their dose, and their frequency of administration.

A. **The MAR is the best place to find out exactly what medications your patient has been prescribed and how they are being administered.** On occasion, the nurse or pharmacist will incorrectly interpret the physician's order. If there is a discrepancy between what was ordered and what was delivered to the patient, you will find it here. The MAR is especially useful when completing discharge prescriptions, which can be transcribed from the list in the MAR.

B. The MAR may be in the patient's chart or kept in a folder on the ward (with the MARs of other patients). Ask the nurse for its location.

XI OLD CHARTS

The old chart is a complete record of a patient's medical past. Old charts are often measured in pounds, not pages; they can be unwieldy without a method for extracting the information you need. Use the following method:

A. Look for the most recent hospitalization.

B. Look for the discharge summary. A good discharge summary will tell you what you need to know to manage your current patient. Table 14-1 will help you judge the quality of a discharge summary.

C. If there is not a good discharge summary, turn your attention to the progress notes and order sheets from the most recent admission or clinic visit.

1. If the discharge occurred less than 1 week ago, start with the admission note for that hospitalization and work forward, reading the progress notes. In the interest of being efficient, it is appropriate to ignore orders, vital sign data, and nurses' notes.
2. If the discharge occurred more than 1 week ago, read the admission note and skim through the progress notes quickly, looking for an off-service or transfer-of-service note. These notes are essentially discharge summaries reviewing all progress to that point. Starting with one of these will relieve you of having to read the progress notes before that note. Read the off-service note, then the progress notes forward from there. If there is no note, start with the last progress note and read backward until you have a sense of what transpired during the patient's hospital stay.

D. Track down old ECGs and radiology reports if they are applicable. See Chapter 13 VII C for advice on how to determine which old test reports should be obtained and recorded in the admission note.

E. Have the discipline to put down the old chart. Extract what you need, then return to your patient. Old data is important, but what

TABLE 14-1. Components of a Good Discharge Summary.

1. Reason for hospitalization and results of hospitalization.
2. List of important test results (e.g., echocardiogram, cardiac catheterization, CT, biopsy).
3. List of important treatment interventions (e.g., surgeries, cancer staging procedures, most recent chemotherapy).
4. Medications on discharge.
5. List of active medical problems.

really matters is what is happening now. Your patient is still the best source for this information.

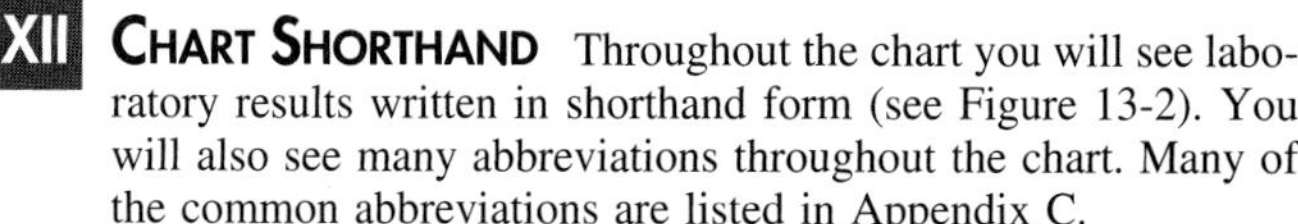

XII **CHART SHORTHAND** Throughout the chart you will see laboratory results written in shorthand form (see Figure 13-2). You will also see many abbreviations throughout the chart. Many of the common abbreviations are listed in Appendix C.

15. Other Written Notes

I Introduction

A. All team members are rarely in the same place at the same time; notes in the medical chart are the way different team members communicate with each other. The entire team takes its directive from the physician's progress note, especially the assessment and plan (A&P).

B. **A good note of any kind contains *only* relevant data.** As in all forms of communication (see Chapter 16), **relevance is defined by what the other person needs to know.** As you write your progress notes, put yourself in the place of the night-float physician; think about what you would want to know about this patient to ensure that optimal care is not interrupted. Provide only this data—anything extra will only obscure the relevant data.

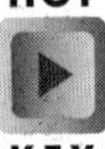

All notes are relevant only in the context in which they are written. Always include the time and date in your notes. This allows readers to interpret your findings in the proper context.

II Function of Notes

A. Major functions

1. **Communicate data that have been obtained** (e.g., results of the history, physical examination, and laboratory studies).
2. **Document what has been done** (e.g., medication doses, procedures or surgeries performed).
3. **Establish a plan for patient care.** Notes serve as the "map" for the patient's course through the hospital. The best map is one that clearly articulates the physician clinical reasoning so other team members can make good decisions when unexpected events occur.

B. Minor function. Notes also have a **medical-legal** purpose. They document any deviation from the standard of care (e.g., patient refusal of therapy that would ordinarily be given or a physician not offering a standard therapy because of a clinical circumstance).

III Admission Note (see Chapter 13)

IV Progress Note

A. The purpose of the daily progress note is to ensure that your patient receives continuity of care when you are not there. Think of the progress note as a letter to the physician who cares for your patient when you leave the hospital (e.g., night-float, consultant). This physician must quickly and easily be able to see what you have found and done and, most importantly, what you think is wrong with the patient and what you are doing to help her. Remember that this physician has never seen your patient, so your note must provide a sense of the patient's baseline condition.

B. Subjective-Objective-Assessment & Plan (SOAP) format

1. **Subjective findings** (Figure 15-1)
   a. Progress of symptoms (e.g., has the abdominal pain improved?)
   b. Any new complaints
2. **Objective findings**
   a. **Physical examination**
      (1) Focus your physical examination documentation on the relevant positive and negative findings other team members need to know. **Use the differential diagnosis to decide what physical examination maneuvers are relevant.**
      (2) For example, in a patient with heart failure, documenting the heart and lung examination is essential each day. The admission note should have documented the results of the tier I examination (other organ systems, see Chapter 21); there is no need to restate these results each day.
      (3) If the diagnosis has been established, focus on physical **findings that would suggest response or failure to therapy** (e.g., Are the crackles and S_3 still present in a patient diagnosed with heart failure receiving diuresis?). Focus also on those **findings that might suggest a complication of therapy** (e.g., Is there blood in the stool by rectal exam if the patient is on a blood thinner?).
      (4) Record the numerical values of the vital signs. This will help the cross-covering physician determine if there is a deviation from baseline when he receives a cross-coverage call.

HOT KEY

Highlight examination findings that would help you manage this patient if you were the night-float or consulting physician. Do not dilute important data with useless information.

When you write a progress note, record what *you* found. Do not record a murmur your intern heard if you did not hear it.

   b. **Results of laboratory tests and other studies.**
      (1) Record results of new laboratory tests and studies, as well as any changes in old laboratory tests (e.g., a change in blood culture results).

2/14/04 Medical Student Progress Note- Medicine

Subjective: She notes her headache has greatly diminished. No further photophobia.
The neck stiffness is still present, but greatly reduced. No fever.

Objective: BP: 120/82; HR: 90; RR 15; Temp. 37.2°C; 98% Sat. (RA)
Her head and neck examination is normal with the exception of minor neck stiffness with flexion.
Her lungs are clear to auscultation; the heart examination remains normal.
Her abdomen is soft and non-tender. Normal bowel sounds.
The neurologic examination remains normal.
The rash has reduced in intensity; some lesions remain but are resolving. There are no new lesions.

137	101	11	
3.8	26	0.8	98

227 > 11.7 / 35 < 11.9

74% P/ 1% B/ 25% L

Blood cultures: NGTD
Urine cultures: NGTD
Lumbar puncture: Culture positive for *Neisseria meningitidis*

Assessment & Plan:

1. Meningitis. The causative agent has been confirmed to be *Neisseria meningitidis.* She is responding well to ceftriaxone, and we will continue this for a seven-day course. She has demonstrated no signs of adrenal insufficiency, but we will continue to be alert for signs of hypotension or hyponatremia. Her family and day-care contacts have been notified and will receive antibiotic prophylaxis.
2. Discharge planning: She will return home following the completion of her antibiotics. She requires no placement assistance or home health care. We anticipate discharge on 2/19/04.
3. Health Care Maintenance. She has been scheduled a clinic appointment on March 1st for follow-up and to further schedule her mammogram and colonoscopy.

FIGURE 15-1. Sample progress note.

(2) Do not continue to record data of past laboratory tests and other studies each day. The reader can access this information by flipping back to previous progress notes or the admission note. If these data are important to the current management (e.g., vegetation seen on an earlier echocardiogram), provide a reference to direct the reader to data in previous notes.

(3) Use laboratory shorthand to present data concisely (Figure 13-2). It is not necessary to write the units of measurement (e.g., write troponin 0.01, not troponin 0.01 pg/dl).

(4) If you wish, indicate particularly important abnormal results by circling them or using an asterisk. Be judicious in your circling: circling every abnormal result defeats the purpose of highlighting the data.

3. **Assessment and plan (A&P).** This is the critical part of the note. The A&P establishes the course for the rest of the team. Use the following guidelines:
   a. **Identify solvency issues.** These can be symptoms (e.g., shortness of breath), physical findings (e.g., broken hip), laboratory values (e.g., hyponatremia), or, if you are certain, diagnoses (e.g., myocardial infarction).
   b. **Organize the A&P by solvency issues.** Begin with the most important problem that needs to be solved as problem No. 1. Additional problems are labeled as problem No. 2 and so on.
   c. If the **diagnosis is certain,** list the diagnosis and focus your discussion only on the treatment plan.
   d. If the **diagnosis is not certain:**
      (1) Note the one diagnosis you think is most probable and why. Then note the other diagnoses you are considering. For example, "Problem No. 1: Shortness of breath. We believe this is due to a pulmonary embolism. We are also considering pneumonia and congestive heart failure."
      (2) Address any new data and how this affects your assessment. "The V/Q scan shows low probability for pulmonary embolism, but given the patient's symptoms and history of a pulmonary embolism, clinical suspicion remains high."
   e. **Present your plan.** Start with diagnostic strategies and then address treatment plans. Diagnostic plans are necessary only when the diagnosis is not certain; if you know the diagnosis, skip the diagnostic plan. "Our plan is to order a high-resolution CT scan of the chest today. The patient will continue to receive enoxaparin 90 mg bid, and we will begin Coumadin 5 mg/day." Include the specific dose and schedule for medications.
   f. **Repeat this process for each solvency issue.**

1. **Patient name and number:** **Owen Meany; #99525511**
2. **Date of admission:** **11/16/2004**
3. **Date of discharge:** **11/20/2004**
4. **Service:** **Medicine. Demming MD, Attending; Miller MD, PGY-3; Cash, MS (555-1212)**
5. **Descriptive Line:**
   "The patient is a 54-year-old man who presented on November 11, 2004 with shortness of breath. He was diagnosed with pneumonia and GI bleed.
6. **Reference the HPI:**
   "See the HPI for full details of the patient's symptoms and condition at the time of presentation."
7. **Hospital course by problem:**
   "Shortness of breath." Give details on the studies that were done, their results, how the patient was treated, and how he faired. Focus on the diagnosis, the degree of success of therapy, and any adverse events that occurred.
8. **Procedures performed and findings**
9. **Discharge diagnoses list:** For chronic diseases, include laboratory values (e.g., creatinine if the patient has chronic renal failure, hemoglobin if the patient has chronic anemia, CD4 count if the patient has HIV) that will help future physicians assess whether the patient's subsequent presentations are a departure from his baseline condition.
10. **Discharge medications (include the dose and schedule)**
11. **Recommended diet**
12. **Recommended activity level (e.g., as tolerated, no heavy lifting, bed rest for 1 week, etc.)**
13. **Disposition:** Include where the patient will go and the next clinic follow-up.
14. **Prognosis**

FIGURE 15-2. Outline of a discharge summary.

g. Always end your A&P by noting the patient's code status (DNR/DNI or full code).

V DISCHARGE SUMMARY

DISCHARGE SUMMARY This note is designed to communicate the most important aspects of the patient's hospital admission to physicians who will subsequently care for the patient. If you are asked to do a discharge summary, follow the formula in Figure 15-2.

VI PREOPERATIVE NOTE

PREOPERATIVE NOTE A preoperative note must be written before each surgery (Figure 15-3). This note documents the condition of the patient before the procedure and the preoperative data that have been obtained.

VII POSTOPERATIVE DICTATION

POSTOPERATIVE DICTATION A postoperative dictation must be written after each surgical procedure. Its purpose is to describe the events of the procedure from start to finish. The note is gener-

Pre-op DX:	Symptomatic cholelithiasis
Procedure planned:	Laparoscopic cholecystectomy
Surgeons:	Dr. Halsted, attending; Dr. Kelly, PGY-IV; K Hude, MS4
Anesthesia:	GETA
Lab results:	List the CBC, BMP, PT/PTT
CXR:	Normal
EKG:	Normal
Blood:	2 units PRBC typed and crossed (A+/−)
Meds:	MS04 2mg q2hours IV/SQ Phenergan 12.5mg IV q8hoursPRN: nausea/vomiting Cefotetan 1 gm IV on call to the operating room.
Diet:	NPO
IVF:	LR @ 125cc/hour

The risks and benefits of the procedure were discussed with the patient. The procedure and possible complications were explained and his questions were answered. The patient agrees to the procedure. A full consent form has been signed and is on the chart.

FIGURE 15-3. Sample preoperative note.

Pre-op Dx:	Appendicitis
Post-op Dx:	Appendicitis
Procedure:	Appendectomy
Surgeons:	Dr. Halsted, Dr. Kelly, K. Hude, MS4
Anesthesia:	GETA
IVF:	Total 250cc LR
EBL:	40cc
UOP:	Total 150cc
Drains placed:	None
Specimens:	Vermiform appendix and mesoappendix
Complications:	None
Findings:	Dilated and inflamed appendix
Disposition:	To PACU in stable condition

FIGURE 15-4. Outline of the postoperative note.

ally dictated by the first or second assistant surgeon, and it follows the same formula as for the postoperative note (Figure 15-4). The surgeon will describe each step of the procedure, including the manner in which the surgical area was prepped and draped, each layer of incision (e.g., skin, subcutaneous tissue, fascia, muscle, etc.), the method of dissection and extraction, the findings of the procedure, and the closure of the wound. In addition, the dictation will document the instrument and sponge count to ensure that no foreign bodies were retained during the procedure. The best way to learn this skill is to listen carefully to your senior residents as they dictate operative reports; note that no detail is too small to be excluded.

VIII **POSTOPERATIVE NOTE** Because the postoperative dictation usually takes 2 days to return from transcription, a postoperative note is also written in the chart to keep the team informed during this 2-day gap (Figure 15-4). The postoperative note is a summary of the postoperative dictation without the detailed description of the procedure. It allows all members of the healthcare team to know what took place during the surgery in case the patient has postoperative complications.

IX PROCEDURE NOTE (Figure 15-5)

A. The procedure note is similar to the surgical postoperative note and is used on all services where procedures are performed (e.g., medicine, obstetrics, pediatrics, etc.). It provides the rationale for the procedure, the events of the procedure, and the outcome (findings). This

Consent:	The patient consented to the procedure. A signed consent form is on the chart.
Prep:	Area prepped and draped in the normal sterile fashion
Anesthesia:	3 cc of Lidocaine 1% injected under the skin
Procedure:	A spinal needle was advanced to the spine until spinal fluid was returned.
Findings:	The opening pressure was 15 mmHg. 10 cc of clear, straw-colored fluid was obtained. The spinal needle was removed and the area was bandaged. Fluid was sent for protein, glucose, cell count, Gram-stain, and culture.
Complications:	The patient tolerated the procedure without complications.

FIGURE 15-5. Sample procedure note.

note communicates the information to other team members who were not present for the procedure but must make decisions based on the outcome.

B. Before performing the procedure, make sure that signed informed consent has been obtained and this is documented in the preprocedure note.

HOT
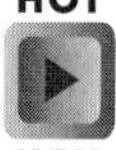
KEY

Never alter or change a note after it has been written. If new information becomes available, make an addendum in the chart.

X VETERANS AFFAIRS (VA) COMPUTER SYSTEM

A. Computerized patient record system (CPRS). All VA notes are written using the CPRS. This system has unique features.

1. **"Cut and paste."** Because all patient notes are available on the computer system, you can "cut and paste" portions of old notes into new notes. Be careful, however. Cutting and pasting the wrong information can result in wrong decisions. Solvency issues will change as the hospital course progresses; keep your notes focused on the current situation.

2. **Templates.** You can save a template on the CPRS computer for commonly used notes (e.g., progress notes, procedure notes, surgical notes).
   a. Choose a note under one of the fictitious test patients. (Your computer access officer can tell you the name and number of the fictitious test patient.)
   b. Create your template under this name.
   c. Access your template when you need it. Fill in the data pertinent to your current patient. Choose "save as" from the file menu. Save under the patient you are currently treating.

16. Spoken Case Presentation: Basic Principles

I DETERMINING WHAT SHOULD BE IN THE ORAL PRESENTATION

A. After you collect your patient's historical, physical examination, and laboratory data, you will be asked to present these data to your attending. Time is limited; you will not be able to present all the data you have collected, nor will you want to. Less vital data will only obscure the vital information you have to present.

B. **The best spoken presentation is composed of only the data relevant to diagnosing and treating the patient;** everything else can be archived in the admission note. **Distinguishing relevant from irrelevant data is the key to a great presentation.**

C. **Identifying relevant data.** In all forms of communication, excellence is achieved by **identifying what your audience needs to know and speaking only to this.** What does your attending need to know? The same information you needed for your clinical reasoning (Chapter 10). Namely, she needs to know the character and time course of the chief complaint in order to construct a differential diagnosis of her own. She also needs the information applicable to evaluating each diagnosis on that list (Chapter 10).

1. As you present the character and time course of the patient's chief complaint, your attending will be formulating a differential diagnosis, just as you did when you obtained the history. Nothing must come before the time course and character of the chief complaint, because without this the attending will not have a differential diagnosis to process subsequent data.
2. With the differential diagnosis in mind, she will then be listening for additional information to help her assess which of those diagnoses is the most probable explanation for the patient's complaint. Believe it or not, it is highly likely that her differential diagnosis is the <u>same</u> as yours (perhaps in a different order, but the same diagnoses nonetheless). **Provide only the historical information that applies to the diagnoses on your differential diagnosis.** This will help your attending in assessing the probability of each diagnosis on her differential diagnosis. This data should be the second portion of your oral presentation of the history.
3. For the remainder of the presentation, use the following standard to determine what is and what is not relevant: **any data that help the attending evaluate the diagnoses on her differential diagnosis is relevant.**

4. In sum, all of the information included in your presentation should focus on your differential diagnosis. You need not explicitly state your differential diagnosis until you reach the assessment and plan (A&P).

II FEATURES OF A GOOD PRESENTATION

Your success depends on how much information your audience retains from your presentation, not upon how much you say. To maximize audience retention, each presentation must be characterized by three key qualities:

A. **Fluent and articulate.** Do not let the fear of leaving out a piece of information disrupt your fluency; in fact, count on leaving something out. There will be time for questions after the presentation is over to fill in the gaps. It is better to deliver 60% of all that you have to present fluently than to try to present 100% nonfluently as you try to recall each detail.

B. **Engaging.** The attention span of the audience is limited. If listeners are not paying attention for even a few seconds, they will miss important data.

C. **Concise.** Presentation of less-than-essential data obscures essential data. If you have seen the movie *Raiders of the Lost Ark,* you will remember that the safest place to hide the Ark of the Covenant (the most prized possession in the world) was in a regular wooden box, nestled among thousands of similar-appearing wooden boxes. So it is with important clinical data in your presentation: if you nestle the valuable (relevant) data among copious irrelevant data, your attending will not be able to find it. **Focus only on relevant data (that which pertains to your differential diagnosis).**

HOT
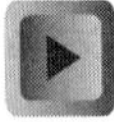
KEY

A formal attending rounds presentation should last no longer than 5 minutes.

III PRESENTING THE FIRST LINE

The first line tells your audience that you mean business, setting the tone for the remainder of the presentation. Look your attending in the eye and speak with confidence; momentum and confidence are vital. Do not be deterred by the fact that of all the people in the room, you may know the least about your patient's disease. The presentation is about your *patient*, and you know more about your patient than your audience does.

A. The first line should contain the patient's age and occupation (or past occupation) and the duration and nature of the chief complaint. For example: "Mr. Wolfe is a 60-year-old retired brake repairman who presents with 3 days of shortness of breath and pleuritic chest pain." Include the patient's race or ethnicity only if you feel it is relevant to your differential diagnosis (e.g., you are considering sickle cell anemia (African-American), or cystic fibrosis (Caucasian), etc.). The patient's gender will be captured by the Mr. or Ms. that begins the line.

B. Past medical history should be excluded from the first line unless you believe it completely changes the differential diagnosis for the chief complaint. For example, in a patient with headache, the differential diagnosis will be very different for an HIV-positive versus an HIV-negative patient. In this case, it would be acceptable to include HIV in the first line (e.g., a 54-year-old, HIV-positive auto mechanic presents with shortness of breath). In contrast, a history of hypertension and gout does not generate a different differential diagnosis for shortness of breath; it should be presented later with the past medical history.

HOT

KEY

Confidence is essential to an effective oral presentation. Practice the opening line of your case repeatedly. Use a similar first-line format for each case so that you become comfortable during the initiation of each presentation.

IV PRESENTING THE HISTORY OF THE PRESENT ILLNESS.

Presentation of the history of the present illness (HPI) is divided into two sections, paralleling your clinical reasoning (Chapters 10 and 11) and your admission note (Chapter 13) (Table 16-1).

TABLE 16-1. How the History Defines the Presentation of the HPI

History	Presentation of the HPI
Identify chief complaint.	First line.
Characterize chief complaint.	*First section:* Description and time course of chief complaint.
Mentally generate a differential diagnosis (Chapter 10) and ask the patient questions about these diagnoses.	*Second section:* The answers to the questions you asked.
Past medical history: Is there any past medical history that would make one of these diagnoses more likely?	*Third section:* Past medical history pertinent to diagnoses considered.

A. **First section (analogous to paragraph 1 of the admission note; Chapter 13 III A and B).** This section should provide:
   1. **Description of the chief complaint/symptoms.** Describe the character of the chief complaint using the FAR COLDER mnemonic in Chapter 11.
   2. **Time course of the chief complaint.** Begin with when the symptom(s) first appeared and what has happened up until the time of admission. Your goal is to tell a story that captures the progression of the chief complaint. Constructing a story will make the patient's history more memorable to you (making it easier to present the patient's data from memory) and your attending.

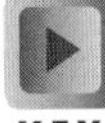

Always express time in relation to date of admission, because this makes it easier for your audience to consider the progression of the symptoms. For example, 3 days before admission is better than last Wednesday or March 3.

B. **Second section (analogous to paragraph 2 of the admission note; Chapter 13 III C).** Use your differential diagnosis to determine what further data is relevant to the case. The second section of the presentation is composed of the answers to these questions you asked to evaluate each diagnosis on your differential. Past medical and social history useful in evaluating the differential diagnosis should be included here as well.

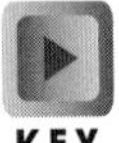

The presentation of the history of the present illness should contain only information that helps evaluate the diagnoses being considered.

V Presenting the Review of Systems

The review of systems reveals additional complaints not elucidated in the history of present illness (Chapter 11 VI). The oral presentation of the review of systems should be very brief. **Any symptoms revealed during the review of systems that relate to your differential diagnosis should be included in the second section of the history of the present illness (see above). Symptoms that do not appear to relate to your differential diagnosis should be briefly noted after the presentation of the HPI; do not elaborate.** Questions the audience might have about these symptoms can be answered at the conclusion of your presentation.

VI Presenting the Past Medical and Social History

A. The presentation of the past medical and social history should be very brief (less than 30 seconds). Do not repeat past medical history that has been presented in the HPI. Begin by stating, "Past medical history in addition to that already presented, includes" (see Chapter 11 V C).

1. Drugs and drug allergies. State the drug name; specific doses can be excluded unless the dose has an impact on the case (e.g., the patient suspected of being dehydrated recently increased his furosemide dose from 40 mg to 80 mg). For example, "He describes no allergies, and his current medications include furosemide, atenolol, and digoxin" (see Chapter 11 V B).
2. Any alcohol, tobacco, or drug use. Example, "He has a 40 pack-year tobacco history; he drinks three beers per day, and he does not use illicit drugs (see Chapter 11 V D).

B. The social history should be very brief unless it has a bearing on the diagnoses being considered. For example, including a history of living in shelters would be important if tuberculosis is in the differential.

VII PRESENTING THE PHYSICAL EXAMINATION

A. Present the examination findings you discovered at the time of admission to the hospital. Section XIII gives guidance for presenting a physical examination that dramatically changes from the time of admission to the time of your oral presentation.

B. Vital signs. Every presentation should include vital signs at the time the patient presented to the hospital. Vital signs should always come first and should be presented in terms of numbers (e.g., "The blood pressure was 150/80," not, "The blood pressure was stable").

C. Organ system approach. Present the physical examination using an organ–system approach (Table 16-2).

1. Give greatest attention to the presence or absence of physical findings that suggest or refute the diagnoses on your differential diagnosis list. For example, if the most probable diagnoses are

TABLE 16-2. Organ System Approach for Presentation of Physical Examination Data.
Head and neck
Lungs
Heart
Abdomen
Genitourinary/pelvic
Extremities
Neurologic
Breast

pneumonia, congestive heart failure, and pulmonary embolism, focus on the presence or absence of fever, elevated neck veins, signs of consolidation, leg edema, and S_3.

2. To save time, group organ systems that do not help to evaluate the diagnoses on your differential diagnosis list and refer to them as normal (if they arc in fact normal). For cxample, in the above case, the relevant positive and negative findings are found in the lung and heart examination. After presenting these organ systems, note that the abdomen and neurologic examinations are normal.
3. If there is an additional examination abnormality that does not appear to pertain to your differential diagnosis (e.g., a skin rash), it should still be presented.

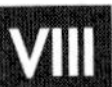

HOT KEY: It is redundant to list an organ system as normal ("The lung exam was normal.") and follow it with a description of its normalcy (". . .there were no crackles, wheezes, or egophony."). Choose one or the other.

VIII Presenting Laboratory and Other Studies

Use your differential diagnosis to decide which laboratory values should be included in your presentation. The following guidelines also apply to other studies, such as the ECG, CXR, and urinalysis. The range of normal values should be presented only when the test is likely to be unfamiliar to the audience (e.g., "The TSH was 0.04; normal is between 0.1 and 1.4.").

A. All laboratory values, both normal and abnormal, that help to evaluate the diagnoses on your differential diagnosis should be presented.
B. All significantly abnormal laboratory values should be presented, even if they do not pertain to the differential diagnosis.
C. To save time, all other laboratory values should be listed en bloc as normal. For example, "The creatinine, complete blood count, and coagulation studies were normal."

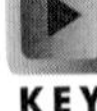

HOT KEY: It is redundant to interpret common laboratory values when you present them. Saying that a patient with a hematocrit of 30% has anemia wastes precious presentation time. Merely state the laboratory value. Uncommon laboratory values (e.g., luteinizing hormone) may be interpreted, because the audience may not know the range of normal.

IX Problem-Based Assessment

A. Throughout the oral presentation, your differential diagnosis determined what data was included in the presentation. The A&P is the time to explicitly state what diagnoses comprise your differential diagnosis list and which of these is the most likely.

B. Presenting the assessment

1. **Identify the first problem** (usually the chief complaint) **and present your leading diagnosis** (e.g., "Problem No. 1: Shortness of breath. I believe this is due to congestive heart failure."). Having the correct answer is not as important as committing to a diagnosis, because this establishes a common point of discussion from which learning and advice can originate. Stating a hypothesis forces each team member to respond to it. Like a scientific study, this keeps the conversation moving forward toward resolution.
2. **Then present the evidence that supports this diagnosis.** "The patient's dyspnea, leg swelling, and CXR are consistent with this diagnosis."
3. Next, present the other diagnoses on your differential diagnosis and a list of historical, physical, and/or laboratory findings that support or refute these diagnoses. For example, "Other possibilities include pulmonary embolism and pneumonia. However, the lack of fever, the normal white blood cell count, and the absence of a history of prolonged stasis or blood clots argues against these diagnoses."

HOT
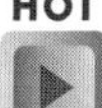
KEY

The three or four most likely diagnoses are usually the only ones that need to be presented. The probability that subsequent diagnoses are correct is so small that it is not worth using presentation time to mention them.

X Presenting the Plan

A. The plan for each problem should be presented only after the assessment of the first problem has been completed. This will put all plans for further diagnostic testing into context.

B. Clearly state the planned diagnostic tests and the sequence in which they will take place. Be committed and decisive. Decisive statements (e.g., "We will obtain an echocardiogram. If this is normal, we will then order a spiral CT of the chest.") encourage the listeners to either agree with or refute each point of the plan. Either way, a decisive plan will prompt action.

C. Then state the therapeutic measures you have taken (or plan to take) to treat the primary diagnosis. Again, be committed and decisive. "We will begin diuresis with 40 mg of furosemide twice a day. He has been given an aspirin and 90 mg of enoxaparin twice a day."

XI When the Patient Has More Than One Problem

A. Identify the primary problem using two questions:

1. **Does a medical problem imminently threaten the patient's life?** If the patient complains of a swollen ankle but is found to

have a myocardial infarction on examination, the primary focus of the presentation should be the myocardial infarction, not the swollen ankle. If no problem imminently threatens the patient's life, the chief complaint is the primary problem.

2. **Has the diagnosis been previously established?** For example, for a patient admitted for a second round of chemotherapy for leukemia, problem No. 1 can be presented as a diagnosis instead of a symptom (e.g., "Problem No. 1: Leukemia."). In this situation, you can skip directly to the plan, as no further diagnosis need be established.

B. Although many patients have multiple medical problems, the majority (80%) of the A&P should focus on the primary problem. Other less active problems (e.g., hypertension and gout in a patient with myocardial infarction) can be deferred to subsequent discussions.

XII How to Allocate Presentation Time

Table 16-3 presents the time allotments for historical, physical, and/or laboratory findings for both 5-minute and 2-minute presentations. The 2-minute presentation should be used for hallway or telephone conversations, where the audience's attention span is even more limited. The structure of the presentation is the same; focus on the HPI and the A&P.

XIII Presenting a Patient Who Has Had a Sudden Change in His Condition

A. The condition of most hospitalized patients will not significantly change from the time you first interview them (i.e., on call) to the time you present their data to the attending (i.e., postcall). On occasion, however, a patient's condition may greatly change from the

TABLE 16-3. Allocation of Presentation Time.

Component	5-Minute (Standard) Presentation	2-Minute Presentation
History of present illness	1–2 minutes	30 seconds
Past medical history	10–30 seconds	5–10 seconds
Social history	5–10 seconds	5 seconds
Physical examination	1–1½ minutes	30 seconds
Laboratory tests/other studies	30 seconds	10 seconds
Assessment and plan	1–1½ minutes	15–30 seconds
TOTAL	**4–6 minutes**	**2 minutes**

time of admission to the time of presentation. When it does, use the strategy described in the next section.

B. Present the history, physical examination, and laboratory studies using the standard method above. Present all of the data as you found it at the time of the initial interview; mentally block out all that subsequently transpired between that time and now.

C. Before the A&P, make a break by stating, "That was his condition until 9 PM last night (i.e., the time the patient's condition suddenly changed). Let me tell you what then transpired".

D. Then present a mini-HPI that describes the events that occurred between the time of admission and the time of presentation. Characterize the patient's symptoms only if they are different from the initial presentation (e.g., if the chest pain character remained the same, just state the character of the pain was unchanged).

E. Then present a mini–physical examination and laboratory update, focusing only on changes in the physical examination and laboratory values during this interval time period.

F. Then present the A&P in full, integrating both the initial and subsequent history, examination, and laboratory data into your clinical decision making. Follow the same formula you used in the standard presentation.

XIV **THE DAILY PRESENTATION** On the days following admission, you will be asked to present the patient and his progress. This presentation should mirror the SOAP method of writing a progress note (Chapter 15).

A. It is important to begin the presentation with a brief reminder of the patient, "This is hospital day No. 2 for Mr. Roark, our 52-year-old patient who presented with shortness of breath." If the diagnosis has been established, substitute the diagnosis for the chief complaint "This is hospital day No. 2 for Mr. Roark, our 52-year-old patient with pneumonia."

B. Note his symptoms and how they have subjectively changed over the course of the last day. "His cough is less, and he feels as if his breathing is easier." If there has been no change, simply note that there has been no change in his symptoms. "There has been no change in his cough and shortness of breath."

C. Next, note the physical examination data that are relevant to his care. Remember, relevance is defined by your differential diagnosis.

1. Begin with the vital signs presented as numbers (e.g., not "stable"). This will allow the team to see trends in the vital signs.
2. If the diagnosis is still uncertain, note the absence or presence of physical findings useful in assessing each diagnosis still being considered (just as you did with the admission presentation).
3. If the diagnosis has been established, focus the presentation on those physical findings that would suggest improvement or wors-

ening of his disease and those that would identify side effects from his therapy.

4. By day 2, it is likely that you will have implemented treatment for the patient. Think about what physical findings might herald success or identify side effects of the treatment. For example, if you gave furosemide to the patient, you might want to comment on whether the S_3, peripheral edema, and crackles have resolved. If you gave a blood thinner, you might want to comment on the absence of neurologic abnormalities (e.g., he has not had a brain hemorrhage as a result of the anticoagulation).

D. Present the laboratory and study data using the same method as you did for the physical examination.

E. Present the A&P. Follow the same method used in presenting the admission case presentation. If the diagnosis has been established, focus the presentation on the plan for the patient's therapy.

XV **DEALING WITH INTERRUPTIONS** Expect that your attending will interrupt your presentation with questions. Do not let the interruption destroy your momentum. There will be two types of questions:

A. Clarification of data presented. The temptation will be to apologize for not including the detail or to break completely and allow the attending to ask all possible questions. Do not succumb to the temptation; when this happens, quickly answer the question and immediately continue your presentation.

B. Jumping ahead. For example, during your presentation of the history, the attending may jump ahead to ask about a laboratory test. The easiest way out is to simply reply with the laboratory test result and immediately pick up where you left off with the history.

C. Do not take the interruption personally. Some people are just impatient.

HOT
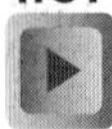
KEY

Gradually wean yourself from the paper, progressing to a memorized presentation.

17. Spoken Case Presentation: Troubleshooting

I Introduction

The structure of the oral presentation is described in Chapter 16. Equally important to your effectiveness as a communicator is your style. This chapter addresses the six most common problems of presentation style.

II The Five-Step Approach to Improve Your Presentations

A. Step 1: Videotape one of your presentations.
B. Step 2: Review the six most common errors of presentation style:
  1. Problem 1: Use of distracting expressions (e.g., "uh," "um," "like")
  2. Problem 2: Boring style
  3. Problem 3: Lack of eye contact
  4. Problem 4: Poor time management
  5. Problem 5: Poor Assessment and Plan
  6. Problem 6: Excessive nervousness

C. Step 3: Even if your presentation has more than one problem, select only the major problem. Focus on improving this problem first.
D. Step 4: Use the techniques in this chapter to solve the problem.
E. Step 5: After practicing these techniques several times, re-videotape your presentation.

III Problem 1: Use of Distracting Expressions

A. Description of the problem. The presentation is marred by frequent "uh's," "um's," and "like's."
B. The Risk. The audience's attention is drawn away from the content because of the annoying interruptions. "Uh's" and "um's" also lengthen the presentation time.
C. The root cause of the problem: The presenter is having a difficult time thinking and talking simultaneously.
D. Techniques to improve the problem
  1. Develop an ability to tell stories. Memorizing a random set of facts is difficult, and the "uh's" and "um's" appear when the presenter is trying to recall these random facts as he talks. A story allows you to sequence the facts so that each fact prompts the next fact, and so on.

a. Practice organizing patient data in a story format. See Chapter 11 IV A 2.
b. Practice telling stories (unrelated to medicine) to friends and family. Developing this skill in nonclinical situations will carry over into clinical presentations.

HOT
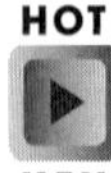
KEY

The best way to develop clinical storytelling ability is to ask your patient to provide the clinical data in a story format as you take the history. Interrupt when necessary to ensure that the patient gives you data in a chronologic format.

2. Relinquish the idea that all patient data must be given in the oral presentation. The fear of leaving something out causes frequent pauses as you ask yourself, "Have I forgotten something?" Not all data are equally important; presenting 60% of the most important information and neglecting some less important information is unlikely to change the presentation substantially. Focus on what you do remember and relinquish what you have forgotten.
3. Become comfortable with pauses in the presentation. Unlike a normal conversation, you are unlikely to be interrupted if you pause. In fact, your listeners may appreciate a break, because it allows them to catch up on the material you have presented.
   a. Practice taking planned pauses between sentences.
   b. Identify the important parts of the presentation by highlighting your admission note. After each important segment, take a 2-second pause to emphasize the content.
4. Aversion training (last resort). Find a friend to serve as your coach. Ask him or her to stop you every time you use an "uh" or an "um." Penalize yourself 3 seconds every time you are stopped, and then continue the presentation.

IV Problem 2: Boring Style

A. **Description of the problem.** The presentation is boring.
B. **The Risk.** If you do not engage the audience, what you say will not be heard. The onus of communication rests with you.
C. **Root causes of the problem**
   1. Failure to create a story
   2. Speaking in a monotone voice
   3. Not using gestures or not being animated
   4. Not being convinced that the case being discussed is interesting
   5. Being overwhelmed or intimidated by the environment and being boring to suppress this nervousness
D. **Techniques to improve the problem**
   1. Develop storytelling ability (see III D 1).
      a. Before presenting the case, organize the information into a story and write it down. The mere act of writing it down will improve your organization.

b. Then choose five interesting features of the case and underline them. When you come to one of the underlined items as you present, emphasize its importance by establishing eye contact with the attending physician, speaking louder, and opening your hand. Lead into the interesting data with, "Now the interesting part about this case is..."

2. Practice using gestures as you speak. Place your hands on the table as you present. When you come to an important piece of data, raise your hand about 6 inches and extend it slightly toward your audience. Supinate your wrist to show your open hand with fingers extended (as if you were offering your audience a pearl in your palm).
3. Practice your presentations in front of a mirror.

V Problem 3: Poor Eye Contact

A. **Description of the problem.** The presenter does not maintain eye contact with the audience.

B. **The Risk.** If you do not engage your audience's attention, communication will be lost. By engaging the audience using eye contact, you increase their interest in what you have to say.

C. **Root causes of the problem**
1. Fear of the audience
2. Fear that the audience's movements will distract your concentration
3. Dependence on use of index cards or notes

D. **Techniques to improve the problem**
1. Practice the presentation in a mirror. Stay focused on the reflection of your own eyes as you present. This will increase your comfort with direct eye contact as you speak and, with practice, will increase your ability to maintain concentration even with movement of the audience.
2. Practice presenting to other students or residents. Focus less on what you say and more on becoming comfortable looking them in the eye as you talk.
3. Wean yourself from the dependence on note cards. Phase into the "no note card" presentation as follows:
   a. Presentations 1–5. Use note cards.
   b. Presentation 6. Present the history of present illness without note cards. Use your notes for the remaining presentation.
   c. Presentation 7. Present the history of present illness and assessment and plan (A&P) without the note cards. Use your notes for the remaining presentation.
   d. Presentation 8. Present the history of present illness, physical examination, and A&P without the note card. Use your notes for the remaining presentation.

e. Presentation 9. Make the entire presentation without using note cards.

VI PROBLEM 4: POOR TIME MANAGEMENT

A. Description of the problem. Your presentations arc consistently longer than 5 minutes.

B. The Risk. Presenting patient data is like trying to carry too many birthday gifts all at the same time: you are likely to drop them all. It is far better to make several trips. If your presentation is longer than 5 minutes, your audience is likely to lose focus. Even though you have presented 100% of the data, they are likely to retain very little.

C. Root cause of the problem

1. Fear of not presenting all the patient data
2. Poor prioritization of information
3. Unnecessary commentary throughout the presentation

D. Techniques to improve the problem

1. Use the "60% rule": 60% of the patient's data presented fluently is better than 100% presented nonfluently. Most patients remain on the clinical wards longer than 1 day, so you will almost always have a "day 2" to present additional data you did not introduce in your first presentation. Also, questions will follow each presentation to pick up what you did not present.
2. Prioritize data
   - **a.** Not all data contributes equally to understanding the patient's current admission. Become comfortable leaving out data that are not crucial. See Chapter 16 for determining which data are most relevant. Data that are occasionally expendable from the oral presentation include:
     - **(1)** Review of systems
     - **(2)** Some past medical, social, or family history
     - **(3)** Some aspects of the physical examination
     - **(4)** Normal laboratory values
   - **b.** To improve your prioritization of data, look at the admission note. In the left hand margin, write down the differential diagnosis. Now go through the admission note and highlight the data that help the audience address the diagnoses on your list. These are the data that are crucial; all other data are fine for the admission note but expendable for the oral presentation.
3. Videotape yourself presenting. Watch for sentences that are there solely to explain other sentences. For example, "He has not taken his insulin for 2 days. *I say that only because his glucose when he came in was 220, which is much more than his usual blood glucose per his report.*" The second sentence is unnecessary; why you noted the noncompliance with insulin will become apparent to your audience when you present the laboratory results.

4. Time each segment of the presentation as you watch your videotaped presentation. Use the values presented in Table 16-3 as a general rule for the length of each segment.

VII Problem 5: Poor Assessment and Plan

A. **Description of the problem.** The presentation is good until the A&P, which is disorganized and noncommittal.

B. **The Risk.** An oral presentation without an assessment and plan is like a scientific study without a hypothesis: there are copious data, but no one knows what to make of the information. Your responsibility is to not only present the data but also to give a "first pass" at synthesizing it. Generating a hypothesis (the assessment and plan) starts the discussion that will move patient care forward.

C. **Causes of the problem**
   1. Reporting but not synthesizing the data.
   2. Not taking a stand on a diagnosis for fear of being incorrect

D. **Techniques to improve the problem**
   1. Use clinical reasoning from the outset of the presentation. A good A&P begins as you present the history of present illness (see Chapter 10).
   2. Begin the assessment with authority. Speak with confidence, even when you are not. Follow the method in Chapter 16 IX.
   3. Present the plan (Chapter 16 X). Be as specific and committed as possible.
   4. If you have a coach, ask him to watch your presentation. Ask him to interrupt you after each major section of the presentation and ask you what your differential diagnosis is at each point and why. This will train you to think about the data as you are presenting them.

VIII Problem 6: Nervousness

A. **Description of the problem.** The presenter is too nervous to present the data fluently. Symptoms include cracking or shaking of the voice, sweating profusely, or "freezing" in midsentence.

B. **The Risk.** No one finds this degree of anxiety enjoyable. When you are nervous, so is the audience. When everyone is nervous, communication is impaired.

C. **Root causes of the problem**
   1. Impostor syndrome. You feel as if you are masquerading as a physician. You feel that the audience knows more than you do, and they are waiting for you to make a mistake.
   2. Fear of failure. If you do not present well, your colleagues will think you are inept.

D. Techniques to improve the problem

1. Address the impostor syndrome head-on. It is true that your audience is likely to know more about diabetes mellitus than you do, but it is unlikely that they know more about your patient. With regard to your patient's history and condition, you are the expert. Before you begin your presentation, tell yourself, "No one knows more about my patient that I do. I am the expert here."
2. Visualize yourself presenting successfully. This is an easy way to gain experience. Have you ever had a dream that seemed so real you wonder if it actually happened? The mind has a difficult time distinguishing between pure mental visualization and what has actually occurred. Visualize yourself successfully delivering patient presentations. One hundred dreams about successful presentations are the same as 100 successful actual presentations.

HOT
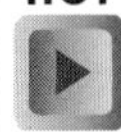
KEY

If you visualize failure, you are likely to fail.

3. Practice presenting.
4. Remind yourself that everyone has bad presentations. The repercussions of one bad presentation are small; it is only when presentations are consistently bad that patient care is compromised.
5. Make sure the conditions are suitable before you present.
   a. Take a few minutes to get organized.
   b. Do not begin when you are out of breath (e.g., if you have just run up a flight of stairs).

HOT KEY

If you are out of breath before a presentation, ask your attending physician a question; it doesn't matter what the question is. This will force the attending physician to talk, giving you time to catch your breath.

18. Spoken Case Presentation: Intensive Care Unit

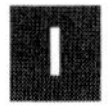

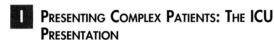

Presenting Complex Patients: The ICU Presentation

A. The "ICU format" is used when presenting patients in the ICU, because most critically ill patients have multiple systemic abnormalities. If you happen to have an ICU patient with only one main abnormality, stay with the standard presentation described in Chapter 16.

B. The initial admission history and physical examination for a patient in an ICU should be presented exactly like those of any other patient (see Chapter 16).

C. The ICU format is used for daily presentations after the patient has been admitted. It uses the same clinical reasoning to identify the relevant information; even though the information is organized by organ systems, it is still the differential diagnosis that defines what data are relevant to include in the presentation.

D. Instead of breaking the presentation into history, examination, laboratory data, and assessment and plan (A&P) sections, the ICU format groups all data relating to an organ system together. All historical, examination, and laboratory data are presented for the cardiac system; then the same is done for the pulmonary system, and so on through each organ system. A problem list is generated *after* all organ systems have been presented. An A&P is presented for each item on the problem list.

E. Begin with a brief (one sentence) overview of the patient. It is useful to remind your audience how long the patient has been in the hospital. For example, "This is the 12th hospital day for Mr. Roark, a 48-year-old man with acute pancreatitis complicated by acute respiratory distress syndrome, acute renal failure, hyperglycemia, and sepsis."

HOT KEY

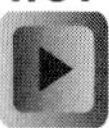

There are two approaches commonly used to organize the presentation in the ICU setting: "Top to Bottom" and "Ending on a High Note." Ask your resident or intern which approach the ICU attending prefers.

F. Organization Method 1: "Top to bottom" approach. Begin with the "top" of the patient (neurologic examination) and work your way down, following this list: neurologic, cardiovascular, pulmonary, gastrointestinal/nutrition, renal/electrolytes/fluids, hematologic/infectious disease. Use the "SEEMS Approach" to describe each organ system (see below). If there is nothing relevant to say about an organ system, merely note that it is normal (e.g., "there are no gastrointestinal issues").

G. **Organization Method 2: "Ending on a high note" approach.** This approach ends with the most active organ system. For example, if the patient has multilobar pneumonia, the presentation would begin with the less-active organ systems and end with the pulmonary system. Begin with the neurology report, and progress as you did with the top to bottom approach, ending with the pulmonary report. The advantage to this approach is that it allows for an easy segue into an A&P focused on the most active organ system.

The following information "**SEEMS**" relevant to each organ system.
Subjective symptoms
Events in the past 24 hours
Examination
Medications
Studies

II Information That Should Be Included for Each System (Table 18-1)

A. **Neurologic system**
1. **S**ubjective symptoms: headache, strength, sensory loss, mental status (obtunded, sedated, confused, alert and oriented)
2. **E**vents that occurred during the past 24 hours: seizures, new stroke, loss of consciousness
3. **E**xamination: findings on neurologic examination
4. **M**edications that could affect mental status or are being used for treatment: narcotics, benzodiazepines
5. **S**tudies that focus on the brain or spinal cord: MRI, CT, EEG

B. **Cardiovascular system.** This is the appropriate place to report pulmonary artery or central venous pressure catheter results.
1. **S**ubjective symptoms: chest pain, shortness of breath, palpitations
2. **E**vents over the past 24 hours: changes in blood pressure or heart rate, telemetry events, episodes of chest pain
3. **E**xamination: heart rate, blood pressure, findings on cardiac examination
4. **M**edications with cardiovascular effects: vasopressors, antiarrhythmics
5. **S**tudy results for cardiac tests: catheterizations, ECGs, echocardiograms

C. **Pulmonary system**
1. **S**ubjective symptoms: shortness of breath, cough, hemoptysis

TABLE 18-1. Part 1 of the Presentation in the ICU: Delivering the Data in a Systems-Oriented Format.

Example Patient: A 48-year-old man

System	Content
Neurologic	Sedated but arousable Moving all extremities and following commands Fentanyl drip: 75 mcg/hr Lorazepam dose: 8 mg in intermittent boluses throughout the day
Cardiovascular	Heart rate: 110–130 in atrial fibrillation Blood pressure decreased yesterday to 70/40 but then increased to 90/60 after dopamine was restarted. There are no murmurs, rubs, or gallops. There is 1+ bilateral lower extremity edema. Dopamine: 8 mcg/kg/min
Pulmonary	He remains intubated. His ventilator settings are SIMV at a set rate of 12 breaths/ minute. His actual rate is 18 breaths/minute. Tidal volume is 600 ml; spontaneous tidal volume is 300 ml. FIO_2 is 0.6 PEEP is 7 cm H_2O ABG this morning was: pH 7.31, PCO_2 54, PO_2 68, with a 92% O_2 saturation. There are bilateral basilar crackles. CXR this morning: endotracheal tube correctly placed; diffuse bilateral infiltrates unchanged compared with yesterday; no pneumothorax He continues on ipratropium MDI 3 puffs q4h.
Renal/fluids/electrolytes	In: total 2000 ml; TPN 1200 ml; medications 800 ml Out: total 900 ml; urine 600 ml; stool 100 ml; NG tube 200 ml Na^+ 144, K^- 4.1, Cl^- 103, CO_2 29, Ca^{2+} 7.8, PO_4 2.5, Mg^{2+} 1.2; glucose 214 Urinalysis: 1+ protein, 5–10 WBCs, 3–5 RBCs, 0–5 epithelial cells

(*Continued*)

TABLE 18-1. Continued

Example Patient: A 48-year-old man

System	Content
	BUN: 70, creatinine: 2.9; BUN and creatinine have increased from 62/2.2 yesterday
Gastrointestinal/nutrition	No abdominal pain One stool yesterday, guaiac negative Bowel sounds hypoactive, abdomen soft but moderately distended Continues TPN at 50 ml/hr Liver function: bilirubin 1.4, AST 90, ALT 80, alkaline phosphatase 110, albumin 2.7 Medications: Insulin sliding scale Ranitidine 50 mg IV q8h for stress ulcer prophylaxis
Hematologic	WBC: 14,000; increased from 11,000 yesterday; 89% neutrophils Hemoglobin: 9.8 mg/dl Received 2 units packed RBCs yesterday Platelets: 78 (decreased from 110 yesterday) PT 13.2, INR 1.2, PTT 68
Infectious disease	Temp max 38.7°C Temp currently 37.6°C 2/2 blood cultures from 3 days ago grew methicillin-resistant *Staphylococcus aureus*. Repeat cultures drawn yesterday are pending. Medications: Vancomycin 1 g IV q24h day 3 Imipenem-cilastatin 1 g IV q8h day 3
Other ICU issues	Foley catheter is in place; day #12. NG tube is on low-intermittent wall suction; day #12. Right internal jugular central venous catheter, day #7, appears clean. His left forearm has a 20-gauge IV, day #3. He is on heparin 5000 units subcut bid for prophylaxis of deep vein thrombosis.

2. **E**vents over the past 24 hours: oxygen requirements, changes in ventilator settings. If the patient is being mechanically ventilated, ventilator settings should be described first because it is difficult to interpret the physical examination without knowing this information.
    a. Mode of ventilation: assist-control (AC) or synchronized intermittent ventilation (SIMV)
    b. Rate of ventilation: set number of machine-initiated breaths and the total number of breaths (i.e., machine-initiated plus patient-initiated)
    c. Tidal volume
    d. FIO_2: the percentage of oxygen delivered
    e. Positive end-expiratory pressure and pressure support settings (if any)
    f. Evaluation of ventilation
        (1) Arterial blood gas numbers (pH, PCO_2, PO_2, O_2 saturation)
        (2) Minute ventilation (respiratory rate $\times$ tidal volume)
        (3) Peak and peak plateau pressures
3. **E**xamination: findings on pulmonary examination
4. **M**edications
5. **S**tudies: results of recent CXR and other studies

D. Gastrointestinal/nutrition

1. **S**ubjective symptoms: nausea, vomiting, diarrhea, constipation, abdominal pain
2. **E**vents over the past 24 hours: tolerating oral feeding, feeding tube or intravenous feeding issues, number of stools, change in quality of stool (blood in the stool, diarrhea), episodes of vomiting (blood in the vomitus?)
3. **E**xamination: abdominal rigidity, bowel sounds
4. **M**edications/source of nutrition: histamine antagonists, proton pump inhibitors, nasogastric feeding, TPN
5. **S**tudy results: hepatic enzymes, albumin, abdominal CT or ultrasound, endoscopy

E. Renal/electrolytes/fluids

1. **S**ubjective symptoms (usually there is nothing to report)
2. **E**vents over the past 24 hours (intake volume, urine output, daily weight, response to dialysis)
3. **E**xamination (usually there is nothing to report)
4. **M**edications with renal effects (diuretics, IV fluids, electrolytes).
5. **S**tudy results (electrolytes, BUN/creatinine, urinalysis)

F. Hematology/infectious disease. These are grouped together to facilitate presentation of the CBC, which has both hematologic and infectious disease implications.

1. **S**ubjective symptoms: fever, cellulitis, pain, cough. Present symptoms only if they have not been presented earlier.
2. **E**vents over the past 24 hours: temperature changes, new bleeding, transfusions

TABLE 18-2. Part 2 of the ICU Presentation: Assessment and Plan as a Problem List.

Example Problem	Example Plan
Acute pancreatitis	We will continue supportive management; pain control via fentanyl and TPN for nutritional support. If his condition worsens, we will obtain a repeat abdominal CT scan to evaluate hemorrhagic pancreatitis or an infected pseudocyst.
Acute respiratory distress syndrome	We will switch his tidal volume to low-volume, high-cycle ventilation. Oxygen will be decreased once the saturation remains consistently above 95%.
Sepsis, with *Staphylococcus aureus* bacteremia, persistent fever, and new hypotension	We will continue the vancomycin and imipenem-cilastatin. Antibiotics will be dose-adjusted based on the creatinine. I will check the results of yesterday's culture today. The dopamine will be continued to maintain mean arterial pressure >60 mm Hg.
Acute renal failure	I suspect this is related to pancreatitis, sepsis, and hypotension, but vancomycin toxicity is possible. We will check the vancomycin level and send urine electrolytes and creatinine.
Anemia	The likely cause is anemia of chronic disease (also known as "anemia of active inflammation"), because his hemoglobin has been stable over the last few days. I have a low suspicion for gastrointestinal bleeding or hemorrhagic pancreatitis. He received 2 units of packed RBCs yesterday.
Thrombocytopenia	I suspect this is related to sepsis. Heparin-induced thrombocytopenia is possible but unlikely.
Nutrition	We will continue TPN.
Hyperglycemia	This is due to pancreatitis. We will continue the insulin sliding scale.
ICU issues	We will begin compression stockings for deep vein thrombosis prophylaxis. We will continue ranitidine.

3. **E**xamination: temperature
4. **M**edications: antibiotics, chemotherapy
5. **S**tudy results: blood cultures, CBC

G. **Prevention of complications in the ICU.** A few miscellaneous ICU issues should be addressed every day.
   1. Any indwelling intravenous lines or catheters (e.g., Foley catheters, nasogastric tubes, feeding tubes). Note how many days the line or catheter has been in place (this ensures that unnecessary catheters are removed).
   2. Prophylactic medications (e.g., subcutaneous heparin or enoxaparin for deep vein thrombosis, pharmacologic agents to prevent stress-related upper gastrointestinal tract bleeding) should be reported if not already addressed.
   3. Any new decubitus ulcers should be reported.

H. Describe the A&P in the form of a problem list (Table 18-2), using the same approach you used for the standard ward presentation. If there are multiple problems, the assessment and plan for each can be discussed immediately following the presentation of each organ system's "SEEMS" issues.

III FURTHER TIPS FOR THE ICU PRESENTATION

A. Expect to feel a sense of discontinuity between the organ systems; this discontinuity is expected by your audience. You do not need to compensate for this discontinuity by using transitions such as "That is all for the neurologic system." After you have presented the previous organ system, simply move to the next organ system.

B. Avoid using terms such as "cardiovascularwise" or "pulmonarily speaking." Although it seems natural to identify the next organ system, the data will make the system being discussed perfectly obvious.

C. Present information only once. If the CXR was described in the cardiac system, you do not need to discuss it again in the pulmonary system. Do not refer to information that has already been presented (e.g., "I presented the CXR above.").

D. Proceed quickly. Do not wait for the attending physician to respond to each piece of information.

E. Be prepared. The patient in the ICU requires greater pre-round preparation than a patient on the wards.

19. Writing Orders

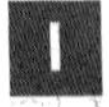

INTRODUCTION **Active participation is the key** to getting the most from your third and fourth years of medical school. You will advance slower if you merely follow along. The act of actually writing the orders is important, even though your orders must be co-signed by a physician. It will force you to make decisions, and it will teach you the subtleties of writing a proper order: one that results in exactly what you intended.

HOT KEY

Ask to write orders. This will teach you to think of the consequences of each decision you make before you make it.

WRITING MEDICATION ORDERS

A. Components of a medication order

1. Drug
2. Dose
3. Method of administration
4. Frequency
5. Modifiers (e.g., PRN, hold orders)
6. Duration. If this is not specified, the patient will receive the drug indefinitely until you stop the order.

B. Example: acetaminophen 500 mg PO every 12h PRN for pain (translation: 500 mg of acetaminophen to be given every 12 hours as needed for pain).

C. Clarity. Take the time to write medication orders neatly. A misinterpreted drug or dose can be disastrous for your patient.

1. Use generic drug names whenever possible. This will allow the pharmacist to substitute another brand if the first is not available. It also allows the patient to choose among cheaper generic formulations at the time of her discharge.
2. Whenever possible, write the *dose* instead of the number of tablets. For example, instead of "aspirin one tablet every 12 hours," write, "aspirin 81 mg PO every 12h."
3. The decimal point is sometimes difficult to see, so all decimals should be preceded by a number. For example, instead of "digoxin .125 mg," write "digoxin 0.125 mg." This will prevent your patient from receiving 125 mg of digoxin.
4. Write each order on a separate line.

5. Write in blue or black ink only. All other colors fade. Pencil is an absolute no.

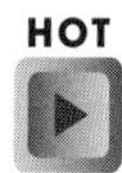

HOT KEY Any drug that ends in "-cet" contains acetaminophen (e.g., Darvocet, Percocet). Be mindful of the total acetaminophen dose you are prescribing (e.g., <3 g/day for patients with normal liver function; <2 g/day for those with compromised liver function).

D. Commonly used abbreviations (Table 19-1)

III ADMISSION ORDERS

The admission orders set the course for the patient's hospitalization. See the example in Figure 19-1.

TABLE 19-1. Common Abbreviations Used in Medication Orders.*

Abbreviation	Latin Derivation	Meaning
Frequency		
q**		*Quodque* Each
d	*Die*	Day
qwk	—	Once each week
qac	*Quodque ante consumption*	Before each meal
qhs	*Quodque hora somni*	Before bedtime
bid	*Bis in die*	Twice each day
tid	*Ter in die*	Three times each day
qid	*Quater in die*	Four times each day
q4h		Every 4 hours
PRN	Pro re nata	As needed
a	*Ante*	Before
p	*Post*	After
c	*Cum*	With
s	*Sine*	Without
Method of Administration		
PO	*Per os*	Oral
IV	—	Intravenous
Sub-Q, subQ, subcut	—	Subcutaneous
IM	—	Intramuscular

* The degree sign (°) is sometimes used to designate "hour."
** "q" is still a commonly used abbreviation, though it is now prohibited by JCAHO.

MEDICAL CENTER OF LOUISIANA AT NEW ORLEANS
DOCTORS ORDER FORM

IMPRINT PATIENT INFORMATION BELOW

- Admit: Internal Medicine. Attending: E. Dantes; Resident: H. Long; MSIII: H. Melville 555-1212
- Diagnosis: Meningitis
- Condition: Stable
- Allergies: Sulfa drugs (rash)
- Vitals: per routine
- Activity: Ad lib
- Nursing: Foley catheter to gravity drainage
  Please place a peripheral IV
  Seizure precautions
- Diet: Regular diet
- IV Fluids: $^{1}/_{2}$ NS at 100 cc/hr.
- Meds: Ceftriaxone 2 gm IV q 12 hours
  Omperazol 10 mg po q d
  Acetominophen 500 mg po q 8 hours prn
  Colace 100 mg po q d
  Metoprolol 50 mg po BID; Hold for SBP less than 110 or heart rate less than 50.
  Dilantin 300 mg po q HS
- Labs: Check CBC and Electrolytes now and q am
  Obtain blood cultures x 2 now
  Obtain urinalysis and urine cultures now
  Obtain head CT with contrast now.
  Send CSF for glucose, protein, cell count, VRDL, gram stain and cultures.
- Notify house officer for: SBP < 110 or > 170;
  HR < 50 or > 110;
  Temp > 38.5°C;
  RR < 10 or > 25

Date:	Time:	M.D.

FIGURE 19-1. Sample admission orders (see Chapter 14 IV).

HOT  **KEY**

The mnemonic "**ADCA VAN DISML**" can be used to remember the standard approach for writing admission orders on all services.

A. *Admission service*

1. Note the **service** to which the patient is admitted.
2. Note the **attending physician**, the **resident or intern**, and **your name**. It is especially important that you include **your pager number** if you wish to be the first contact for patient issues. The number you write will be the one nursing staff will call to report information about the patient.

B. *D*iagnosis. Note the suspected diagnosis. This tells everyone on the team why the patient is in the hospital.

C. *C*ondition. This tells the nursing staff how closely the patient should be observed.

1. Critical. The patient should be in the ICU.
2. Guarded. This alerts nurses so they pay more attention to the patient and perhaps reduce the nurse-to-patient ratio.
3. Good. Synonyms for "good" (e.g., fair, stable) are not helpful. These terms all have the same meaning: the patient does not need closer observation than other patients.

D. *A*llergies

1. Note any allergies and the specific type (e.g., "Allergies—penicillin: rash").
2. If there are no allergies, write NKDA (i.e., no known drug allergies).

E. *V*ital signs

1. Tell the nurses how often you want the vital signs checked. Order what is necessary, but do not tax the nurses unnecessarily. Doing so will only divert their attention from other patients. Patients who require vital signs checks more frequently than every 4 hours should be in the ICU.
2. Note any special vital signs, such as "neurologic checks" for neurology patients.

F. *A*ctivity. Examples are bed rest, out of bed with assistance, and ad lib (*ad liberatum* = at the patient's discretion).

G. *N*ursing orders. Note any specific tasks for which you want assistance from the nursing staff (e.g., Foley catheter, surgical drains).

H. *D*iet. Designate a special diet if necessary. Unless designated, the patient will receive a normal diet.

1. NPO *(non per os)*. The patient will receive no food. A patient should be NPO at 12 midnight before any procedure or test the following day if the test could potentially involve aspiration of food into the lungs (e.g., any procedure involving anesthesia).
2. American Diabetes Association 2500-kcal diet. This is standard for patients with diabetes mellitus.
3. Low-salt diet. This diet is used for patients with heart failure or hypertension.
4. Soft-mechanical diet. This diet is used for patients with impaired pharyngeal muscles (e.g., stroke). Solids cannot be swallowed, and liquids do not provide sufficient stimulation to ensure closure of the glottis and prevention of aspiration.

HOT

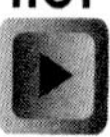

KEY

Do *not* give liquid or pureed diets to patients with pharyngeal dysfunction.

5. Pureed diet. Pureed food is useful only for patients who cannot chew.
6. Liquid diet. This diet is the best place to start for patients who have not eaten recently (e.g., postsurgical patients or those recovering from pancreatitis). The order can be followed with the instruction to "advance as tolerated" if you believe the patient will tolerate the liquid diet.

I. *IV* fluids. Designate the type of fluid and the rate. If you want IV access but do not want the patient to receive volume, order either: "Heplock the IV" or "TKO" ("to keep open"). A TKO order is equivalent to 10 ml/hr of fluid. Both options keep the IV from clotting.

1. Normal saline or lactated Ringer's solution. Use for all situations in which you want to increase intravascular volume (preload). All other fluids have inadequate osmotic strength to remain in the intravascular space. Lactated Ringer's solution is used on surgical services where large-volume (>10 L) infusions are common. Normal saline is used on medical services where large-volume infusions are rare.
2. D51/2 normal saline. Use this for maintenance fluids (i.e., to replace what patients would ordinarily require if they could eat and drink normally). The rate should be around 86 ml/hr. This will give 1 L of fluids every 12 hours, which meets daily requirements and corresponds to the nursing shift schedule (i.e., a liter will finish at the end of each 12-hour nursing shift). Usually, you will see the specified hourly rate vary between 50 ml/hr and 100 ml/hr depending on the size of the patient.
3. D5W. Use for hypernatremia but only after normal saline has filled the intravascular space. Remember that most cases of hypernatremia are due to dehydration. Use normal saline until the serum sodium has declined to 154 mEq/L (the concentration of normal saline); then switch to D5W to further decrease the sodium to normal levels (i.e., 140 mEq/L).

HOT
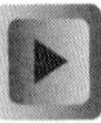
KEY

If you give IV fluids to replenish the intravascular space (e.g., to increase renal perfusion or improve hypotension), there are only two choices: normal saline or lactated Ringer's solution. Albumin solutions have no benefit over normal saline, and they cost much more ($232/1 vs. $2.32/1).

J. *Special orders*

1. Note any special precautions (e.g., for falls, seizures, suicide, neutropenia, aspiration).
2. Note any special orders for patients with diabetes mellitus.

a. Glucose checks tid. Sliding scales should be avoided (see VIII A).

b. Oxygen administration

(1) Nasal cannula (2 to 8 L/min). Each liter provides approximately 3% of additional O_2. That is, 4 L of O_2 increases room air oxygen of 21% to 33% ($21 + 4 \times 3$).

(2) Face-mask. A face-mask with 100% oxygen can increase the FIO_2 to 50%.

(3) Venturi mask/nonrebreather. FIO_2 may become as high as 60%.

K. *M*edications (see II above)

L. *L*aboratory tests

1. Note the laboratory test and how often you want it checked (e.g., "electrolytes every AM," "CBC every 8h").
2. Designate any special timing requests. "Check the gentamicin level 30 minutes before administering gentamicin."

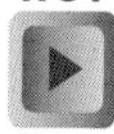

HOT KEY
Set finite limits on laboratory orders. For example, CBC daily × *3* days. This will prevent serial phlebotomy long after it is useful.

IV "As Needed" Orders

PRN (*pro re nada:* as the situation requires) orders are written to anticipate simple symptoms that might arise. A PRN symptom should be one of minimal significance that does not require a physician to see the patient. A common pitfall is writing PRN orders for symptoms that are warning signs of negative future events (e.g., anxiety may be a warning sign for myocardial infarction). Do not write PRN anxiety orders unless you know that anxiety is an expected feature of the patient's disease (e.g., alcohol withdrawal, primary anxiety disorder). A patient with new-onset anxiety should be evaluated by a physician to ensure there is not an underlying cause of the anxiety. Generally acceptable PRN orders are listed in Table 19-2

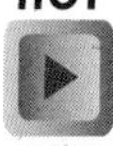
HOT KEY
It is very difficult to expel extremely soft stool. Stool softeners are satisfactory for chronic constipation, but in acute situations, always combine them with lactulose or Senokot to expel the stool.

V Hold Orders and Notification Orders

A. Hold orders. All medications that could affect the hemodynamic system (e.g., blood pressure medications, opiates) should have "stop" parameters (i.e., vital sign threshold below which the medication is

TABLE 19-2. Examples of "As Needed" (PRN) Orders.

Symptom	Drug and Dose
Fever	Acetaminophen 500 mg PO every 8h
Pain	Acetaminophen 500 mg PO every 8h
Diarrhea	Imodium one tablet PO every 8h
Constipation	Lactulose 30 ml PO every 8h
Insomnia	Diphenhydramine 50 mg PO every 8h
Itching	Diphenhydramine 50 mg PO every 8h
	Atarax 10 mg PO every 8h
Nausea and vomiting	Phenergan 10 mg PO every 8h

not to be given). For example, "metoprolol 25 mg PO bid; hold for SBP <110 or HR <50."

B. Notification orders. Give the nurses the criteria (vital signs) for which you want to be called. For example, "call house officer for: T >38.5°, SBP <90/50 or >180/100, RR <10 or >30."

VI Verbal Orders

Verbal orders should be used only when it is important that the order occur immediately (e.g., patient needs a Foley catheter for sudden urinary obstruction), and you are unable to be at the bedside immediately. All verbal orders must be signed within 12 hours.

VII "Do Not Resuscitate" Orders

DNR orders tell the nursing staff and cross-covering physicians the patient's desire in the event she stops breathing or has a cardiac arrest. They have no bearing on other therapy or whether the patient is a candidate for the ICU. These orders are always a result of having a discussion between the physician and the patient regarding the patient's wishes, and this discussion should be documented in the progress notes. A DNR order requires the co-signature of an attending physician within 24 hours.

VIII "Sliding Scale" Orders

Sliding scale orders tell the nurse how much drug to give based on a measured parameter.

A. Insulin. Sliding scales are no longer indicated in the management of diabetes. Instead, estimate the amount of daily insulin needed (e.g., the patient's outpatient insulin dose), check glucose levels three times a day, and adjust the daily doses based on the glucose levels. Extremely strict glucose control is beneficial provided the nurse can quickly identify signs of hypoglycemia and provide glucose to correct it (e.g., in the ICU). This tight response loop is not available on the general wards, however; aggressively tight glucose control frequently leads to hypoglycemia.

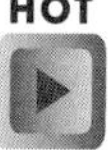

HOT KEY In ward patients with diabetes mellitus, your attending physicians will likely dislike hyperglycemia but *despise* hypoglycemia.

B. Heparin. IV heparin has largely been replaced by low-molecular-weight heparins, which have more reliable bioavailability. The use of IV heparin has been largely limited to two circumstances: to provide quick anticoagulation while waiting for the effects of low-molecular-weight heparin to begin or when it is beneficial to be able to quickly stop the heparin (e.g., a surgical procedure is planned in the next day or two). When IV heparin is used, the dose should be adjusted based on the PTT (measured every 6 hours).

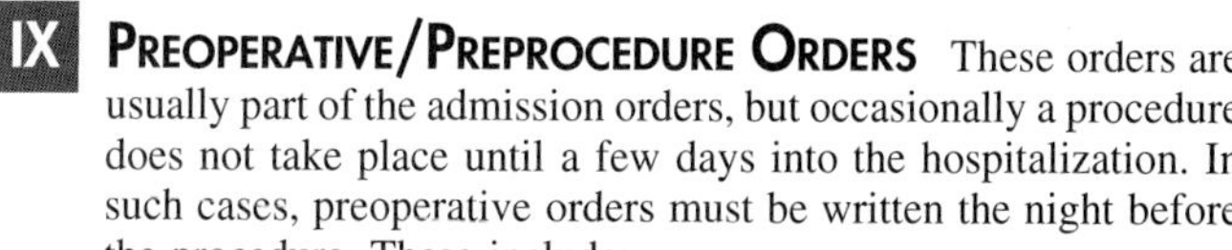

IX Preoperative/Preprocedure Orders

These orders are usually part of the admission orders, but occasionally a procedure does not take place until a few days into the hospitalization. In such cases, preoperative orders must be written the night before the procedure. These include:

A. NPO. No food should be given after midnight; medications may be given.

B. Hold orders. Hold all diabetic medications (sulfonylureas, insulin, etc.). The patient will be NPO; insulin without food intake will result in hypoglycemia.

C. Laboratory tests

D. IV fluids

E. Bowel preparation. For surgeries or studies (e.g., CT) that involve visualizing the bowel, the bowel must be cleaned of stool. Common bowel preps include:

1. Magnesium sulfate (e.g., Milk of Magnesia). Do not give magnesium-containing bowel preps to patients with renal failure; they have no way of expelling the high magnesium load.
2. GoLYTELY. Give 1 gallon the night before the procedure.

X Postoperative Orders

Postoperative orders are rewritten after each surgery as if the patient was being newly admitted to the ward. The format follows that used for admission orders (see III), except as noted:

A. Nursing

1. Strict I&O and daily weights. Fluid shifts are common in surgical procedures; this information is vital to make fluid management decisions.

2. Incentive spirometry. Patients given general anesthesia will have some degree of alveolar collapse (atelectasis) following the procedure, because the anesthetic washes out the nitrogen in the alveoli that keeps them open. This can cause low-grade fever and hypoxemia. Incentive spirometry keeps alveoli open.
3. Drains and tubes. Output of all drains should be recorded.
   a. Foley catheter: gravity drainage
   b. Nasogastric tube: low, intermittent suction
   c. Jackson-Pratt drain: bulb suction
   d. Chest tube: 20 ml suction
   e. Hemovac drain: suction
   f. Ostomy bag: straight drainage

B. Diet. NPO is ordered.

C. IV fluids

1. Calculate the IV fluid rate using the following method:
   a. Read the anesthesiology note for the I&O during the procedure.
   b. Start with the IV fluids given during the procedure and subtract the amount of fluid lost. For every 1 ml of estimated blood loss (EBL), multiply by 3. For example,

$$\text{Fluid deficit} = \text{IV fluids} - \text{urine output} - (\text{EBL} \times 3).$$

2. Replace the fluid deficit in addition to maintenance fluids. (Maintenance fluids = 2 L/day.)

D. Medications

1. Resume preoperative medications. Convert all oral medications to intravenous formulations until the patient can tolerate oral intake.
2. Give pain medication, stool softeners, antibiotics, and deep venous thrombosis prophylaxis (e.g., enoxaparin 30 mg subcut bid or heparin 5000 units subcut bid), if necessary. Deep venous thrombosis prophylaxis is indicated only if the risk of bleeding from the procedure is low.

E. Laboratory tests and other studies. Order laboratory tests immediately on arrival to the floor if there has been significant blood loss or fluid shifts. An ECG and chest radiograph should be ordered the following morning.

XI TRANSFER ORDERS

Each time a patient transfers services, a new set of admission orders should be written by the receiving physician. Although this may seem inconvenient, it ensures that the new team of physicians knows exactly what medications the patient is receiving, thereby preventing drug interactions.

XII DISCHARGE ORDERS

To discharge a patient, write the following orders:

A. Ask the clerk to schedule follow-up appointments.
B. Remove devices such as IVs and catheters.
C. Order any appliances the patient will receive from the hospital before to going home (e.g., wheelchairs, canes).
D. Write the order to discharge the patient.

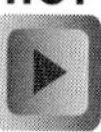

Discharging a patient from the hospital is a high-risk procedure. Make sure the discharge paperwork—especially medications and follow-up appointments—is completely accurate.

XIII Ventilator and ICU Orders

A. Mode of ventilation (AC, SIMV, PS). This tells the machine how to deliver the breaths to the patient.

1. AC (Assist-Control). This mode will deliver a fixed number of breaths per minute, with a fixed tidal volume per breath. If the patient initiates a breath (even if it is a weak effort), the machine senses this and delivers the prespecified tidal volume to the patient. This is useful in patients who are not initiating spontaneous respirations, because any patient-initiated breaths (even hiccups) will initiate full machine-driven breaths (on top of the set machine rate) with the set tidal volume. The risk is overventilation or barotrauma. The normal values are AC 10 with TV 700 (see below for TV).
2. SIMV (Synchronized Intermittent Mechanical Ventilation) This mode is exactly the same as assist control, except that the machine will not augment any patient-initiated breaths with tidal volume. Whatever the patient pulls in, the patient gets. Machine-initiated breaths will receive the set tidal volume (see below). This is a good weaning mode, because it allows the physician to slowly dial down the number of machine breaths and gradually let the patient take over.
3. Pressure support. The machine will deliver no set number of breaths; whatever the patient initiates is what the patient gets. Each time the patient takes a breath, however, the machine provides some inspiratory pressure to help the patient take a larger tidal volume.

B. Rate of ventilation (respiratory rate). Usually this is 5 to 10 breaths per minute.
C. Tidal volume (usually 5 to 10 ml/kg ideal body weight)
D. Oxygen concentration (FIO_2). Always start with 100% FIO_2 and wean it down as quickly as possible. High oxygen tension (>60%) leads to oxygen free radicals that may cause (in the order of a week or two) pulmonary fibrosis.

E. PEEP (positive end-expiratory pressure) is sometimes added to keep alveoli from collapsing during exhalation. The normal parameters are 5 to 10 mm Hg.

F. Pressure support is sometimes added to augment the patient's spontaneous tidal volume. Pressure support increases oxygenation, thereby decreasing the FIO_2 required.

20. Organizing Patient Information

I INTRODUCTION There are small windows of opportunity on the wards. For example, catching the attention of a consultant as she passes through the hall can be the difference between having a consultation performed today instead of tomorrow. If you are well organized and have relevant data on each of your patients at your fingertips, you are in a position to deliver a presentation about your patient at any given moment.

HOT
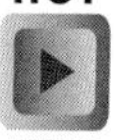
KEY

Chance rewards the prepared mind.

II THE IMPORTANCE OF A GOOD PATIENT DATA SYSTEM You cannot remember all of the details about your patients. Therefore, it is important to have a data-tracking system. A good data system will offer you the following benefits:

A. Revealing data trends. The rate of change of any given clinical variable is more important than the absolute number. For example, a sodium that has changed from 145 mEq/L to 130 mEq/L in 1 day is more worrisome than a sodium of 120 mEq/L that has been present for a week. The body does not adapt to small changes that are introduced suddenly as well as it adapts to large changes that are introduced gradually. **Your data-tracking system must be able to detect these sudden changes. It must also reveal trends in laboratory values and physical examination findings** (e.g., the blood pressure has steadily increased since stopping the beta blocker).

B. Portability. Your patient data tracking system should fit in your pocket so that your hands are free to examine your patient and interact on rounds. Do not burden yourself with large clipboards or charts.

C. Independence from carrying progress notes. It will initially be tempting to copy the progress notes from the chart and use these as a template for your oral presentations. This method, however, has drawbacks.

1. It is not possible to view trends.
2. Taking progress notes from the chart (even for the few minutes it takes to find a copy machine) prevents other team members (e.g., nurses, consultants, social workers) from using these notes to guide their decisions.

D. External discipline. When the wards are busy you will become tired and have difficulty concentrating, making mistakes more likely. A good data-tracking system will keep you disciplined so oversights do not become mistakes. A good system will prompt you to fill in every vital sign, laboratory value, and culture result each day. This process will make you more disciplined and thorough, even when you are tired.

III Components of a Data Card

The data card should focus on the important details that a consultant or other physician might need to know at a moment's notice. Extraneous details deprive the data card of clarity and obscure the important information. The place to provide all the details of the patient's care is the admission or progress notes in the chart. Figure 20-1 shows an example of a data card.

A. Identifying information. Note the patient's name, age, and race, as well as the medical record number and the patient's hospital room number.

B. Highlights from the history of present illness. For the most part, you should strive to memorize your patients' clinical story; this will keep you from depending on your card during oral presentations. The first box on the card is for recording highlights of the story to prompt your memory should you forget.

C. Past medical history. Focus on past medical history that may be pertinent to the current diagnostic and management decisions. Use your differential diagnosis to decide what might be relevant to your patient's care (see Chapter 10). Disorders such as congestive heart failure, diabetes mellitus, renal insufficiency, and drug allergies are examples of diagnoses worth noting. Diagnoses such as gout or allergic rhinitis may not need to be included.

D. List of medications. List all active medications. It is important to list the doses and, for antibiotics, the date they were started. This allows you to assess response to therapy and the completion date. Do not include PRN medications such as acetaminophen and diphenhydramine. When a medication is discontinued, scratch it off the list.

E. Social history. List past social history that may be useful in the patient's current management (e.g., social habits such as alcohol, nicotine, or narcotics that may result in withdrawal) or useful in discharge placement.

F. Physical examination

1. Vital signs are included on the other side of the card; this allows you to see trends in the vital signs from one day to the next.
2. The front box on the card is for noting only the abnormalities present on the initial physical examination. As abnormal findings

Name CAULFIELD, H	25	C	M	# 9842315

History
SOB began 4 d ago.
DOE at 1 block
Assoc. orthopnea and PND
No fevers; No cough.
Recently stopped medications
Noted rash 1 wk ago

Meds: (Admit)
1. Lasix 40 q d
2. Digoxin 0.25 q d
3. KCl 10mEq q d
4. Albuterol puffs BID
5. Septra DS q d

(NEW)
6. ~~6.~~
7. ~~7.~~
8. Penicillin 1.6 M units
9. Lasix 40 mg BID
10. Septra DS q d
11. Digoxin 0.25 q d
12. KCl 10 mEq q d
13.

PMH: CHF (EF% = 30% on 4/2003)
COPD
HIV (CD4 = 52 on 4/2003)

All: Ø ETOH: 4 becas /d Tob 10 pk/yrs Drugs Occ. cocaine

Physical Exam 110/54; 120; 37°; 22; 92%
Bilateral crackles 1/2 up ⓑ; PMT lateral & down.
IVP 10 cm; Ø murmurs;
2^+ Edema; Macular rash on hands & feet

Problem/Assessment

1) SoB	2) Rash	3) HIV	4)	5)
* ? CHF * ? COPD * ? PCP * ? Pneumonia *	? Drug Allergy ? Syphilis			

Day 1	Day 2	Day 3
☑ Echo ☑ Increase lasix ☑ Order CD4 Count ☑ Spirometry ☑ RPR	☐ Start Penicillin ☐ Urine electrolytes	
Day 4	**Day 5**	**Day 6**

Date	4/23	24	25				
BP	110/54	105/50	110/58				
Pulse	120	110	90				
T max	37°	36°	37^2				
RR	22	20	16				
Sat %	92%	94%	98%				
Weight	70	69	67				
HCT	30	32	33				
WBC	4.1	4.0	4.2				
PLT	156	170	164				
PT/INR	13/1.0	—	—				
PTT	32	—	—				
CD4	—	(26)					
Na+	131	133	135				
K+	4.1	4.0	4.0				
Cl–	100	102	100				
HCO3–	26	27	27				
BUN	12	13	13				
Creat	0.8	0.8	0.9				
Gluc	102	100	95				
Trop							
RPR	—	(1:640)					
AST	35						
ALT	32						
Alk. P	40						
T. bili	1.1						
UA	1.02/Ø cells						
Cultures	⊖	⊖					

Echo: 25 EF%
Normal values
No vegitations

Cath: ___ LAD
___ RCA
___ Circ

CT:

NL
Cephalization

FIGURE 20-1. Sample data card.

resolve, delete them from your card. If new ones appear, add them to the right on the card.

G. Problems. Keep a running problem list. There is limited space, so **focus on the solvency issues:** those issues that have to be solved before the patient can go home. As new problems occur, record them in the numbered squares. Below each square are asterisks; insert the differential diagnoses under each problem. Cross off each disease in the differential diagnosis as you exclude it.

H. Scut List. List the to-do list for each patient in the appropriate box.

I. Vital signs. Vital signs are *vital;* record the values each day. Trends are very important here, because a sudden drop from a high value, even if into normal range, can have grave consequences (e.g., a SBP of 180 to 120 mm Hg may result in a hypoperfusion stroke or suggest a sudden gastrointestinal bleed). This section of the card will keep you from missing these important trends.

J. Laboratory tests and other studies

1. **Enter laboratory values for each day.** You may want to customize this portion of the card to the service on which you are working, depending upon which laboratory values are routinely followed on that service.
2. **Check culture results.** Failing to check cultures is one of the biggest pitfalls to which a disorganized medical student or resident is subject. Include a row on the patient data card for cultures, and put an "X" in each box every day after you have checked to make sure the cultures remain negative. Do this until the laboratory reports the cultures as definitely negative.

HOT
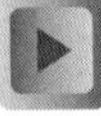
KEY

An initially "no growth to date" culture result may later be changed to a positive culture. Check all cultures each day until the laboratory designates the culture as negative.

III WARD TEAM ORGANIZATION: SCUT LIST

In addition to keeping track of your own patient's data on data cards, keep a separate 3 × 5 card for recording the to-do list (scut list) for other patients on your team's service (Figure 20-2).

A. Organize this list by tasks rather than by patients. This will allow you to group patients who require the same task. This will keep you from making multiple trips to the radiology reading room or the laboratory; once you are there you can ask for the results for all of the patients on your team.

B. As work or attending rounds progress, keep track of the scut tasks that still need to be completed for other patients on the team.

1. This will keep you involved with the management of other patients on the team, thus allowing you to step in and help other team members with the management of their patients.

Scut: 2/25/04

Radiology	Laboratory
☑ Roberts (9842356); CXR	☑ Roberts (9842356); Smear
☑ Meany (9923546); CXR	☑ Meany (9923546); UA
☑ Melville (9823114); CT	
☑ Dana (9914365); CT	

Med/Records	Social Work
☑ Walker (9965736)	☑ Sallinger (9928756); Nursing Home
☑ Owens (9984796)	☑ Orens (9998746); Home Health

FIGURE 20-2. Sample ward-team scut list.

2. Other opportunities, such as performing procedures and being in the operating room, will be offered to you once the team knows that you can handle more than just your assigned role. This will also enable you to trade tasks that you cannot perform for tasks that you can easily perform. (e.g., "I need some help putting in this central line. I can take care of the discharge summaries if that would free up some time for you to show me how to do the line.") Remember, each team member has greater effectiveness in some areas, and your goal is to capitalize on that effectiveness.

C. **Prioritize.** Once work rounds have ended, you may want to number the tasks in order of greatest importance (No. 1) to those of least importance (No. 6). Do the highest ranked tasks first.

D. **Meet with the team at the end of work rounds to divide up tasks.** Periodically through the day, compare your list to those of your interns. You can demonstrate what you have done to your interns, as well as avoid doing tasks they have already done.

IV Lists of Telephone Numbers for Hospital Staff

A. Make it a personal rule to look up a phone number only once. Once you look it up, record it on a card. This will require more time up-front, but it will save you time in the long run.

B. Keep a list of residents, attending physicians, consultants, and other healthcare staff such as ward nurses and respiratory therapists with whom you have come in contact. Note pager numbers next to each name, because this information is seldom published in phone books, and operators are reluctant to release it.

V Keeping Your Patient Data Cards

A. The best way to keep your data cards straight is by buying a small three ring binder (the shell of personal organizer) or an ordinary ring binder.

B. The same goals listed above can be accomplished by using 3 × 5 cards with an ordinary ring binder.

C. Personal digital assistants (PDA)

1. PDAs are useful for time management in setting monthly or weekly schedules. They are useful for keeping phone numbers and lists of information.
2. PDAs are less effective in the hour-to-hour schedule of the physician. They are not good for organizing patient data, because writing with pen and paper is still faster than writing with the palm board.
3. Use caution if you choose to use a PDA to organize patient data; they are frequently stolen on the wards.

PART III

Tier I Physical Examination

21. Examination Fundamentals

I INTRODUCTION There is no physician who has the time to do every possible examination maneuver on each patient. Even if there was time, this compulsiveness would be as silly as ordering every possible laboratory test for fear of missing something. **The Tier I/Tier II method will rescue you from these two competing forces (compulsiveness vs. efficiency)** by giving you a method for developing a concise yet thorough physical examination that is tailored to your patient.

II THE TIER I/TIER II METHOD: AN OVERVIEW All physical examination maneuvers fall into one of two categories:

A. **Tier I maneuvers:** those maneuvers that **should be done on every patient** in your practice.

B. **Tier II maneuvers**: those maneuvers that should only be done if:
   1. An abnormality is detected on the Tier I examination that needs further evaluation.
   2. The maneuver is useful in evaluating a diagnosis on the differential diagnosis constructed from the patient's history.

III TIER I PHYSICAL EXAMINATION MANEUVERS: SCREENING TESTS

A. The Tier I examination is a screening examination, looking for abnormalities that the patient may not have reported. **There is no set list for what examination maneuvers should be included in a perfect Tier I examination.** This book gives a few suggestions, but ultimately, you should compose your own Tier I examination based on what maneuvers you think make sense in screening for disease in your patients. Regardless of what examination maneuvers you choose to include in your Tier I roster, all of them should share the following:
   1. Like other screening tests, a Tier I physical examination maneuver should be **highly sensitive,** easily detecting disease if it is present. For example, listening for crackles in the lungs is a much more sensitive test for CHF than listening for an S_3 (even though

an S_3 is more specific). Listening for crackles is a good Tier I maneuver; listening for an S_3 is a good Tier II maneuver.

2. Tier I maneuvers should be **quick and easy to perform.** The Tier I examination should be performed on every patient you see, so choose tests that are time-efficient. Observing the patient's gait as she walks into the room is a quick Tier I assessment of neurologic function. Testing strength in each limb requires much more time; it is therefore a Tier II maneuver.
3. The Tier I examination should **focus on diseases that are prevalent** in your patient population. For example, routine breast examinations are a good Tier I examination maneuver because breast cancer is relatively common; palpating for a renal mass is not a good Tier I maneuver because renal cell cancer is uncommon.

B. Perform the same Tier I maneuvers on every patient. The repetition of the same method from patient to patient will make you efficient and proficient.

C. If an abnormality is found on a Tier I maneuver, other Tier II maneuvers should be performed to evaluate the abnormality.

IV Tier II Physical Examination Maneuvers: Answer a Question

Tier II maneuvers should have a **high specificity** for the diagnosis being considered. If the specific test is positive, the diagnosis being evaluated is confirmed. A patient found to have a murmur on Tier I examination, for example, should have additional Tier II maneuvers (e.g., hand grip, squatting) to evaluate which valve is involved (see Chapters 25 and 31).

V General Method of the Physical Examination

Osler noted two common features of all great physicians: good methods and thoroughness in application of these methods.

A. With the exception of the abdominal examination (see Chapter 26), the components of the physical examination always follow this order:

1. Observation
2. Palpation
3. Percussion
4. Auscultation
5. Contemplation

B. Religiously following this sequence will vastly improve your examination, because early parts of the examination (e.g., observation of a PMI) will improve the sensitivity of subsequent parts (i.e., where to palpate the PMI).

VI Observation

Obvious physical abnormalities may be missed unless you carefully observe the patient. Begin by looking at the patient and asking yourself, "Does anything appear abnormal?"

A. Ask the patient to undress during the admission examination. This allows you to observe all parts of the patient at least once. In so doing, you will never be surprised (and embarrassed) by finding an enormous decubitus ulcer on the buttocks of a patient admitted for fever of unknown cause after 3 days of inpatient evaluation.

B. Have the patient get out of bed and walk. This will reveal previously unseen abnormalities.

C. Always position yourself where you can observe the patient.

   1. When you auscultate the heart and lungs, stand at the patient's side so you can see her face. This allows you to see if the patient is following your breathing instructions and if there is pain or labored breathing (e.g., nasal flaring).

   2. When you palpate, watch the patient's face for signs of pain (e.g., grimacing during palpation of the abdomen).

D. Turn on the lights and open the window shade. Natural light sometimes reveals subtle findings that you may miss under fluorescent lighting (e.g., jaundice).

E. Train yourself to be observant even when not in the hospital. While you are sitting in a coffee house, standing in a grocery line, or watching a football game, look carefully at the people around you. Do you see abnormalities? This will also train you to be observant without being obvious.

F. Learn to interpret facial expressions and body language. Watch television sitcoms without the volume and try to figure out the dialogue or plot. Listen to the last 5 minutes to see if your interpretation is correct.

VII PALPATION

A. If you see something abnormal, use touch to characterize it. Use the "real-estate" rule of palpation:

   1. What is its location?

   2. How big is it?

   3. Is it raised or flat?

B. For small lesions, the fingertips are best. For larger findings (e.g., PMI), use the palm of your hand; the palm is more discriminating that the fingertips.

C. Once you have found what you wish to palpate, close your eyes. This maximizes sensory input from your fingers.

D. As you palpate a mass, note its consistency, firmness, mobility, and size.

E. Measure your hand and stop carrying a ruler. Use landmarks on your hand as measures of distance (e.g., 8 cm = across MCP joints; 6 cm = across PIP joints; 1 cm = fingernail).

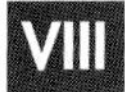

PERCUSSION Percussion is not an innate skill. It takes considerable practice to improve percussion skills.

A. **Practice percussing your own liver edge.** This will put your hands in a position that encourages good percussion technique.
   1. Place your left hand on your right upper abdominal quadrant with your fingers pointing to your right. Press down lightly with the DIP joint of your left middle finger to obtain a good seal. This seal is important; if the seal is slack, the energy from the percussion note is absorbed by the vibration of your left finger, and no sound will be liberated.
   2. Good percussion begins with extension and flexion of the wrist. By placing your left hand on your liver and percussing with the right hand, you will be forced to extend and flex the right wrist to generate a strong percussion note. Bend your right middle finger slightly at the PIP joint. Fold the 2nd, 4th, and 5th fingers into your hand. Maximally extend the wrist and then tap as the wrist is flexed. Aim for the DIP joint of your left middle finger.

B. **Practice, practice, practice.** You are not born with a neuron that connects the position sense of the right and left middle fingers. To percuss successfully, however, these two fingers must always know there the other's position is located. Ultimately, you should be able to percuss without watching your hands. (When you percuss your own liver, the left DIP is out of sight and forces the fingers to "find" each other.) You lose momentum in percussion if you have to aim the right finger to hit the left.

C. **Only percuss three notes at a time.** No sound is diagnostic alone; the merit of percussion is in comparing one percussed note to neighboring percussed sounds. To do this, you have to remember the last percussed notes in comparison to the currently percussed notes. You can reliably remember only the last three percussed notes for comparison to the next three notes.

D. **Do not stand too close to the patient's bed if you are percussing on that side of his body.** This will lock you into a cramped position in which it is hard to extend and flex the wrist. Take a step back so that your wrist has room to flex; remember, the percussion note comes from flexion of the wrist.

IX Auscultation

A. **Obtain a good seal.** Auscultation requires a tight seal between the stethoscope and the patient's skin. Even small friction between a mobile stethoscope and the skin or moving clothing can sound like a murmur.
   1. If you are auscultating the anterior chest of a seated patient (e.g., heart), stand to the patient's right side and place the stethoscope on the skin with your right hand (Figure 21-1) Place your left hand on the patient's back to stabilize him. This allows you to provide pressure with the stethoscope without pushing over the patient. For the reclining patient, the bed will stabilize him as you press.

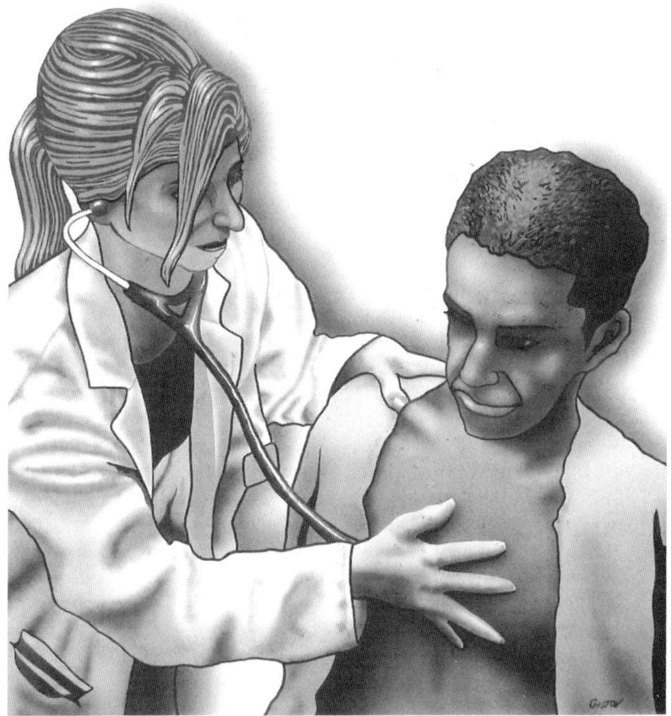

FIGURE 21-1. Cardiac auscultation.

2. Place the stethoscope in the palm of your hand and press hard. Allow your fingers to touch the patient's skin to stabilize the stethoscope.
3. **The bony chest.** If the patient has a bony chest, sound from the room will enter through the air space between your stethoscope and the ribs. To prevent this, you may want to place a 100-ml bag of saline on top of the chest, and press your stethoscope through the bag to the chest wall. This forms a barrier to outside noise.
4. **Hairy chest.** You must press very hard, because any hair moving under the stethoscope head will sound like a murmur.

B. Be in a good position. When auscultating the heart or lungs, always be in a position to watch the patient's face as he breathes.

C. Place the stethoscope correctly in your ears.

1. Use hard rubber tips. Floppy rubber tips can fold over on themselves, thereby obscuring the sound.

2. Open your mouth slightly. This opens the eustachian tubes, decreasing pressure in the middle ear, allowing your eardrum to vibrate more with each sound.
3. If it is still difficult to hear, move the metal Y-part of the stethoscope in front of your face (like a face mask of a football helmet). This better positions the earpieces in your ears.

D. **Close your eyes.** This optimizes the sense of hearing.

E. **Do not auscultate through clothing.** Clothing dampens sound.

F. **Make the room quiet.** Turn off the television, beeping monitors, and fans. If you are in a noisy environment (e.g., emergency department), repeat your examination when you get to a quieter floor.

G. **Use the diaphragm of your stethoscope** unless you are listening for the low-frequency sounds of an S_3, S_4, or the diastolic rumble of mitral stenosis. The diaphragm augments high-frequency sounds by extinguishing low-frequency sounds. If you use the bell of the stethoscope, *do not press hard;* this tenses the patient's skin, forming a new diaphragm over the bell.

H. **When listening to lung sounds, have the patient breathe in and out through the mouth.** Lung sounds come from airflow rate. The nose creates a resistance to expiratory flow, thereby diminishing expiratory lung sounds. Stand or sit to the side of the patient so that you can see that he is following your instructions. Place one hand on the anterior shoulder to stabilize his chest; this will allow you to put firm pressure on your stethoscope on the back of the chest (Figure 21-2).

I. **Take care of your stethoscope.** Alcohol wipes are fine for cleaning the head, but they will dry and crack the rubber tubes.

X CONTEMPLATION

Know what to expect for a given disease. The absence of an expected finding (e.g., no egophony in the setting of pneumonia) can often provide clues to the etiology of the disease.

XI IMPORTANT EXAMINATION TIPS

A. **Look for patients with known disease. Practice your physical examination on these patients.** If you learn of a patient on the ward who has echo-proven mitral stenosis, listen to that patient until you are certain that you can hear the murmur associated with mitral stenosis. If you have a patient with a known central venous pressure (as assessed by a subclavian catheter venous pressure monitor), look for the JVP at that height above the clavicle.

B. **See other students' patients.** Always ask your colleagues for permission to see their patients. This will allow you to maximize your physical examination experience without appearing competitive.

C. **Share your own physical findings with other students**. Your colleagues will ultimately care for as many patients as you do. The

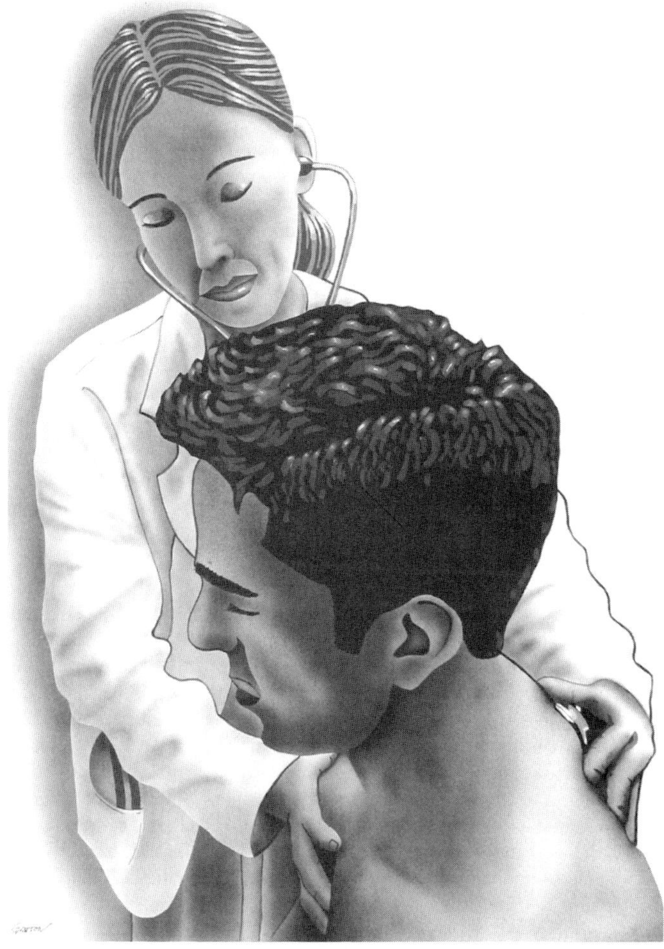

FIGURE 21-2. Pulmonary auscultation.

better they are, the better their patients will do. Once other students and physicians know you are truly interested in the physical examination, they will begin to alert you to physical examination abnormalities in their patients.

D. Know what normal is. To appreciate abnormalities, you must be familiar with the normal findings. The "range of normal" changes as patients age, so you must become adept at knowing what is normal at a given age by examining many normal patients. This range is available to you on the wards, but only if you invest the time to examine all of your patients fully.

E. **Report *your* examination findings, not a colleague's.** The only way to improve your examination technique is to present what you find. If your attending physician hears something different, he will correct you. This will allow you to refine your examination.

F. **Do not underestimate the social power of the physical examination.** Patients crave physician interaction and **they expect to be examined.** Even if the examination is not diagnostic, it contributes to role congruence (i.e., doing what a patient expects a physician to do) and thereby facilitates trust. Routinely performing a physical examination also ensures that you come to the bedside each day. You never know what you might find (e.g., a bag of salty chips hidden under the blanket of a patient with refractory hypertension). You will also be more likely to notice a serious event at an early stage.

XII The Most Important Examination Tip

Think about what you expect to find before you do the examination. Physical findings do not just present themselves; you must have an idea of what you are looking for in order to find it ("seek and ye shall find"). The following tips will help:

A. **Use your differential diagnosis to guide you.** Before you begin your examination, think about what physical findings are associated with each diagnosis you are considering.

B. **Know how to perform the maneuver properly.** There are many ways to perform maneuvers. The chapters in Sections 3 and 4 describe ways to increase the sensitivity of your examination.

C. **Know what the sensory input smells/sounds/tastes/feels like.**

1. Each sound has a frequency that your ears must be trained to detect (e.g., aortic insufficiency murmurs have a much higher frequency than the S_1 and S_2 heart sounds). It is worth buying a heart-sound or lung-sound CD/tape to familiarize yourself with the frequencies that go with different abnormalities. Chapters 24 and 25 have some additional tips on becoming familiar with these sounds.
2. Each organ has a texture your fingers must recognize. The best way to learn these sensory inputs is to examine as many patients as possible in the company of a physician who knows what she is feeling for.

HOT

KEY

To learn the most from physical findings rounds, be honest about what you do and do not hear, feel, or see. The expert clinician can then help you appreciate the finding.

22. Vital Signs

I **Introduction** The brain needs oxygen to survive. The vital signs are so named because they assess the vital delivery of oxygen to the brain. When oxygen delivery to the brain is inadequate, vital signs provide the essential information to determine the cause. As you read this chapter, use Equations 3 through 7 in Appendix A to help you organize your thoughts. **Vital signs are always a Tier I examination.**

II **General Appearance** The most important "vital sign" is the appearance of the patient. **Learning to identify patients who look sick is the most important lesson to be learned in medical school and internship**. The only way to learn this is to see a variety of patients, both sick and not sick. When in doubt, ask your resident, "Does this patient look sick?" Although it seems like an easy lesson, it is the most difficult to master in the course of an internship. Learning it now will put you well ahead of the game.

III **Heart Rate and Pulse** Learn to multitask. While you are taking the history, place your fingers on the patient's wrist to obtain the pulse. Place your first two fingers parallel to the patient's flexor tendons. Let your fingers slide laterally into the groove between the tendons and the head of the radius. Press lightly; too much pressure extinguishes the pulse, too little will not detect it. The thumb is not sufficiently sensitive to detect the pulse. Feel the pulse for at least 30 seconds. This is enough time to assess the heart rate and discern the quality of the pulse (strength and regularity).

A. **Heart rate.** Interpret the heart rate in the context of the patient's condition. Expect a higher heart rate in the following conditions:

1. **Fever.** Fever increases the metabolic needs of the tissues. To match oxygen delivery to these metabolic needs, the heart rate increases (Appendix A, Equations 3 and 7). Each Fahrenheit degree of temperature is expected to increase the heart rate by as much as 5 beats per minute.
2. **Hypoxemia.** Hypoxemia reduces the oxygen saturation, which decreases the delivery of oxygen to the tissues. To compensate, the heart rate increases to boost cardiac output (Appendix A, Equation 3).
3. **Cardiac dysfunction.** The heart rate increases to compensate for decreased stroke volume due to failing contractility (Appendix A, Equations 4 and 5).

4. **Dehydration or hemorrhage.** The heart rate increases to compensate for a decline in stroke volume due to inadequate preload (Appendix A, Equations 4 and 5).

B. **Heart rhythm.** The pulse should be regular and consistent. Occasional irregular beats suggest premature contractions (atrial or ventricular); consistently irregular beats suggest atrial fibrillation.

C. **Strength of the pulse.** The strength of the pulse corresponds to the pressure generated in a vessel and is an indirect measure of stroke volume (Table 22-1).

TABLE 22-1. Using the Pulse Strength to Assess Stroke Volume.

Pulse Findings	Interpretation
Fast heart rate with a weak pulse	The stroke volume is weak due to low preload (i.e., dehydration). The heart rate is compensating to maintain cardiac output (Equation 4). The stroke volume is weak due to poor contractility (i.e., a myocardial infarction). The heart rate is compensating to maintain cardiac output (Equation 4). An arrhythmia is increasing the heart rate so fast that the ventricle does not have time to fill completely. Effectively, the preload is too low, and this decreases the stroke volume, causing a weak pulse.
Fast heart rate with strong pulse	The strong pulse tells you that the fast heart rate is not due to inadequate cardiac output. The most likely causes are anxiety, fever, anemia, or stimulants.
Slow or normal heart rate with weak pulse	The weak pulse suggests inadequate cardiac output. The heart is unable to increase its rate to maintain cardiac output. Causes include a bradycardic arrhythmia (heart block) or medication overdoses (beta blockers, calcium channel blockers).
Slow heart rate with a strong pulse	The patient has a healthy heart. Despite the low heart rate, his cardiac contractility and/or preload is able to sustain a normal cardiac output.

D. Bounding pulse. The pulse has two components: distention of the vessel wall (part 1: what you feel) and relaxation of the vessel wall (part 2: what you do not feel). A bounding pulse is indicative of a wide pulse pressure: that is, high systolic blood pressure (part 1) and low diastolic blood pressure (part 2). The pulse pressure is the SBP minus the DBP. A **wide pulse pressure** suggests one of several conditions:

1. **Aortic insufficiency.** The aortic valve does not close during diastole; some of the diastolic volume regurgitates into the left ventricle, thereby decreasing the diastolic pressure in the arteries. This extra volume to the left ventricle increases left ventricular preload and thus increases systolic stroke volume (i.e., the systolic pressure increases with each contraction).
2. **Sepsis.** Sepsis induces peripheral vasodilation; a greater percentage of arterial volume is transferred to venous volume. The DBP decreases due to decreased systemic vascular resistance; the SBP increases due to the increased venous volume (preload).
3. **Anemia.** The decline in hemoglobin decreases delivery of oxygen. To compensate, heart rate and contractility increase to optimize cardiac output (Appendix A; Equation 3). This increases the SBP. The peripheral vessels dilate to help the cells extract more oxygen; this decreases the DBP.
4. **Thyrotoxicosis.** Thyroid hormone can be considered a "spark plug" for each cell in the body; when levels of thyroid hormone are high, the cells increase their metabolic rate. This requires more oxygen delivery to meet the increased metabolic demands of the cells (Appendix A, Equation 7). To compensate, heart rate and contractility increase to optimize cardiac output (Appendix A, Equation 3). This increases the SBP. The peripheral vessels dilate to help the cells extract more oxygen; this decreases the DBP.

IV BLOOD PRESSURE

The blood pressure cuff estimates the pressure inside a vessel by measuring how much external pressure is required to occlude the artery.

A. Physiology. Understanding the physiology involved will prevent potential pitfalls.

1. The artery is a hollow tube that remains open when the pressure inside the artery is greater than the pressure outside the artery (Figure 22-1A). The inside pressure is the perfusion pressure to the tissues.
2. Hearing sound over the artery depends on turbulence. Turbulence is increased when blood **flow is increased** or the vessel **area is decreased.**
   a. When blood flow through an artery is unimpeded, the blood makes no sound, because there is no turbulence (Figure 22-1A).

$$\textbf{Sound} = \textbf{turbulence} = \frac{\textbf{Flow}}{\textbf{Area}}$$

A

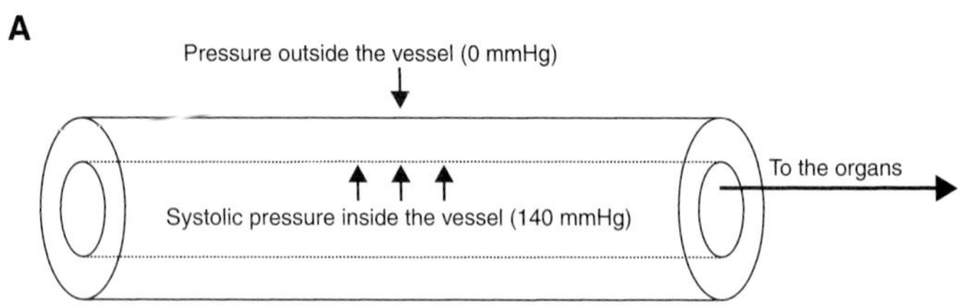

B

Pressure outside the vessel (150 mmHg)

To the organs

C

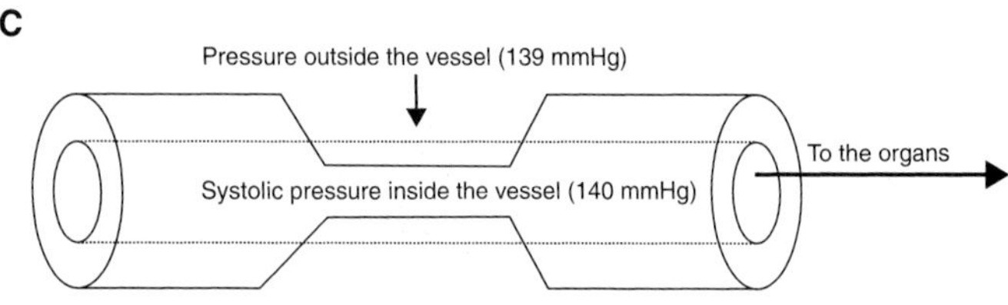

FIGURE 22-1. The physiology underlying the blood pressure assessment. **A, The blood pressure cuff is applied but not inflated.** Flow through the artery is maximal, but the area inside the vessel is large. Thus, there is no turbulence, and thus no sound is heard. **B, The blood pressure cuff maximally inflated.** The inside area of the artery is very low due to outside pressure of the cuff. However, there is also no flow through the artery. Thus, there is no turbulence, and thus no sound is heard. **C, The blood pressure cuff is gradually deflated.** At the point where the pressure inside the artery overcomes the pressure exerted from the cuff, flow resumes. The area inside the artery is decreased by the pressure of the cuff, and the combination of increased flow and decreased area creates turbulence. This results in the first sound that signifies the **systolic blood pressure**. The sound will persist until the area inside the vessel re-expands (as the cuff pressure is released). The point at which the sound goes away signifies the **diastolic blood pressure (see A).**

b. When blood flow through an artery is completely occluded, which occurs when the blood pressure cuff is inflated over the pressure inside the artery, there is no flow because the artery is occluded. Therefore, there is no turbulence, and no sound is heard (Figure 22-1B).

3. As the pressure is decreased, flow resumes, but the cross-sectional area of the vessel is still less than normal. Flow with decreased area creates turbulence, and this creates sound. The pressure at which sound is first heard is the SBP (Figure 22-1C).

4. When the pressure is further decreased so that the pressure in the artery completely overcomes the external pressure, the cross-sectional area of the artery returns to normal. Although flow is at a maximum, the area is maximal again, and there is no turbulence to create sound. The pressure at which sound ceases is the exact point at which the inside vessel pressure balances the outside cuff pressure. The cuff pressure at this point is the DBP.

B. Method

1. Attach the blood pressure cuff to the proximal arm and feel the radial pulse. Sit where you can see the blood pressure dial. Place the stethoscope over the brachial artery in the antecubital space. It may also be useful to drape the patient's arm over yours, so that you can balance holding the stethoscope head with one hand while pumping up the blood pressure bulb with the other (Figure 22-2).

2. Inflate the cuff until you feel no radial pulse. The absence of the pulse tells you that the cuff pressure is well above the artery pressure. Listen with your stethoscope; you should hear no sound at this point, because there is no flow to induce turbulence (Figure 22-1B).

3. Deflate the blood pressure cuff slowly. At some point, the pressure in the artery will exceed the pressure produced by the cuff. In this example, the pressure in the artery is 140 mm Hg; flow will begin to return when the pressure produced by the cuff drops below 139 mm Hg. This will cause turbulence and thus sound (Figure 22-1C). The sounds correspond to each heart beat (each heart beat raises the intra-arterial systolic pressure). **The pressure at which you first hear heart sounds is the systolic blood pressure (SBP).**

4. Continue to deflate the blood pressure cuff until the sounds stop. At this point, the intra-arterial pressure completely exceeds the pressure produced by the cuff. Although there is flow, the larger cross-sectional area in the artery reduces turbulence so that there is no sound. **This is the diastolic blood pressure (DBP).**

C. Pitfalls

1. Large arm. A small cuff on a large arm may lead to a falsely elevated blood pressure. The small cuff has less surface area, so it must exert greater than normal pressure to compress the artery

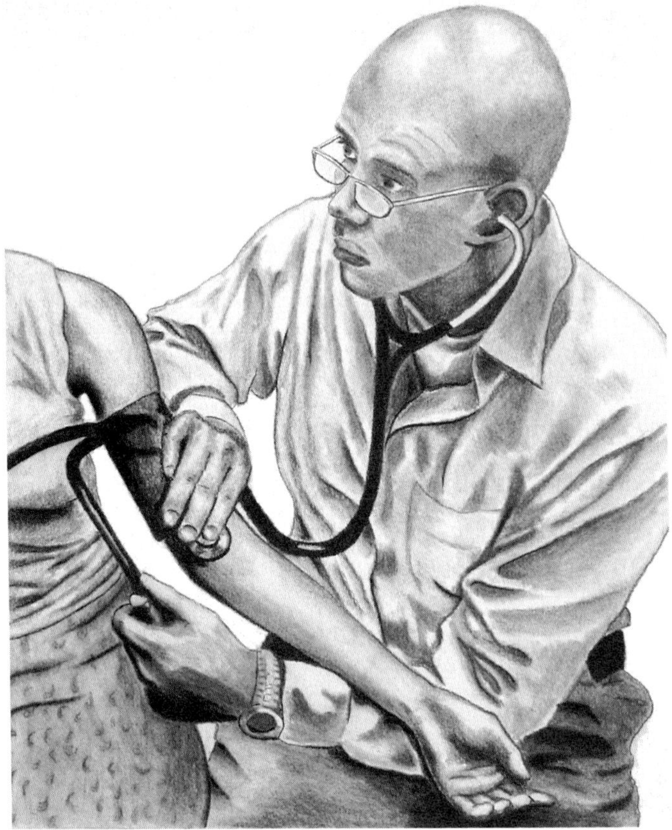

FIGURE 22-2. The ideal position for taking the blood pressure.

within the thick arm. This will give you a falsely elevated estimate of the pressure required to overcome the arterial pressure. When in doubt, always use a large cuff, especially if the patient's arm is large. There are no published accounts of false readings associated with using a large cuff.

2. **Ausculatory gap.** This results from large amounts of venous blood trapped in the arm distal to the blood pressure cuff. This may occur in three circumstances: following many failed attempts at taking the blood pressure, when the cuff has been placed on an arm in a dependent position, or when the cuff has been inflated very slowly on an arm with large amounts of adipose tissue. The spurious reading occurs as follows:

a. Systolic blood pressure will be accurately assessed as the cuff is deflated to below the systolic pressure within the artery (see IV B 3 above).

b. At some point in the middle of testing, the large venous pressure from the trapped blood distal to the cuff exerts a back-pressure on the arterial pressure. The back-pressure from the trapped venous blood distends the arteries from below, increasing the cross-sectional area of the artery. This eliminates turbulence and thus the systolic sounds will cease. You will be fooled into thinking the diastolic pressure has been reached (see IV B 4 above). However, continued reduction of the cuff pressure releases the venous blood that has been trapped by the cuff. Now the artery is less distended from below, and the cuff pressure again pinches on the artery. Systolic sounds resume, and continue until the true DBP is reached (Figure 22-3).

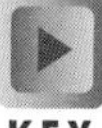

To avoid finding the ausculatory gap, always decrease the cuff pressure to zero before determining the DBP.

3. Vessel wall stiffness. If an artery is very stiff (due to calcifications, atherosclerosis, or fibrosis), its occlusion will require increased pressure. Imagine inflating a blood pressure cuff over a lead pipe. The stiffness of the pipe wall, not the pressure in the pipe, opposes the pressure produced by the blood pressure cuff. The blood pressure inside the artery will appear to be higher than it actually is.

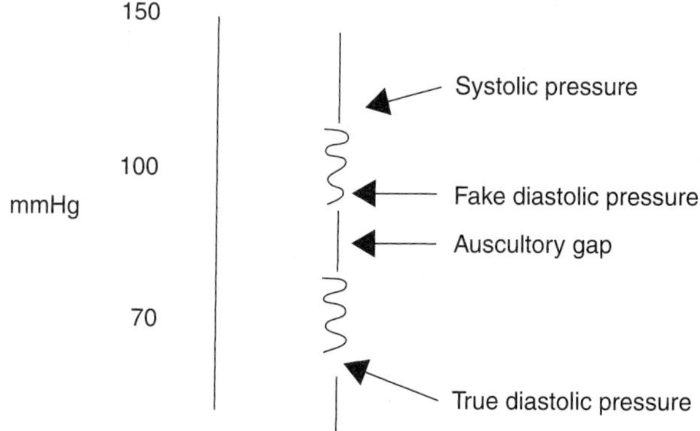

FIGURE 22-3. Ausculatory gap.

a. The method described in IV B will keep you from being fooled by this phenomenon (Osler phenomenon).

b. If you still feel the radial artery (a hard cord) after completely inflating the blood pressure cuff, the vessel wall is keeping the artery in an open position (like a lead pipe) even without blood pressure inside the artery. In this situation, measure the blood pressure in another limb, or interpret the results with caution.

D. Differences in blood pressure between the extremities. Blood pressure may vary between the two arms. Because the driving force behind the blood pressure is the heart, the blood pressure should be equal in all extremities. A difference of >10 mm Hg between the two arms suggests that there is an obstruction in one of the arms (the one with the smaller blood pressure).

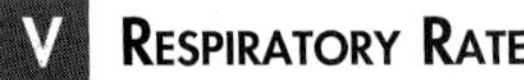

V Respiratory Rate

A. Method. The patient will change his breathing rate if he knows that you are measuring the respiratory rate. To avoid this, assess the respiratory rate while you are measuring the pulse rate. Spend a total of 1 minute taking the pulse: 30 seconds measuring the heart rate and 30 seconds pretending to measure the heart rate but actually measuring the respiratory rate.

HOT
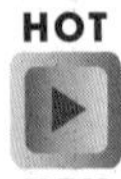
KEY

It is also useful to estimate the patient's tidal volume. The easiest way is to talk with him. The speech of patients with a small tidal volume is broken into segments (as if he had just hiked up a flight of stairs).

B. Signs of respiratory distress

1. **Accessory muscle movement.** The primary muscles of respiration are the intercostals and the diaphragm. The neck muscles are accessory sources for expansion of the chest. Use of these accessory muscles suggests that the primary muscles are fatigued or nonfunctional (see Chapter 30).
2. **Paradoxical breathing.** The abdomen should rise with inspiration. If the abdomen falls with inspiration, the diaphragm is tiring. This is a sign that the patient may soon stop breathing and require intubation.
3. **Chest wall trauma.** Every part of the chest should expand. If a part of the chest retracts while the remainder expands, this indicates a flail chest (broken ribs) or splinting. When a patient experiences pain in a focal area (above *or* below the diaphragm), she may suppress movement of the chest in that area to reduce the pain (see Chapter 24).
4. **Breathing pattern.** The respiration pattern should be even. Note the following patterns:

a. **Cheynes-Stokes breathing.** Deep, rapid breaths are followed by the absence of breathing, which is followed by a crescendo return of the deep rapid breaths. This pattern suggests congestive heart failure, because the failing heart cannot pump enough blood to the brain. The brain becomes acidotic due to inadequate oxygenation, and this stimulates the lungs to breath rapidly to remove the excess carbon dioxide in the brain. The deep breathing suddenly increases oxygen delivery to the brain and causes a decline in carbon dioxide. This shuts off the stimulus for rapid breathing. The cycle then repeats.
b. **Biot breathing.** Breaths occur very rapidly and have equal intensity. This is usually due to a midbrain infarction or bleed.
c. **Apneustic breathing.** Breaths are irregular and gasping. This is a sign of impending brain death.
d. **Kussmaul respirations.** Breaths are deep and fast. This usually indicates metabolic acidosis as the patient is trying to expel carbon dioxide to normalize the pH. It may also indicate hypoxemia. In this case, the body will attempt to increase the oxygen concentration in the alveoli by decreasing CO_2 from the alveoli (Appendix A, Equations 1 and 8).
e. **Panting.** Breaths are fast and shallow and indicate either hypoxemia or pain. This may also be seen in obstructive airway disease, when the chest is so full of trapped air that it cannot accommodate additional inspiratory volume.

VI TEMPERATURE

A. There are several methods of assessing the temperature. Listed in order from most to least reliable: rectal, tympanic, oral, and axillary. Oral temperatures may be falsely elevated following consumption of a hot beverage (e.g., coffee, tea), or falsely low if the patient is rapidly breathing through the mouth. As a rule, axillary temperatures are 0.5°F lower than the actual core body temperature.

B. The normal temperature range is from 36.8° to 37.4°C. The temperature increases during the late evening, as cortisol levels drop (9 PM to 1 AM), and decreases in the early morning, as cortisol levels rise.

HOT
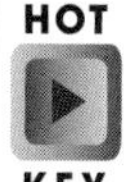
KEY

The regular increase in evening temperature may cause many patients with common illness to have **evening sweats (9:00 PM to 1:00 AM)**. These do not have the same significance as **night sweats (1:00 AM to 6:00 AM)**, which suggest tuberculosis or malignancy.

C. **Hypothermia** (<36°C). Infection may lead to low temperature; in fact, low temperature is as much an indicator of infection as high temperature. Other causes of low temperature include hypothyroidism and environmental exposure.

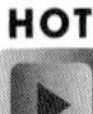

Hypothermia is sepsis until proven otherwise.

D. **Hyperthermia (>38°C).** Fever is usually due to infection, rheumatological disorders, malignancy, drug reaction (allergy), or heat stroke. When interpreting the temperature, use caution with the elderly and with immunosuppressed patients; both may be unable to mount a fever in response to infection. In all patients, be sure they have not recently taken acetaminophen, aspirin, ibuprofen, or cold or pain medications that contain these drugs, because this dampens the temperature response.

E. **Extremely high temperatures.** Temperatures greater than 40°C (105°F) (hyperpyrexia) generally indicate damage to the thermoregulatory apparatus (i.e., a thalamic stroke), or heat stroke due to exposure or anticholinergic poisoning.

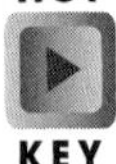

Sound smart in your presentation. Do not say, "The patient does not have a temperature." Everyone has a temperature. You mean, "The patient does not have a *fever*."

23. The Tier I Head and Neck Examination

I THE BIG PICTURE The function of the head and neck is to interact with the environment. Because the primary function is sensory, the conscious patient is usually able to direct the head and neck examination based on symptoms. If the patient has no complaints of pain or sensory deficits, the Tier I head and neck examination may be very brief (Table 23-1). However, if the patient cannot give a good history, a complete Tier II examination should be performed (see Chapter 29).

II STEP 1: EXCLUDE TRAUMA TO THE HEAD AND SPINE A detailed Tier II examination should be performed if the patient complains of head trauma or headache (see Chapter 29), or if there is ecchymosis or tenderness present.

III STEP 2: EXCLUDE MENINGISMUS Ask the patient to touch his chin to his chest. The inability to do so is a sign of inflammation of the meninges (meningitis) due to bacteria, viruses, or a drug reaction. Forward flexion of the head (but not lateral movement of the head) stretches the meninges and prevents the patient from touching his chin to his chest.

IV STEP 3: EXCLUDE FACIAL RASHES AND MALIGNANCIES The face and ears are the most sun-exposed areas of the body. For this reason, skin cancer and photosensitivity rashes are most common on the face. Look for anything that does not look like your face.

A. Skin cancers. Many skin lesions (especially actinic keratosis) will be felt before they are seen. Look and feel carefully over sun-exposed areas. A biopsy should be performed early on suspicious lesions (Table 23-2).

B. Photosensitivity rashes occur when an antigen (lupus antibodies, porphyrins, drugs) deposits in the skin. When exposed to ultraviolet light, the antigen splits oxygen to oxygen free-radicals, damaging the skin.

   1. Lupus. The lupus antibody (ANA) and the nuclear antigen complexes (Ab-Ag) deposit in the skin. When exposed to UV light, oxygen free radicals are formed, which cause the wolflike (*lupus* (L.) = wolf) rash on the cheeks and bridge of the nose (e.g., a butterfly rash).

TABLE 23-1. The Tier I Head and Neck Examination.

Step	Action
Step 1: Examine the Scalp and Spine	Palpate the neck and scalp for tenderness. Look for signs of head trauma.
Step 2: Examine the Eyes	Extraocular muscles Nystagmus Proptosis Conjunctiva, sclera, and cornea
Step 3: Look for Pupil Function	Pupil response to light Pupil size and shape
Step 4: Look in the Pharynx	Cracked teeth Buccal discolorations or lesions Tongue lesions Ulcers Pharyngeal symmetry Gum swelling/gingivitis Pharyngeal infections/ ulcers
Step 5: Examine the Neck	Lymphadenopathy Thyroid size and nodules Meningismus

TABLE 23-2. Skin Diseases Affecting the Face.

Disease	Characteristic Findings
Actinic keratosis	Raised lesions with a clear flaky appearance. These premalignant lesions must be frozen off (liquid nitrogen) if found.
Basal cell cancer	Raised circular lesions with pearly, smooth borders
Squamous cell cancer	Raised lesions with heaped boarders and flaky overlying skin
Melanoma	Lesions with one or more of the **A,B,C,D criteria: a**symmetric **b**orders, irregular or changing **c**olor, change in **d**iameter
Lupus, rosacea, drug reaction	Photosensitivity rash involving the cheeks and bridge of the nose

2. Rosacea (i.e., "adult acne") is similar in appearance to the rash of lupus, but none of the other criteria for lupus are present (Chapter 33). It should be treated promptly (with metronidazole cream) because ocular complications can result if it progresses.
3. Porphyria is similar in appearance and physiology to lupus, except it is the porphyrins (instead of the lupus Ab-Ag complexes) that induce the skin damage when exposed to UV light.
4. Drug reactions.

V STEP 4: EXAMINE THE EXTRAOCULAR MUSCLES

As you take the patient's history, watch how she tracks your movements with her eyes. This method will miss subtle extraocular muscle palsies, but it is sufficient for a Tier I screening examination. Look especially for:

A. **Nystagmus** is rhythmic, jerking movement of the eyes due to vestibular disease or impairment of the extraocular muscles. Two beats of nystagmus are normal; more than two beats require a detailed Tier II examination to discover the cause (see Chapter 29).

B. **Proptosis** is forward displacement of the eye. Ask the patient to look at you normally (i.e., not with the eyes wide open). Proptosis is present if a rim of white sclera is apparent superior to the patient's iris. It most often occurs in Graves' disease as the result of swelling of the extraocular muscles induced by autoantibodies. Other causes include retro-orbital tumors and fungal infections.

C. **Amblyopia** is a lazy eye that is "out of synch" with the opposite eye. Affected patients do not complain of double vision, because the brain eliminates sensory reception from the "lazy eye" during the patient's childhood development.

D. **Disconjugate gaze** is one eye that does not track with the other due to a paralyzed extraocular muscle or a lesion of the medial longitudinal fasciculus within the brainstem. An impaired extraocular muscle is usually neurologic in origin (Chapter 34), but may also be due to entrapment of the muscle from trauma to the face. In both conditions, the patient will complain of double vision, because sensory input to both eyes is still preserved due to the acute nature of the abnormality (unlike amblyopia, which will have been present since childhood).

VI STEP 5: OBSERVE THE SCLERA, CONJUNCTIVA, AND CORNEA

A. **Sclera** ("white of the eye")
1. Yellow (icteric) sclera suggests that bilirubin has been deposited in the scleral membrane. Look only at the sclera superior or inferior to the iris when looking for jaundice; darkening of the sclera on the medial and lateral sides of the iris can be due to natural

oxidization due to exposure to air, causing a brown, ruddy appearance. Overconsumption of carrots can induce a yellow sclera, overconsumption of tomatoes can induce a red sclera, and overconsumption of both can induce an orange sclera. Make sure you evaluate patients under natural light (e.g., near a window), because florescent lights mask a yellow color.

2. **Blue sclera**. If the scleral membrane breaks down, some of the underlying choroid may be revealed, giving the sclera a blue color. This can occur in congenital collagen disorders or in longstanding rheumatoid arthritis.
3. **Red sclera.** Within the conjunctiva (the transparent membrane overlying the sclera) are small blood vessels. If one of these vessels ruptures (following trauma, vigorous coughing, laughing, or vomiting), blood will collect between the conjunctiva and the sclera, creating a *solid* red appearance. This is quite dramatic in appearance, but harmless.

> **HOT KEY** The physical examination can predict the serum bilirubin concentration. Icteric sclera ("**two** eyes") is a bilirubin of ≥**2** mg/dl; icteric sublingual membrane ("**fifth** nerve") is a bilirubin of ≥**5** mg/dl; and icteric tympanic membranes ("**ten**-panic membrane") is a bilirubin of ≥**10** mg/dl. Because hemolytic anemia alone rarely elevates the bilirubin above 3 mg/dl, an icteric sublingual membrane indicates that hepatic or biliary disease is present.

B. **Conjunctiva.** The conjunctiva is composed of two parts: one that lines the inside of the eyelid and one that extends to cover the sclera to the border of the cornea.

1. Eyelid (palpebral) conjunctiva. Grasp the lower eyelid and pull outward. Look just inside of the eyelid. The capillaries are uncovered here, allowing you to see how much hemoglobin is in the vessels. The darker the conjunctiva, the higher the hemoglobin concentration. The color should be red to pink.

> **HOT KEY** The physical examination can predict the hematocrit. A red conjunctiva is a hematocrit >35%; a pink conjunctiva is a hematocrit of 25% to 35%; and a white conjunctiva is a hematocrit of <25%.

2. Scleral conjunctiva. This transparent membrane overlies the eye and is visible only when there is inflammation of the vessels within the membrane (viral conjunctivitis, exposure to the elements, etc.). Conjunctivitis is dilation of these vessels in response to inflammation. Nonvasculitic conjunctivitis will always spare the rim of sclera around the cornea (the limbus), because the conjunctival vessels stop just shy of the cornea. Vasculitis, as

might be seen with lupus and seronegative spondyloarthropathies, will involve both the vessels overlying the sclera and the rim surrounding the cornea (because there is also inflammation in the anterior chamber of the eye underlying the cornea).

3. Conjunctival edema (chemosis). The potential space between the conjunctiva and the sclera can fill with fluid when the venous pressure is elevated (e.g., due to the high intrathoracic pressure of mechanical ventilation opposing venous drainage from the head). Although dramatic in appearance, this eventually abates; no treatment is required other than to keep the eyelids taped shut to protect the cornea from abrasions due to the inability to blink.

C. **Cornea.** This is the tough avascular membrane over the anterior chamber of the eye. Damage to the cornea always induces pain, and the patient with a corneal abrasion will note the sensation of a foreign body within the eye, even if it is no longer there. See Chapter 29 for the Tier II examination of the cornea.

HOT
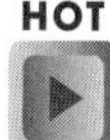
KEY

All bacterial infections of the eye will produce pus, but when gonorrhea involves the eyes, pus flows from the eye like a fountain.

VII Step 6: Pupil Function

A. **Pupillary response to light**

1. The **light reflex** has three components (Figure 23-1):

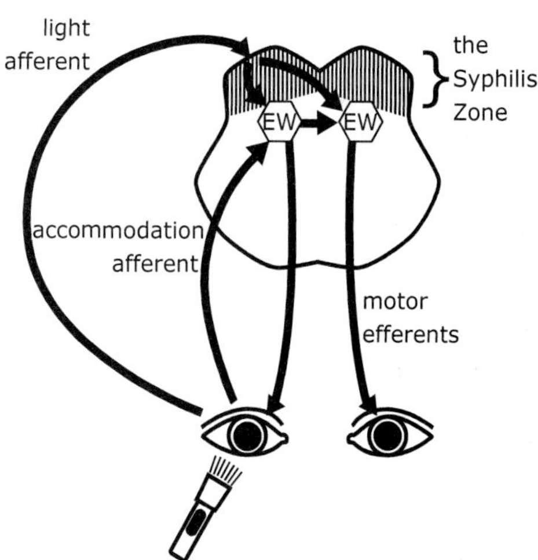

FIGURE 23-1. Light and accommodation reflex arcs.

   a. Sensory component (retina)
   b. Two sensory arcs (first: optic nerve to the dorsal brainstem; second: dorsal brainstem to the Edinger-Westphal nucleus)
   c. Motor component (Edinger-Westphal nucleus to the pupillary constrictor muscle)

2. Method. (Figure 23-2)
   a. Place the palm of your right hand on the patient's forehead (with your thumb pointing down). With your thumb, lift the patient's left upper eyelid. With your index finger, lift the patient's right eyelid (not shown in Figure 23-2). This will keep him from blinking.
   b. Shine a pen light into the left eye. The left pupil should constrict if the sensory and motor arcs to the left eye are intact. If the brainstem and right motor component are intact, the right pupil should also constrict (Figure 23-3).
   c. It will be difficult to see the right pupil, however, because your light is focused on the left eye. To see the right pupil, quickly swing the light to the right eye.
      (1) If the sensory and motor tracks to the right eye are normal, this pupil should already be constricted (because it was

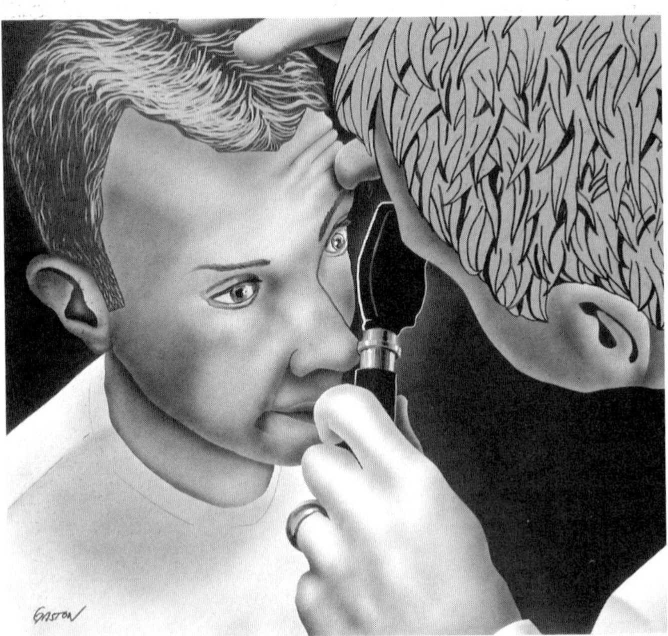

FIGURE 23-2. Examining the pupils.

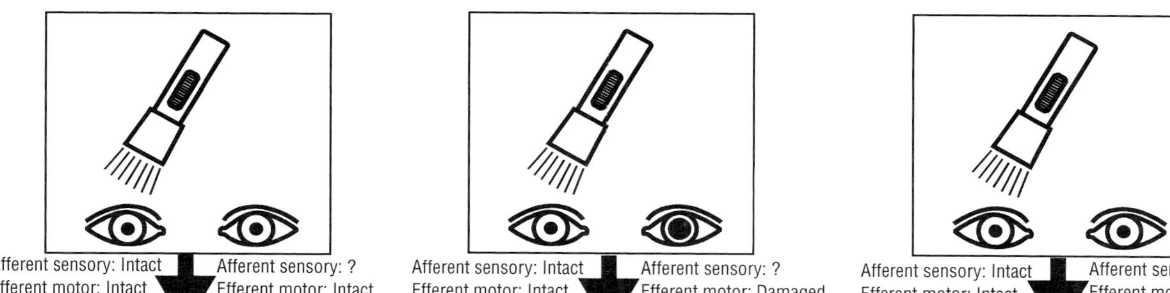

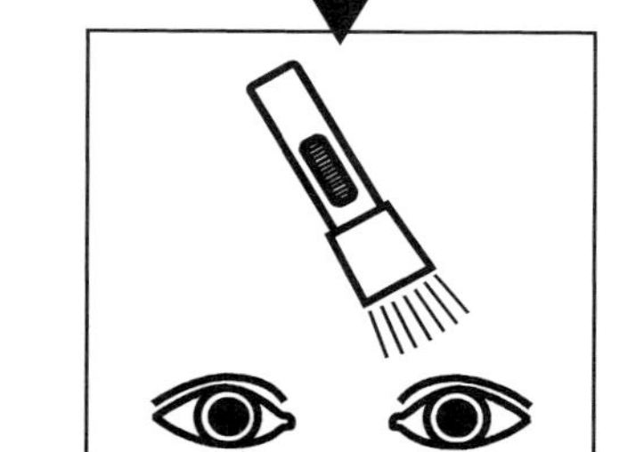

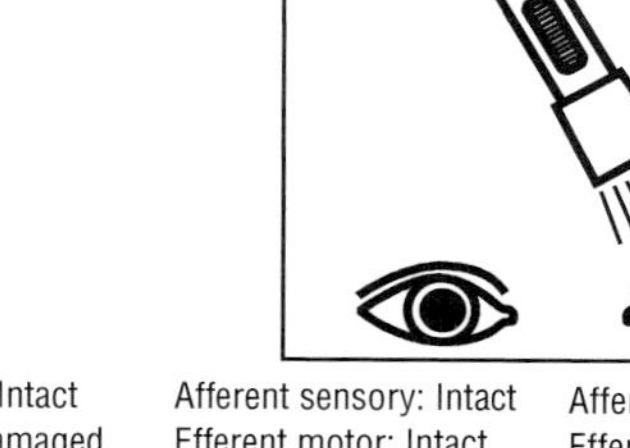
Afferent sensory: Intact
Efferent motor: Intact
Afferent sensory: ?
Efferent motor: Intact
Afferent sensory: Intact
Efferent motor: Intact
Afferent sensory: Intact
Efferent motor: Intact
A
Afferent sensory: Intact
Efferent motor: Intact
Afferent sensory: ?
Efferent motor: Damaged
Afferent sensory: Intact
Efferent motor: Intact
Afferent sensory: Intact
Efferent motor: Damaged
B
Afferent sensory: Intact
Efferent motor: Intact
Afferent sensory: ?
Efferent motor: Intact
Afferent sensory: Intact
Efferent motor: Intact
Afferent sensory: Damaged
Efferent motor: Intact
C

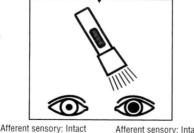

FIGURE 23-3. Normal and abnormal pupils.

receiving motor input from the brainstem when sensory input from the left eye was stimulated by shining the light in the left eye). The right pupil should stay constricted (Figure 23-3 A).

(2) If the right pupil is dilated and stays dilated when you swing the light, you know the motor arc to the right eye is damaged: it does not constrict to sensory input from either eye (Figure 23-3 B).

(3) If the right pupil suddenly dilates, you know that it has been previously constricted due to light into the left eye (i.e., the motor component to the right eye is intact). (Figure 23-3 C). The dilation is due to a damaged sensory arc from the right eye.

(4) If the right pupil constricts when you swing the light to it, you know the right eye's sensory and motor components are intact, but that the brainstem connection has been damaged (i.e., the right eye was not receiving sensory input from the light in the left eye).

3. Pupillary response to accommodation is a Tier II maneuver and should only be done if there is an abnormal papillary response to light. Hold your index finger about 2 feet away from the patient; ask the patient to stare at your finger. Move your finger toward the patient's nose. His or her pupils should constrict to permit focusing on the near object. This reflex has one sensory arc (retina directly to Edinger-Westphal nuclei) and one motor arc (Edinger-Westphal nuclei to eyes). Because this reflex does not involve the dorsal brainstem, it is spared in diseases that damage the dorsal brainstem. Preservation of the accommodation reflex with loss of the light reflex is known as the Argyll Robinson pupil. It is diagnostic of a dorsal brainstem disorder, namely syphilis (see Figure 23-1).

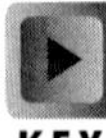

HOT KEY

If the patient can see light, he or she has enough sensory input to constrict the eye. Cataracts are not a cause of sensory impairment preventing papillary constriction.

B. Size and shape. The pupils should be the same size and shape.

1. Anisocoria refers to pupils of different size. The most common causes include:

a. Adie pupil, a congenital difference in pupillary size. The pupil reacts to light and accommodation.

b. Argyll Robinson pupil (see VII A 3)

c. Trauma to the pupil (e.g., after cataract surgery)

d. Damage to the CN III carrying parasympathetic fibers to the eye. One pupil is dilated. Proceed to a Tier II examination of the cranial nerves (Chapter 29).

2. **Poikiloscoria** refers to pupils of different shapes. This is due to damage or inflammation of the iris. The most common causes include:
   a. Inflammation of the anterior chamber (infection, glaucoma) with adhesions pulling on part of the iris. It is very painful when the iris moves, and the patient will be exquisitely sensitive to light (photophobia).
   b. Trauma or prior cataract surgery.
   c. Glaucoma. The elevated pressure in the eye induces an oval shape to the iris.

VIII Step 7: Pharynx

A. Method

1. Have the patient extend his neck ("Look at the ceiling.") and open his mouth. Stand above him and look down into the mouth. This maneuver drops the tongue to the floor of the mouth, exposing the pharynx (Figure 23-4).

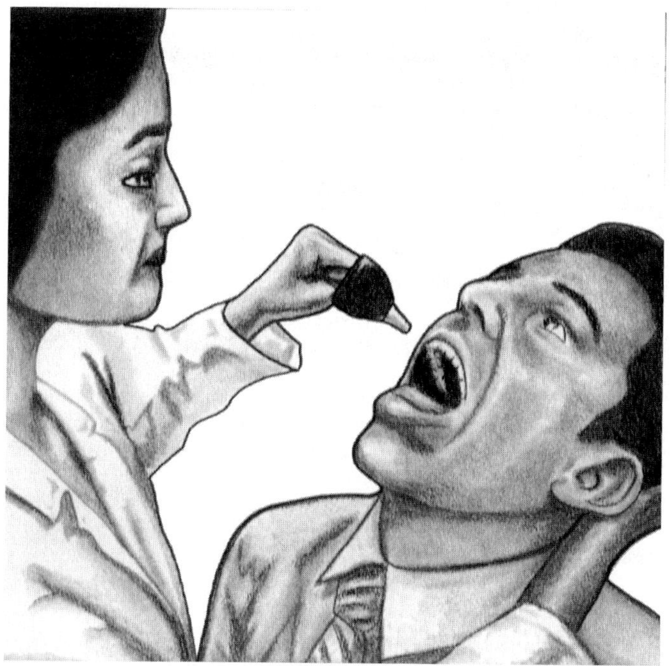

FIGURE 23-4. Examining the pharynx.

2. Alternatively, you can use a tongue depressor to push the tongue down to see the pharynx. If you do, remember that the tongue blade should *pull* the tongue forward and down, *not push* it back into the throat. To reduce gagging, wet the tongue depressor with water and enter the mouth an angle (i.e., not straight back, where anticipatory gagging is the greatest). Aim for about halfway back on the tongue (the gag reflex is greatest in the posterior third of the tongue). Apply downward pressure and use the depressor to pull the tongue down and toward you. If needed, use a piece of gauze to grasp the tongue with your other hand and pull it forward.

B. Interpretation. Things to look for:

1. **Cracked teeth.** A cracked or partially fractured tooth ultimately leads to a dental abscess if not removed or capped.
2. **Buccal discolorations.** It is especially important that you see the buccal and lip mucosa in patients who smoke or chew tobacco. Early cancer begins here. For long-term tobacco users, palpate under the tongue for a mass that may suggest early malignancy.
   - **a.** Petechiae (small purple dots) in the mouth usually indicate that the platelet count is less than 15,000/μl. (Petechiae on the skin suggest a platelet count of <50,000/μl; Chapter 27.) This is a useful finding in the setting of thrombocytopenia, because there is little risk of a spontaneous central nervous system bleed if there are no petechiae in the mouth.
   - **b.** White plaques may represent:
     - **(1)** *Candida* (thrush) invades the mucosa. It is easily scraped off but leaves an erythematous or bleeding lesion beneath the plaque where the fungus has invaded the mucosa.
     - **(2)** Dried saliva easily scrapes off without hemorrhage.
     - **(3)** Oral leukoplakia is a premalignant lesion that does not scrape off. A biopsy should always be performed to exclude malignancy.
   - **c.** Vesicles on the buccal mucosa or pharynx (see VIII B 6 b)
3. **Tongue lesions.** The tongue should be covered with normal papillae.
   - **a.** Geographic tongue. The surface of the tongue may be heterogenous, creating shapes similar to those of the continents. This is a normal finding as long as there are normal papillae on some parts of the tongue.
   - **b.** No papillae. The tongue is the most rapidly regenerating part of the body (thus the reason a scalded tongue from hot soup only lasts for one day). A deficiency of vitamins necessary for rapid cell division (e.g., vitamin B_{12}, folate) results in balding of the tongue, or loss of papillae.
   - **c.** Large tongue extending outside of the mouth. Causes include Down syndrome, angioedema, and infiltrative diseases (e.g., amyloid, hemochromatosis).

d. Black tongue. This condition, which is caused by an incidental fungus, is of no clinical significance. It can also be seen in patients who ingest medicinal garlic or in heavy smokers.

4. **Lips.** The lips are skin without the outer layers of the stratum corneum (and thus they appear red). Because they lack this extra layer, they are a good place to look for dermal disease (Table 23-3).

5. **Gums**
   - **a.** Gingivitis is inflammation and tenderness of the gums, manifesting in either swelling bleeding or recession of the gums.
   - **b.** Gingival hypertrophy occurs early in gingivitis or following drugs such as phenytoin, procainamide, and carbamazepine. Discontinuing the drug results in cessation of the hypertrophy with all drugs except phenytoin, which results in permanent hypertrophy.

6. **Pharynx and uvula**
   - **a.** The pharynx should be a **symmetric** arch, with the tonsils at the base of each arch, and the uvula dangling in the center (Figure 23-5A).
     - **(1)** When the patient says "Ahhhh" both pharyngeal muscles will attempt to lift the uvula (like two people lifting a backpack by each strap) (Figure 23-5B). A stroke involving CN IX paralyzes the pharyngeal muscles contralateral to the side of the brain infarction (i.e., a left-sided cerebral stroke results in right pharyngeal muscle paralysis). Only the intact muscle will lift the uvula, tilting the uvula (like the backpack) to the side of the normal pharyngeal muscle.

TABLE 23-3. Diseases Affecting the Lips.

Disease	Characteristic Findings
Cheilitis	Painful fissures perpendicular to the lip border. This suggests syphilis.
Cheilosis	Painful fissures at radiant angles to the lip border
Peutz-Jeghers syndrome	Pigmented macules on lips and mucosa
Osler-Weber-Rendu syndrome	Red macules/telangiectasia on lips This is a congenital disorder characterized by multiple telangiectasias (an arteriole that comes close to surface of mucosa) existing throughout bowel. Because the vessel is so close to the mucosa, it is a potential source of gastrointestinal bleeding.

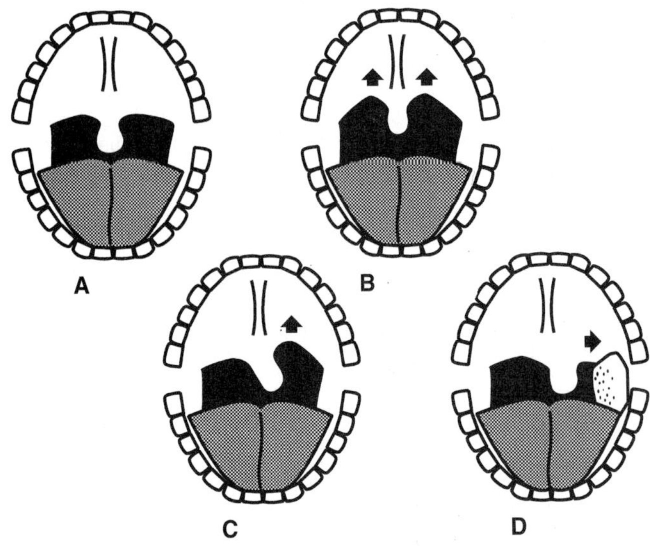

FIGURE 23-5. Appearance of the pharynx. **A,** Baseline. **B,** Normal response to "ahhh." **C,** "Ahhh": right CN IX defect (or left stroke). **D,** Peritonsillar abscess.

Thus, the uvula will point toward the side of the brain infarction (Figure 23-5 C).

(2) A peritonsillar abscess pulls the uvula toward the abscess. **This complication of bacterial pharyngitis is a medical emergency; the abscess must be drained immediately** before it extends into the carotid artery that sits just behind it. (Figure 23-5 D).

(3) Uvulomegaly results from repeated trauma to the uvula, which occurs with heavy snoring. It is dramatic, but harmless. It is also seen with infiltrative disease such as myeloma.

b. Look for erythema, vesicles, or ulcers in the mouth and pharynx. Painless ulcers suggest cancer because the cancer cells are not neurally innervated. Painful ulcers may be due to infection (e.g., HIV, Epstein-Barr virus, adenocarcinoma, histoplasmosis, herpes) or autoimmune disease (e.g., Crohn disease, lupus, aphthous ulcers). Eighty-five percent of patients with acute HIV seroconversion have ulcers in the mouth. Ulcers also may occur due to a drug reaction, known as Stevens-Johnson syndrome, which is at the extreme end of a spectrum of drug reactions. Mortality is greatly increased, because ulcers in the mouth suggest that there is similar epithelial damage throughout the gut. (The surface area of the gut is huge.)

c. Enlargement of the tonsils or adenoids in association with an erythematous pharynx is suggestive of a viral or bacterial infection. Pus on the tonsils, fever, lymphadenopathy, and the absence of upper respiratory tract symptoms (e.g., no cough, rhinorrhea) suggest a bacterial cause (the Centor Criteria).

IX STEP 8: NECK

The neck examination has three components: feeling for lymph nodes, feeling for the thyroid, and ensuring there is no neck stiffness (meningismus). Inspection of the neck veins and auscultation of the carotid arteries is discussed in Chapter 25.

A. Lymph nodes. There are two important lymphatic chains: the anterior and posterior cervical chains. Place your palm on the patient's forehead and ask him to push against your palm; this will make the sternocleidomastoid muscles prominent. The anterior cervical chain is located anterior to the sternocleidomastoid; the posterior cervical chain is located posterior. With your landmarks established, place your fingertips (four fingers) in the "valley" and make small massaging circles as you move from the base of skull to the base of the neck. If you feel a node, characterize it by size, tenderness, mobility and shape.

1. Posterior cervical nodes are more worrisome than anterior cervical nodes, because anterior nodes are almost always due to mouth infections. Posterior nodes are more likely to be due either to systemic infections, collagen vascular diseases (sarcoid, lupus) or cancer. However, a lymph reaction to scalp dandruff is still the most common cause.
2. Matted, nonmobile, flat or irregularly shaped, nonpainful nodes are suggestive of malignancy, because the cancer cells are extending out of the lymph node to attach to contiguous tissue.
3. Lymph nodes also can be palpated under the mandible. Like anterior cervical nodes, these nodes usually reflect gingival or oral infections.

B. Thyroid enlargement. Normally, the thyroid is at the base of the neck, just superior to the clavicles and just lateral to the trachea. The enlarged thyroid may be easier to see than feel. Assess both the size and consistency of the thyroid. After looking for enlargement, stand behind the patient with your hands circling around the neck so that your fingers are just lateral to the trachea at the base of the neck. Ask the patient to swallow; providing water usually helps (Figure 23-6). Swallowing raises the upper part of the thyroid from beneath the sternum up into the neck. You may not be able to palpate a thyroid; this is normal. If you do palpate a large thyroid or a nodule

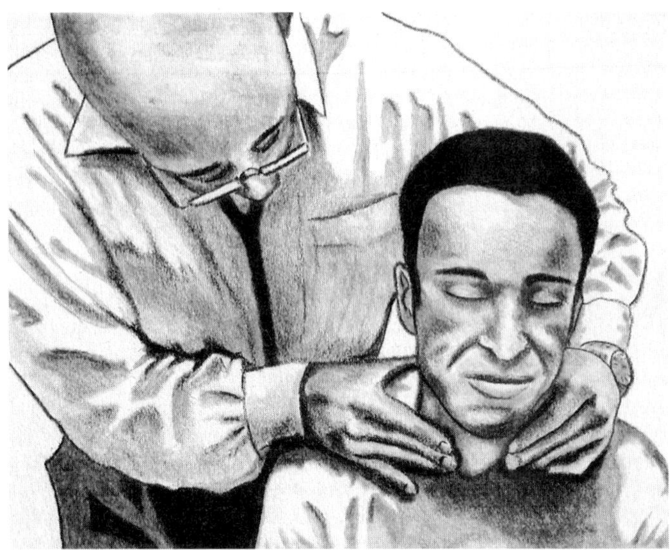

FIGURE 23-6. Palpating the thyroid.

in the thyroid gland, a Tier II examination should be performed (see Chapter 29).

X **STEP 9: EAR EXAMINATION** The ear has two functions: hearing and balance. When examining children, the ear examination should always be saved until last, because it is the most uncomfortable of the head and neck maneuvers.

A. External ear

1. Repeated trauma to the pinna of the ear will result in a thickened, irregular pinna (cauliflower ear).
2. The ears are the most sun-exposed parts of the body, and as such are at the greatest risk for skin cancer. Look for any discolored or raised lesions (see above).
3. Trauma to the pinna can result in a hematoma. Blood is toxic to cartilage; if the hemorrhage is acute, it should be drained.
4. Diseases affecting cartilage (relapsing polychondritis, leprosy) will causes erythema and tenderness of the pinna.

B. Tympanic membrane

1. If the patient can hear you and has no ear complaints (including normal balance), your Tier I examination is complete. If not, conduct a Tier II examination (see Chapter 29).

2. Note that the external auditory canal courses into the head; any head trauma should include a careful examination of the external auditory canal to exclude damage (see Chapter 29).

XI **NOSE EXAMINATION** Evaluation of the nose is almost always a Tier II examination. If the patient has pain or discharge from the nose, perform the examination outlined in Chapter 29.

24. The Tier I Lung Examination

I THE BIG PICTURE

A. The lung has two functions:

1. Transport oxygen to the alveoli and absorb it across the cell membrane into the blood; and

2. Remove carbon dioxide from the blood into the alveoli and transport it out of the body.

B. The Tier I examination detects abnormalities that impair the lung's ability to accomplish these two tasks (Table 24-1). Use the Tier II examination to determine the cause and severity of any abnormalities detected in the Tier I examination (Table 24-2) (see Chapter 30).

II METHOD

Like all Tier I examinations, the Tier I lung examination is designed to be efficient. You should be able to complete it in less than 1 minute. To perform it successfully, however, you must train your ears to listen for four different sounds simultaneously.

A. Step 1: Observe the thorax front and back for abnormalities. Look for anything that does not look like your thorax (see III A and Table 24-2).

B. Step 2: Place both palms on the posterior thorax. **Feel** for focal warmth or tenderness.

C. Step 3: Percuss the posterior thorax.

1. Stay within the midclavicular lines, percussing at four areas on each side (Figure 24-1).

2. No one sound is special; each sound is meaningful only in comparison to the percussion sound below and on the contralateral side of it. All percussion notes should sound the same. If one note is more resonant or dull than the others, proceed to a detailed Tier II examination to investigate its cause (see Chapter 30).

3. To improve your percussion skills, see Chapter 21 VIII.

D. Step 4: Auscultate the posterior thorax using one of the methods in Figure 24-1. Stay within the midclavicular line to keep your percussion focused on the aerated lung tissue. Anterior and lateral auscultation are part of the Tier II examination.

1. Listen for the absence of breath sounds, crackles, wheezes, and bronchophony. These findings are described in section IIIC.

2. If you hear any of these abnormalities, perform a detailed Tier II examination (see Chapter 30).

TABLE 24-1. The Tier I Lung Examination.

Step	Action
Step 1	Observe the thorax for abnormalities: Splinting Accessory muscle use Accessory muscle hypertrophy Skin discolorations or rashes Spinal curvature abnormalities Abnormal breathing patterns
Step 2	Feel for warmth and tenderness
Step 3	Percuss for dullness or tympani
Step 4	Auscultate for: No breath sounds Crackles Bronchophony Wheezes

HOT  KEY

When you describe a physical examination, avoid words that are subject to multiple interpretations. *Rales* and *rhonchi* are two such words. To avoid confusion, use the specific word for each: **rales** = **crackles** and **rhonchi** = **wheezes**.

III INTERPRETATION (see Table 24-2)

A. Observation

1. **Splinting** is the act of holding one part of the chest motionless during inspiration. Patients with pain in the right lower lung field, for example, will tilt the chest down and to the right to keep this portion of the thorax from moving to reduce the pain. Splinting may occur with pleural inflammation, pneumonia, or trauma.
2. **Accessory muscle movement.** When the diaphragm weakens, the neck muscles (sternocleidomastoids) are recruited to raise the upper portion of the thorax to maintain the chest expansion required for inspiration. This is an ominous sign that the patient's primary respiratory muscles are fatiguing and the patient may soon need intubation and respiratory support.
3. **Accessory muscle hypertrophy.** Hypertrophy of the sternocleidomastoid muscles (the diameter of the muscle is larger than the caliber of the patient's thumb) is a sign that the patient regularly relies upon these muscles for respiratory support (the patient may have chronic emphysema or asthma).
4. **Ecchymosis** suggests local trauma to the area.

TABLE 24-2. Interpretation of the Tier I Lung Examination.

Finding	Interpretation
Step 1: Observation	
Splinting (not moving part of the chest during inspiration)	Pleural inflammation, pneumonia or trauma
Accessory muscle use	Respiratory muscle fatigue
Skin abnormalities	Herpes zoster, ab igne
Curvature of the spine	Scoliosis
Tripod body position	Obstructive lung disease
Abnormal breathing patterns	See Chapter 30.
Obvious trauma	
Obesity	
Step 2: Palpation	
Focal warmth	Pleural inflammation, pneumonia
Tenderness	Herpes zoster, trauma, consolidation
Step 3: Percussion	
Dullness	Consolidation or pleural effusion
Hyper-resonance	Pneumothorax
Step 4: Auscultation	
Bronchophony	Consolidation
Crackles	Consolidation, heart failure, or chronic bronchitis
No breath sounds	Pleural effusion, consolidation, or pneumothorax
Wheezes	Obstructed airways or CHF

5. **Skin discoloration.** Patients with long-standing pleuritic pain may resort to placing hot towels or water bottles on the area. This may induce ab igne, a lacy, spider-web appearing rash. Reactivation of herpes zoster may also be observed on the chest.
6. **Curvature of the spine.** Kyphosis is forward curvature of the spine (the patient will look hunched over). Scoliosis is lateral curvature of the spine (in the form of an "S"). The combination of both, especially when severe, may lead to respiratory impairment.
7. **Position of the patient.** Patients with chronic obstructive lung disease trap air in the alveoli because the floppy bronchioles collapse on expiration and oppose expiratory flow. This trapped

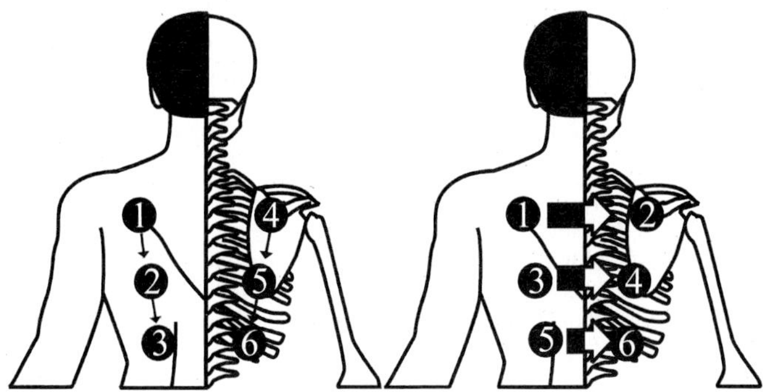

FIGURE 24-1. Two methods of percussing and auscultating the lungs.

air pushes down and flattens the diaphragm. The patient will lean forward with his elbows on his knees (like a tripod) to push abdominal contents into the diaphragm to re-form the normal curvature of the diaphragm (see Chapter 30).

8. **Breathing patterns.** Look for a breathing pattern that is unlike yours. See Chapter 22 (VB4) and Chapter 30 for an interpretation of abnormal breathing patterns.
9. **Obesity.** Obese patients arc at great risk for obstructive sleep apnea, or periods of hypoxemia during sleep due to upper airway obstruction from compression by the obese body habitus. The hypoxemia and lack of deep sleep can lead to pulmonary and arterial hypertension, daytime somnolence, and irritability.

B. Palpation

1. **Focal warmth suggests underlying pleural inflammation or consolidation.** Hippocrates described the practice of putting a wet slurry of clay on the patient's thorax. The warmth from a focal infection would accelerate the drying of the clay overlying that area.
2. **Tenderness** to very light palpation suggests an early outbreak of **herpes zoster infection;** tenderness may occur before the vesicles. Tenderness is also seen with **trauma** (broken ribs, pleural contusion) or an underlying **pneumonia.**

C. Percussion

1. **Causes of dullness to percussion**
   a. **Consolidation.** The normal air-filled lung consolidates into a solid mass when bacteria and the resulting inflammation fill the alveolar spaces.
   b. **Effusion.** Pleural effusion is fluid between the lung and the chest wall. This will cause dullness to percussion, unlike fluid in the alveoli or pulmonary interstitium (due to congestive heart failure, for example) that will not exhibit dullness.

2. It is impossible to tell the difference between consolidation and effusion on the basis of percussion. A Tier II examination is required to differentiate these two conditions (see Chapter 30).

D. Auscultation

1. **Normal breath sounds.** To appreciate abnormal breath sounds, you first must be able to identify normal breath sounds. Listen to as many normal lungs as you can to gain this appreciation (friends, family, healthy patients).
   a. **Alveolar breath sounds** are generated as air moving into the lungs sequentially opens waves of alveoli: proximal alveoli first, then distal alveoli. This creates a large, steady inspiratory sound. The increased pressure in the chest during exhalation squeezes every alveolus simultaneously, resulting in a short burst of sound at the beginning of exhalation (Figure 24-2A). Alveolar sounds are also known as **vesicular sounds** (vesicle = "little bag"). It is normal to hear alveolar sounds in all peripheral lung fields.
   b. **Bronchial breath sounds** are generated by air flowing in and out of the large-diameter bronchi and are normally heard in the middle upper third of the posterior chest (i.e., where the bronchi are located). Airflow is constant during both inspiration and expiration, creating an equal sound during both phases (Figure 24-2B). Because of the large diameter of the bronchi and the speed of airflow through the center of the tube, small eddy currents form along the sides of the bronchial tubes creating a hollow, haunted house–like sound. **Bronchiolar sounds have the same volume and character in both inspiration and expiration.** In contrast, alveolar sounds have a strong inspiratory component but a quick expiratory component. This difference in expiration is the easiest way to distinguish bronchiolar sounds from alveolar sounds.
2. **Abnormal breath sounds**
   a. **Bronchophony** is hearing bronchial breath sounds (strong, hollow expiratory sounds) where there are no bronchi (i.e., in the peripheral part of the lung). This implies that the normal air-filled lung has consolidated and become solid (e.g., pneumonia has filled the air spaces of the alveoli). The bronchiolar sounds generated in the central part of the chest travel through the solid to the periphery (Figure 24-3).
   b. **Crackles** are the "popping open" of small alveoli. **Take a lock of hair and rub it between your thumb and finger next to your ear.** This is the sound of crackles. Normally, surfactant keeps the alveolar air space open. When bacteria or other foreign material enter the alveoli and stimulate an immune response, the surfactant is neutralized. The alveoli collapse on expiration and "pop open" on inspiration. Crackles imply one of the following conditions:

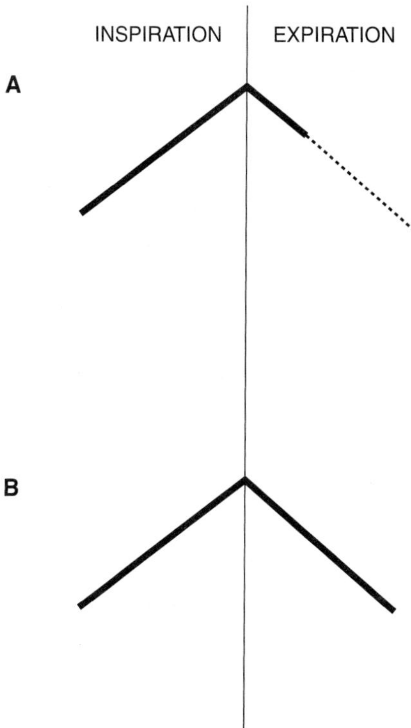

FIGURE 24-2. Alveolar and bronchiolar breath sounds. The caliber of the line represents the loudness of the sound. The expiratory component is the key to differentiating alveolar from bronchiolar sounds. **A,** Alveolar breathing sounds: a short, soft expiratory burst is alveolar. **B,** Bronchiolar breath sounds: a drawn out, hollow-sounding (haunted house) expiratory sound is bronchial.

(1) Consolidation due to pneumonia (organisms in the alveoli)
(2) Congestive heart failure (fluid in the alveoli)
(3) COPD. The mucus in the terminal bronchioles causes the bronchioles to "pop open" during inspiration. Because bronchi pop open before alveoli, crackles due to bronchiolar secretions occur earlier in the inspiratory cycle than crackles due to alveolar secretions.

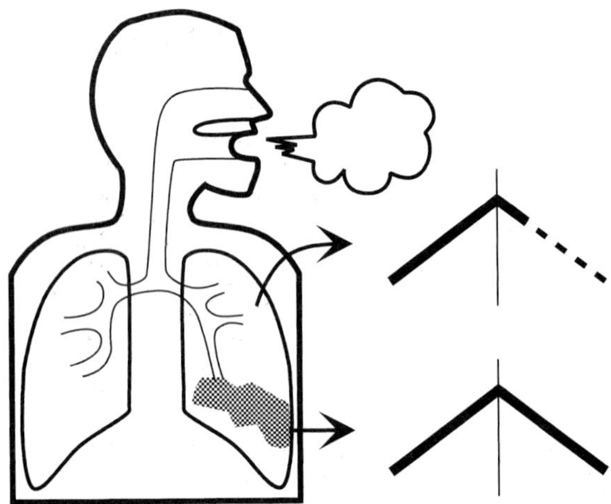

FIGURE 24-3. Consolidation and bronchiolar breath sounds.

c. **No breath sounds** implies the lung has been densely consolidated into a solid (e.g., due to pneumonia) or that fluid has collected around the lung, displacing the normal air-filled tissue. No breath sounds implies a **dense consolidation, pleural effusion, or pneumothorax.**

d. **Wheezes** are expiratory sounds that result when the bronchi are obstructed due to either **COPD or asthma.** Expiratory flow vibrates the small airways when they are obstructed. In this way, the airways act like a reed in a clarinet. Causes of wheezes are discussed in Chapter 30.

25. The Tier I Heart and Vascular Examination

I THE BIG PICTURE

A. The function of the heart is to move blood in a forward direction. Three abnormalities can impair this forward flow:

1. **Muscle failure:** damaged left ventricle, producing signs of heart failure (see Chapter 31)
2. **Valve failure:** blood going in the wrong direction, producing signs of valve failure (see Chapter 31)
3. **Obstructed arteries:** prevent blood flow to the tissues (see Chapter 33)

B. The Tier I heart and vascular examination identifies abnormalities in these three areas (Table 25-1). This chapter describes a seven-step method for performing a Tier I heart examination and how to interpret the findings and determine which Tier II examinations are indicated (Table 25-2 and Table 25-3).

II STEP 1: OBSERVE AND PALPATE THE POINT OF MAXIMAL IMPULSE (PMI)

The PMI provides information about the size and shape of the left ventricle (see Table 25-2).

A. Physiology. The heart is normally shaped like an upside-down cone (Figure 25-1A). The base of the cone is at the second intercostal space on either side of the sternum; the apex of the cone is normally at the fifth intercostal space in the midclavicular line. **The PMI is the point at which the ventricle is squeezing the hardest: the apex of the cone.**

B. Method. Position the patient at a 30-degree angle and remove the patient's shirt. Move close to the patient (1 foot away from the chest) and observe the left anterior and lateral chest. Look for pulsations on the chest wall. If you see a pulsation, put your fingers on it. Assess its location and size.

1. **Location.** The PMI should approximately be at the fifth intercostal space in the midclavicular line. **A PMI that is lateral to the midclavicular line** is due to either a **hypertrophied left ventricle** or a **dilated left ventricle** (Figure 25-1B and C).
   a. Place your entire right hand on the patient's left chest so that your hand cups the chest wall (just under the breast) (Figure 25-2). If the patient has large breast tissue, use the back of your left hand to lift the breast tissue up, and place your right

TABLE 25-1. Tier I Heart and Vascular Examination.

Step	Action
Step 1	Observe and palpate point of maximal impulse.
Step 2	Observe jugular venous pulsations.
Step 3	Palpate for left ventricular heaves.
Step 4	Listen for the S_1 and S_2 to establish systole and diastole.
Step 5	Note the loudness of S_1 and S_2 heart sounds.
Step 6	Listen for split heart sounds.
Step 7	Listen for murmurs.

hand on the chest wall under the breast. The web between your thumb and first finger should be just below the patient's fifth intercostal space, and your fingers should extend toward the midaxillary line.

b. Do *not* use the nipple as the landmark; as patients age, the nipples may descend laterally. Take the time to identify the midpoint of the clavicle and draw an imaginary line from there to the 5th intercostal space.

c. Close your eyes. What part of your hand is feeling a vibration? Take your time; it may take several seconds for the vibration to become apparent.

d. Once you feel a vibration, use one finger to pinpoint that location. **Although not feeling a vibration may be due to lack of experience, it may also signify a heart too weak to create a vibration.** Take note of the absence of this finding.

2. **Size.** The **PMI should be smaller than a quarter.** A PMI greater than the size of a quarter implies that the ventricle has assumed a spherical shape and suggests dilated cardiomyopathy (Figure 25-1C). **If the heart is dilated, the impulse is diffuse and the PMI is large.** Use the Tier II heart failure examination to confirm this finding (see Chapter 31).
3. **Clinical tip.** This method prevents you from mistaking a left ventricular heave (see Section IV) for a PMI. A left ventricular heave on the medial chest may fool you into believing that the vibration from the left ventricular heave is the PMI, when the true PMI is resting far lateral. When a left ventricular heave is present, the cup method described in II B 1 will detect both vibrations: one at the base of the palm (the left ventricular heave) and another at the tips of the fingers (the PMI).

C. Interpretation

1. **Lateral PMI:** If the left ventricle is subjected to a prolonged period of high pressure (e.g., hypertension, aortic stenosis, idiopathic hypertrophic subaortic stenosis), the ventricle hypertro-

TABLE 25-2. Observation and Palpation in the Tier I Heart and Vascular Examination.

Finding	Interpretation	Tier II Follow-up
Observation		
Lateral PMI	Hypertrophied left ventricle	Listen for S_4.
	or	
	Dilated cardiomyopathy	Listen for signs of heart failure: S_3, crackles, soft S_1. Look for elevated JVP, pulsus alternans.
Inferior/lateral PMI	Dilated cardiomyopathy	Look for signs of heart failure (see above).
JVP		
Not seen (e.g., below the clavicle)	The JVP is <5 cm.	Normal
See above the clavicle. (e.g., 7 cm above the clavicle).	The JVP is 12 cm (5 + 7 = 12).	Look for signs of heart failure (see above) or fluid overload.
Step 2: Palpation		
Laterally displaced PMI	See above.	
Interior/laterally displaced PMI	See above.	
PMI larger than a quarter	Dilated cardiomyopathy	Look for signs of heart failure
Heave left of sternum	Hypertrophied left ventricle	Listen for S_4.
	or	
	Left ventricular aneurysm	Look for signs of heart failure

JVP, jugular venous pulsations; PMI, point of maximum impulse.

TABLE 25-3. Auscultation in the Tier I Heart and Vascular Examination.

Finding	Interpretation	Tier II Follow-up
<u>Loudness of Heart Sounds</u>		
Louder than expected	High closing pressure	
S_1	Strong ventricular contraction	Normal
S_2	Aortic or pulmonic hypertension	Obtain blood pressure. Listen for signs of pulmonary hypertension (S_2 louder in pulmonic space than aortic space).
Softer than expected	Low closing pressure	
S_1	Poor ventricular contractility	Look for signs of heart failure.
S_2	Hypotension, calcified heart valve Slow heart rate	Listen for murmurs. Take pulse.
<u>Split heart sounds</u>		
S_2 is split on inspiration, but single on expiration.	Normal	No further examination.
S_2 is split on expiration, but single on inspiration.	Aortic valve is closing late	Listen for murmurs (VSD, pulmonic/aortic stenosis).
S_2 is split on expiration <u>and</u> split on inspiration.	Pulmonic valve is closing late	Assess blood pressure. Listen for signs of pulmonary hypertension (S_2 louder in the pulmonic space than aortic space). Obtain an ECG.

(Continued)

TABLE 25-3. Continued

Finding	Interpretation	Tier II Follow-up
Murmurs		
Systolic: Front door	Aortic sclerosis or stenosis; IHSS	Listen while the patient squats. Increased murmur = aortic stenosis/sclerosis. Decreased murmur = IHSS.
Systolic: Back door	Mitral or tricuspid insufficiency	Listen during hand grip (increase = mitral) or during inspiration (increase = tricuspid).
Diastolic	Aortic insufficiency; mitral stenosis	See Chapter 31.

IHSS, idiopathic subaortic stenosis.

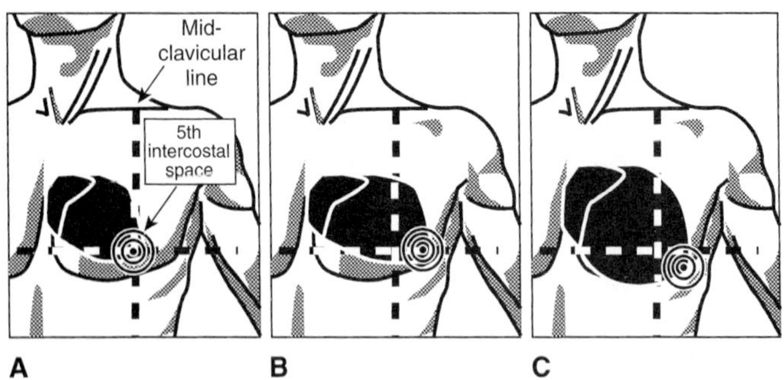

FIGURE 25-1. The point of maximal impulse (PMI). **A,** Normal PMI. **B,** Laterally displaced PMI. **C,** Inferiorly and laterally displaced PMI.

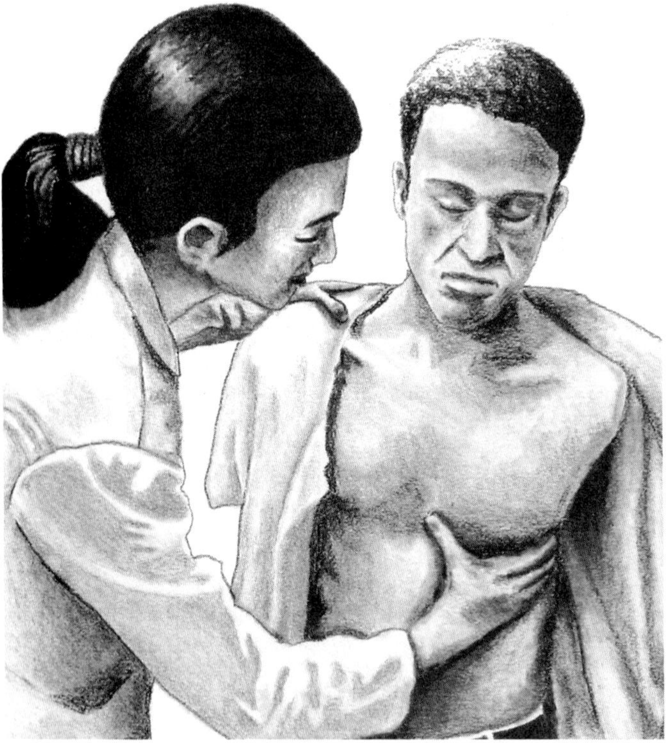

FIGURE 25-2. Palpating the PMI.

phies and the PMI (i.e., the apex of the cone) shifts laterally (Figure 25-1B). Equation 10 in Appendix A explains why this happens.

2. **Lateral and down or diffuse PMI**: If the left ventricle muscle is damaged (e.g., following a myocardial infarction or viral cardiomyopathy), it loses its contractile force and the cardiac output decreases. This decreases blood flow to the kidney, and the kidney releases renin. Renin stimulates angiotensin II, which in turn stimulates aldosterone. Aldosterone reabsorbs more salt and water from the kidney; the increased volume (preload) compensates for the decreased contractility. This maintains the cardiac output (to understand why, see Equations 4 and 5 in Appendix A). To accommodate the increased preload volume, however, the cone-shaped ventricle must dilate to assume the shape of a sphere (the shape that accommodates the maximum volume for any given surface area). As the ventricle assumes a spherical shape, the PMI shifts down and outward and becomes more diffuse (Figure 25-1C).

HOT

KEY

Always begin your heart examination by finding the PMI. A displaced or large PMI alerts you to the possibility of left ventricular failure, prompting you to perform a Tier II heart failure examination (Chapter 31).

III Step 2: Observe the Jugular Venous Pulsations

The JVP tells approximately how much blood is "backed up" on the right side of the heart. The JVP is important in diagnosing and treating both hypotension and congestive heart failure.

A. Method

1. Place your hand on the patient's forehead, and ask her to push her head against your hand. This makes the two lower "bellies" of the sternocleidomastoid muscle prominent. The two bellies form a triangle with the clavicle as the base; the apex of this triangle points toward the ear. Between the two bellies is a valley. Along this line, from the valley to the ear, is the best place to see the JVP. Spend the first 10 seconds just looking at the neck. Now see if there is a "waving pulsation" that becomes prominent. That is the JVP.
2. Do not turn the patient's head all the way to the left, because this will tighten the sternocleidomastoid muscles and pinch off the JVP.
3. The venous pulsation has two or three vibrations. For now, do not worry about what is causing the vibrations; that is a Tier II issue (see Chapter 31). Look for the uppermost part of the neck, where you see the vibrations; this is the top of the fluid column.

a. If the patient is sitting upright, the distance from the right atrium to the clavicle is 5 cm. If you cannot see pulsations, the JVP is less than 5 cm in height. If the pulsations are right at the level of the clavicle, the JVP is 5 cm in height. Both of these values may be normal, depending on the clinical situation.

b. If the JVP is higher than the clavicle, measure the distance from the clavicle to the point where you see pulsations. Add this number to the baseline 5 cm; this is the JVP.

c. A word of caution. Patients with severe congestive heart failure may have a JVP that extends into the head, making the pulsations invisible on the neck. Usually, however, there are other signs to suggest this degree of heart failure (see Chapter 31).

4. If you are having a difficulty finding the JVP, you can perform one of two maneuvers:

a. Position the patient at a 30-degree angle. Just like tilting a glass of water at this angle, the meniscus on the backside of the glass rises (Figure 25-3). This allows you to better see the JVP, though you will have to make an adjustment for reporting how high it is. To do this, imagine a line parallel to the floor, originating from the JVP meniscus and extending out to above the second intercostal space. Measure the vertical distance from the atria to this line; this is height of the JVP column.

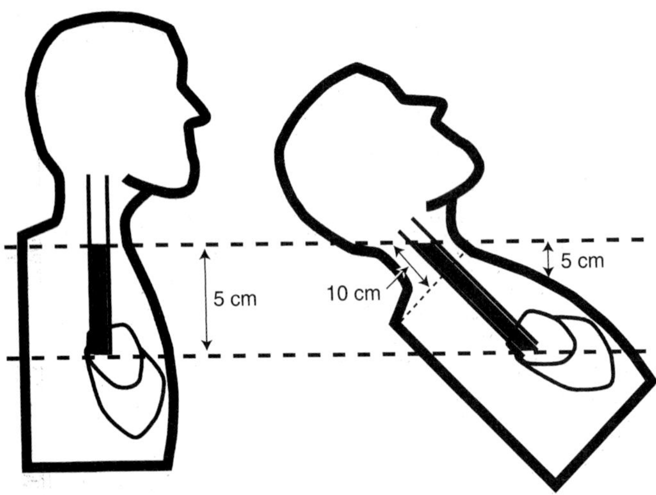

FIGURE 25-3. Tilting the patient to see the JVP.

b. Place your right hand on the center of the patient's abdomen and apply 35 mm Hg of pressure. (Until you are familiar with the amount of pressure required to exert 35 mm Hg, roll out a blood pressure cuff and place it flat on the abdomen. Pump it up until the dial shows 20 mm Hg; then apply pressure over the cuff until the dial reads 55 mm Hg.) This squeezes abdominal blood into the vena cava. Some of this blood "overshoots" the heart, and you see the JVP move up the neck. Moving pulsations are easier to see than stationary pulsations. This is also useful in distinguishing the JVP from a carotid pulsation, because the carotid pulsation does not move. In all patients, this maneuver causes the JVP to increase. In patients without pericardial disease, the right side of the heart compensates for the extra blood it has received, and the JVP decreases to its baseline position within 15 seconds (see Chapter 31). Measure the JVP at the level to which it returns. It is important to warn the patient before you do this maneuver; if the patient is surprised, she will tense her abdominal muscles, increasing pressure in the chest. This will prevent blood from being mobilized from the abdomen into the chest.

5. Be sure the pulsations you are seeing are not the carotid pulsation. The carotid impulse looks like a boxer inside the neck punching his way out; there is one large pulsation. The venous pulsation looks like a small child inside the neck waving at you with three, quick flexions of his fingers. If you are still confused, take the side of one finger and apply slight pressure on the right anterior-lateral part of the neck just above and parallel to the clavicle. **This pressure pinches off the jugular pulsation but does not compress the carotid artery pulsation.** If the pulsation disappears, what you saw was the JVP. If not, it was the carotid pulsation. Alternatively, ask the patient to perform the Valsalva maneuver ("Take a deep breath and then blow out hard, but do not let the air out of your chest.") Venous vibrations will rise up in the neck as blood volume is pushed into the jugular vein; arterial vibrations will not change.

C. Interpretation. The JVP is used to assess three clinical situations:

1. The volume status of the patient
2. The contractile function of the ventricle (e.g., does the patient have heart failure?)
3. To exclude pericardial or tricuspid valve disease by looking at the JVP waves (see Chapter 31)

D. From a clinical point of view, the actual number is not that important. Do not get mired in the details of distinguishing a 7-cm JVP from an 8-cm JVP. Rather, **determine whether it is elevated (>5 cm) or not**. An **elevated JVP can be caused by:**

1. **Too much total volume in the body** (as might occur with renal failure). Look at the rest of the body. Is there evidence of fluid overload (e.g., evidence of peripheral edema or ascites)?

2. **Obstruction of blood flow into the heart.** Perform a Tier II pericardial and valve examination (see Chapter 31).
3. **Poor contractility of the heart leading to an elevated left-ventricular preload.** Visualize yourself caring for a patient with hypotension. What is the cause? If there is no valve obstruction or incompetence between the left ventricle and the vena cava (see Chapter 31 for how to exclude tricuspid, pulmonary, and mitral valve disease) and there is no pericardial disease, the JVP tells you how much preload is in the left ventricle. If the JVP is elevated, the LV preload must also be elevated. If the heart rate is normal, the elevated JVP tells you that low preload is not the cause of the hypotension: the contractility is poor (see Appendix A, Equations 4, 5, and 6).

IV Step 3: Palpate for Left Ventricular Heaves

A. **Method.** Place your hand on the patient's chest, parallel to the sternum, with your fingers pointing toward the patient's head (Figure 25-4). The chest wall will lift your hand if the patient has a left ventricular heave.

B. **Interpretation.** Ventricular heaves **indicate a dilated or hypertrophied ventricle.**

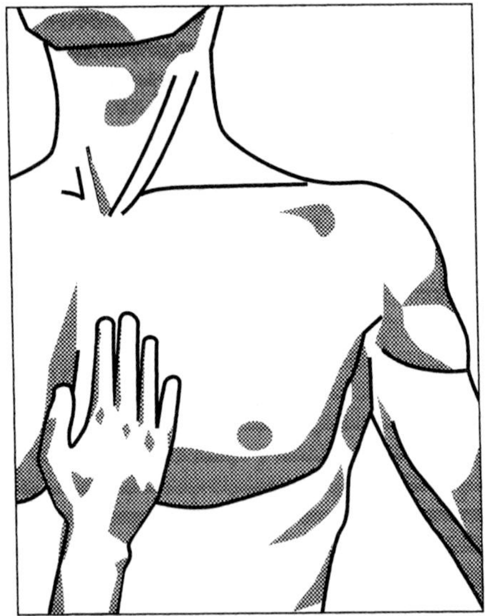

FIGURE 25-4. Palpating for heaves.

1. **Nonsustained ventricular heaves (taps)** are due to a **very muscular ventricle (caused by hypertrophy)** that is contracting vigorously against the chest wall. You can replicate this in yourself by doing 20 push-ups and then feeling your chest wall. This is normal following exercise but not while resting. If you feel a ventricular heave in a resting patient, it implies left ventricular hypertrophy. Because this is the result of the ventricle wall contracting in synchrony with the rest of the ventricle, the impulse is brief and then decreases (nonsustained).
2. **Sustained ventricular heaves** are due to the anterior part of the ventricle wall not contracting in synch with the rest of the ventricle. This is a **left ventricular (LV) aneurysm.** The anterior wall of the ventricle has been damaged from a previous infarction, and the scar tissue that remains does not contract. As the rest of the ventricle contracts, the anterior segment is pushed toward the chest wall (instead of contracting away from the chest wall). The LV aneurysm is displaced until the very end of systole, when the remaining ventricle stops contracting. The heave is sustained throughout systole.

STEP 4: LISTEN FOR THE S_1 AND S_2 TO ESTABLISH SYSTOLE AND DIASTOLE This is the foundation of the heart examination, because all other sounds in the cardiac examination will first be characterized as occurring during systole or diastole.

A. **Physiology.** Sounds heard after S_1 and before S_2 are systolic; sounds heard after S_2 but before S_1 are diastolic.
   1. S_1 is created by the closure of the mitral and tricuspid valves and is the end of diastole and the beginning of systole.
   2. S_2 is closure of the aortic and pulmonic valves and is the end of systole and the beginning of diastole.

HOT 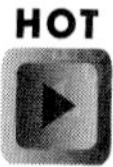 KEY

To appreciate abnormalities on the heart examination, you must have a good grasp of how the normal heart sounds. Listen to your own heart frequently until you are familiar with the normal sound of an S_1 and S_2. Then listen to patients of various ages *without* heart disease to establish what is normal at these ages.

B. **Distinguishing S_1 from S_2**

At slow heart rates, this is not difficult; the first sound of the S_1–S_2 couplet ("lub"–"dub") is S_1 (i.e., S_1 is the "lub."). At faster heart rates, feel the carotid pulse as you listen to the heart. **The sound that occurs at the same time as the carotid pulse is S_1,** because both S_1 and the carotid pulse occur at the beginning of systole.

HOT KEY

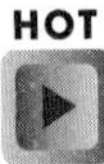

Do not use the radial pulse to determine which heart sound is S_1; use the carotid pulse. The time it takes for blood to travel to the wrist makes the radial pulse correspond more closely with the end of systole, which is closer to S_2.

VI STEP 5: NOTE THE LOUDNESS OF S_1 AND S_2 HEART SOUNDS.

The loudness of the heart sounds is a clue about the pressure that is closing the valve.

A. Listen at the area where you expect the valve in question to be the loudest. S_1 should be louder at the apex of the heart (where the mitral and tricuspid valves are best heard). S_2 should be louder at the base of the heart (where the aortic and pulmonic valves are located).

B. A loud S_2 at the aortic or pulmonic location indicates aortic or pulmonic hypertension, because it is this pressure that is closing the valve. **The higher the pressure; the greater the force closing the valve, and thus the greater the sound.** Because the aortic pressure is normally much greater than the pulmonary artery pressure, S_2 should be louder in the aortic space (right of sternum) than the pulmonary space (left of sternum). If you hear the opposite, pulmonary hypertension is likely.

C. A soft or absent S_2 implies that the cusps of the valve in question are not coming together, because the calcified valve is locked in a fixed position, or that the aortic or pulmonic pressure is very low.

D. A loud S_1 at the apex indicates that the left ventricle is contracting with vigor. This is usually a good sign; it indicates that the left ventricle is healthy. The right ventricle normally has comparatively little contractile force, relying mostly on preload for its stroke volume (see Appendix A; Equation 6). For this reason, the mitral valve contributes most of S_1. A loud S_1 suggests a strong left ventricle.

E. A soft or absent S_1 implies that the contractile force of the left ventricle is impaired, or that the valve is incompetent, with one of the flailing leaflets not coming to a point of closure.

HOT KEY

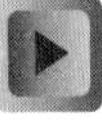

Neophyte physicians often discount their physical examination skill when they cannot hear crisp heart sounds. Although this may be due to inexperience, it may also be a real clue that the heart is not contracting forcibly.

F. A word of caution. The loudness of a heart sound generally corresponds to the pressure closing the valve. (Think of an obnoxious friend who closes the passenger car door a little too hard when leaving your car.) However, there are exceptions to this statement.

1. When the **heart rate is slow,** the valves flutter almost to closure before they are pushed closed. A nearly closed valve (e.g., like a door that is only 1 foot ajar) makes less of sound than one that is forced closed from its point of maximal opening.

2. **All sounds are softer when you listen through an insulated layer**. Patients who are obese, have obstructive lung disease, trapping air between the heart and chest wall, or have pericardial effusions have softer-than-normal heart sounds.

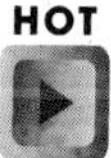

HOT KEY: It is difficult to auscultate through breast tissue. Use the back of your left hand to raise the breast; use your right hand to hold the head of the stethoscope against the chest wall.

VII Step 6: Listen for Split Heart Sounds.

The contraction of the left and right ventricle, and thus the closure of the left and right heart valves, should be almost simultaneous. Thus, the S_1 and S_2 should each be a single sound. If you hear a split sound, this means that one ventricle is closing later than the other. See Chapter 31 for identifying which ventricle is closing later than the other.

VIII Step 7: Listen for Murmurs

A. **Physiology.** Murmurs are simply turbulence created as blood flows over a valve. The intensity of a murmur's sound is proportional to

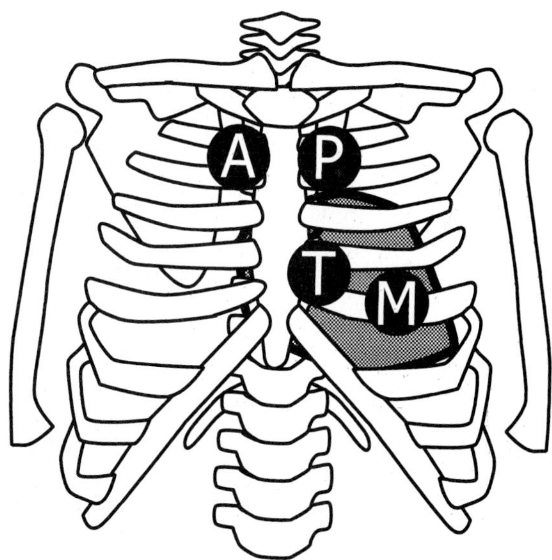

FIGURE 25-5. High-yield cardiac examination locations. *A*, aortic; *P*, pulmonic; *T*, tricuspid; *M*, mitral.

its turbulence. There are two ways to increase the intensity of a murmur: (1) **increase the flow** over the valve or (2) **decrease the valve area.**

B. Method. Listen in the four auscultation areas (Figure 25-5). Be warned, however—although hearing a murmur at one location (e.g., aortic space) is a <u>clue</u> that the murmur is from that valve (e.g., the aortic valve), this is not an absolute certainty. **Murmurs from one valve can be heard at other locations in the heart.** For example, the sound of an aortic valve murmur may radiate through the heart muscle to be heard at the mitral valve space. Use the Tier II examination in Chapter 31 to definitely diagnose the cause.

1. Murmurs at the **base** of the heart may be:
   a. Aortic: second right intercostal space
   b. Pulmonic: second left intercostal space
2. Murmurs at the **apex** of the heart may be:
   a. Tricuspid: fifth left intercostal space at the edge of the sternum
   b. Mitral: fifth left intercostal space at the midclavicular line

C. Interpretation. A heart murmur tells you that there is something wrong with a valve, except in situations in which you know that blood flow has suddenly increased.

> **HOT KEY**
> Be specific in your description of the location of murmurs. Instead of "left lower sternal border" (the entire heart is at the left lower sternal border), describe the location as being at the <u>base</u> or the <u>apex</u>.

26. The Tier I Abdominal Examination

I THE BIG PICTURE.

The abdominal organs may have different functions, but they should not be inflamed and should be normal in size. The Tier I abdominal examination focuses on evaluation of these two features and is summarized in Tables 26-1 and 26-2.

II GENERAL PRINCIPLES OF THE ABDOMINAL EXAMINATION

A. Before performing the examination, undress the patient so that you can see the thorax and abdomen.
B. Have the patient lie flat on the bed, with the knees bent and the soles of the feet flat. This relaxes the abdominal muscles and improves your ability to palpate the abdomen.
C. Observe the patient's abdomen from the side and from the foot of the bed. Pulsations and contours are revealed only at the proper angle, and you must be in different positions to see this.
D. Describe the abdomen as scaphoid, normal, or obese. The only clinical significance of this description is that it tells your audience the sensitivity of the remaining abdominal examination (i.e., abnormalities may not be appreciated in examining an obese abdomen, but should be found if the patient has a scaphoid abdomen).

> **HOT KEY** Observe the patient's facial expressions as you palpate the abdomen. Palpation of a distended organ (e.g., stomach, bowel) induces a vagal response that stimulates a vomiting reflex. The vomiting reflex is usually preceded by raising of the upper lip and lifting of the nose (Elvis Presley snarl).

III STEP 1: OBSERVE THE ABDOMINAL SURFACE

A. **Discoloration.** There are two types of discolorations on the abdomen. Make sure you visualize the flanks and the groins, because these are the places where leaking fluid (e.g., blood, bile) drains.
   1. **Ecchymosis** around the umbilicus or the flanks suggests that bleeding has occurred inside the abdominal cavity. This blood will leak from potential exits: the umbilicus and the inguinal canal. **Cullen's sign is ecchymosis around the umbilicus** (Cullen's sign is seen in the center of the body), and **Grey Turner's sign is ecchymosis at the groins and flanks.** Neither sign is specific for any one diagnosis; both simply imply that there has been a hemorrhage in the abdomen.

TABLE 26-1. Tier I Abdominal Examination.

Step	Action
Step 1	Observe the abdominal surface: Ecchymosis Pulsations Focal splinting Scars Dilated veins Hernias
Step 2	Auscultate bowel sounds. Presence or absence of bowel sounds Borborygmi
Step 3	Exclude abdominal pain with palpation.
Step 4	Exclude abdominal distention, ascites, and masses.
Step 5	Assess liver size.

2. **Greenish discoloration** around the umbilicus is a rare finding that suggests a ruptured bile duct, with bile leaking out around the umbilicus.

B. Pulsations

1. Pulsation in the abdomen is caused by one of the following:
   a. **Right-sided heart failure.** Pulsations are transmitted via the inferior vena cava to a distended liver. The right side of the abdomen will pulsate much more than the left, and the liver will be enlarged (see below). Other signs of heart failure will be present.
   b. **Aortic aneurysm.** A weakened aortic wall bulges outward and transmits pulsation to surrounding tissues (see palpating the abdomen below).
   c. **Normal vibration** of the diaphragm from the left ventricle. The vibrations will be greater on the left side of the abdomen (i.e., nearer the heart).
2. If you see pulsations, perform a Tier II examination (see Chapter 32).

HOT KEY

A pulsatile liver has the same three-phase pulsation as the jugular venous distention. A tongue depressor can help you see these pulsations. Place the end of a tongue depressor over the liver, with the depressor pointing medial and superior at a 45 degree angle. Lightly hold it to the abdomen so that only the tip touches the skin. Watch the vibrations of the other end; you should see the three vibrations associated with venous pulsations (see Chapter 31).

TABLE 26-2. Interpretation of the Tier I Abdominal Examination.

Finding	Interpretation	Tier II Follow-up
Step 1: Observation		
Ecchymosis	Blood in the abdomen	
Pulsations	Heart failure Abdominal aneurysm Diaphragm vibrations	Tier II heart examination Deep abdominal palpation None
Focal splinting	Peritonitis	Guarding; cross palpation
Scars	Prior surgery Risk for small bowel obstruction	Auscultate for borborygmi
Dilated veins	Portal vein obstruction Superior vena cava obstruction	Signs of liver disease Tier II lung examination for lung masses
Hernias	Potential source for small bowel obstruction	Assess whether the mass in the hernia is reducible (able to be easily pushed back into the abdomen)
Step 2: Auscultation		
Presence of bowel sounds	Normal	
Absence of bowel sounds	Inactive bowels	
Borborygmi	Small bowel obstruction	
Step 3: Palpation		
No tenderness	Normal	
Tenderness	Potential peritonitis	Guarding; cross palpation
Step 4: Percussion		
Tympanitic	Bowels full of air	
Dullness with epigastric tympani	Ascites	Liver size Fluid wave Shifting dullness
Diffusely dull	Abdominal mass Stool-filled bowel	Deep palpation
Step 5: Percussion for Liver Size		
8–12 cm	Normal	
>12 cm	Hepatomegaly	
<8 cm	Cirrhosis	

C. Focal splinting. If one part of the abdominal peritoneum is inflamed (peritonitis), the patient will hold this part of the abdomen motionless during deep inspiration (see Chapter 32).

D. Scars. Scars on the abdomen are a clue to prior surgeries (Figure 26-1). More importantly, scars increase the likelihood that small bowel obstruction is the causc of abdominal pain, because this condition is usually due to adhesions.

E. Dilated veins on the abdomen. The veins on the abdomen are anastomoses between the superior circulation (superior vena cava) and the inferior circulation (portal vein draining into inferior vena cava). They are not apparent in healthy patients because there is normally no flow between the two circulations; each circulation drains into its respective vena cava. When there is obstruction to this drainage (e.g., obstruction of the portal vein due to cirrhosis of the liver, or superior vena cava obstruction), the high venous pressure opens up the connection to the other circulation; the veins become prominent as they fill.

1. **Caput medusae refers to veins that *originate from* the umbilicus** (so named because the veins originating from the umbilicus look like the snakes that made up Medusa's hair). **Caput medusae always refers to obstruction of flow of the portal vein.**
2. **Caput "Wiese" refers to veins on the abdomen that do *not* originate from the umbilicus** (so named because the "bald"

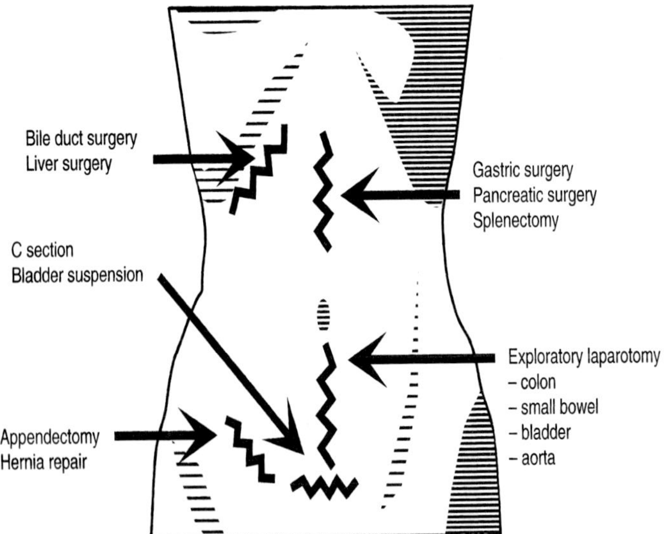

FIGURE 26-1. Scars on the abdomen are a clue to prior surgeries.

umbilicus [i.e., no hair attached] resembles the bald head of Dr. Wiese (Figure 22-2). The veins to either side of the head resemble the strands of loose hair that have fallen from the head. This condition may be due to obstruction of either the **portal vein** or **the superior vena cava.** If you observe caput "Wiese," use the following method to determine where the obstruction is located.

a. Determine the direction of flow by "stripping the vein." Put two fingers together on top of one of the abdominal veins. Apply and hold pressure. While maintaining pressure, spread your fingers apart along the length of the vein for about 1 to 2 cm. Release one finger, and note how long it takes for the vein to fill. Repeat the pressure, and now release the other finger (Figure 26-2). Which side fills more quickly? **The side that fills most quickly is the side with the most pressure.** This is the side from which the obstruction is redirecting the blood flow.

b. If the blood is flowing in an inferior-to-superior direction, the blood is trying to travel to the heart by traveling *superiorly* over the abdomen. The diagnosis is portal vein obstruction.

c. If the blood is flowing in a superior-to-inferior direction, the blood is trying to travel to the heart by traveling *inferiorly* over the abdomen. The diagnosis is superior vena cava obstruction.

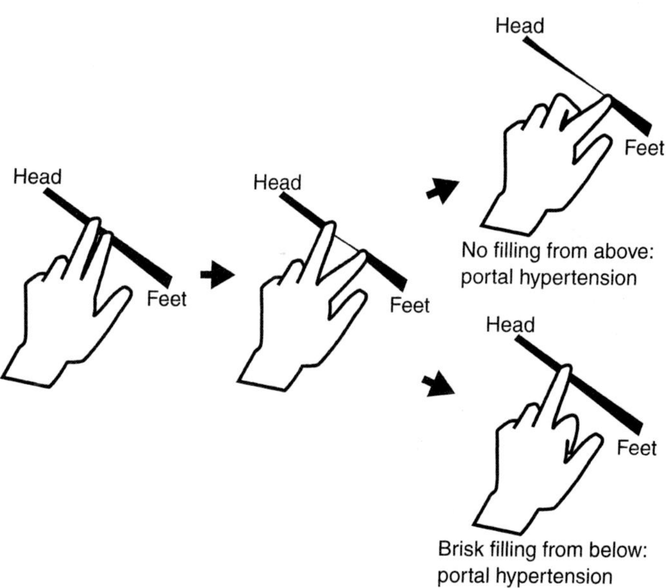

FIGURE 26-2. Stripping veins to determine the site of obstruction.

F. Look for masses or hernias. Any such finding must be investigated. There are four prominent types of hernias (see Chapter 32).

1. Ask the patient to take a deep breath and then exhale forcibly against a closed glottis. Say, "push as if you are going to exhale, but do not let any air out."
2. Look for bulges where the abdominal wall is weakest: the inguinal region, the midline of the abdomen, or around scars.

IV Step 2: Auscultation of Bowel Sounds

The sequence of observation, palpation, and percussion differs in the abdominal examination from that used in the heart and lung examinations. Auscultation comes immediately after observation, because both palpation and percussion can hyperexcite or suppress bowel activity, thereby altering the findings on auscultation.

A. Presence or absence of bowel sounds. There is no clinical significance of hyperactive or hypoactive bowel sounds. **All you can say is that the bowel sounds are present or absent.** If present, the bowels are functional. If absent, the bowels are not moving. Be careful: **to reliably say that bowel sounds are not present requires that you listen for at least 2 minutes.**

HOT  KEY

Sound smart when you present the results of your examination. Bowel sounds are either present or absent, not positive or negative. Pain is something the patient has, and tenderness is what you elicit.

B. Borborygmi. The presence of a special type of bowel sound that sounds like "tinkles and rushes" is a sign of small bowel obstruction (see Chapter 32).

HOT 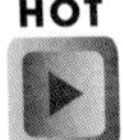 KEY

Bowel sounds are especially important to evaluate in the postsurgical abdomen. Anesthesia or a bowel incision puts the bowels to sleep, and patients cannot be fed after abdominal surgery until the bowels are "awake."

V Step 3: Exclude Abdominal Pain

Palpate in all four quadrants of the abdomen, beginning shallowly, and then if there is no tenderness, palpate more deeply.

A. Shallow palpation: guarding. Lightly palpate all quadrants of the abdomen. If you detect tenderness, use the method described in Chapter 32 to discern the cause.

B. Deep palpation: masses. Deep palpation is not a routine Tier I examination unless the history suggests that cancer or an aneurysm may be present (see Chapter 32).

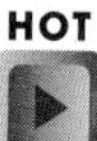

If a patient is too ticklish to allow for palpation of the abdomen, place your hand on the patient's and use it to palpate the abdomen. A patient cannot tickle himself.

VI Step 4: Exclude Abdominal Distention, Ascites, and Masses

General percussion is not necessary unless the abdomen appears distended. Percussion can determine whether distention is due to ascites, stool, tumor, or air-filled bowel. If necessary, **percuss** in all four quadrants, listening for the tone of the sound.

A. **Tympanitic** (i.e., sounds like a drum) indicates distended bowel full of air.

B. **Dullness with an area of tympani between the epigastrium and the umbilicus** (assuming the patient is lying flat) indicates ascites. This tympani is due to air-filled bowels floating on top of the ascites fluid.

C. **Diffusely dull** means that either the bowels are full of stool, or a large mass (tumor) is occupying that space.

VII Step 5: Assess Liver Size

A. **Percussion**

1. Stand at the patient's right side. Stand back 2 feet from the patient when percussing the liver to ensure that your right wrist has enough room to extend and flex during percussion. Do not stand so close that your percussion is hampered (Figure 26-3).
2. Place your left hand flush against the patient's right thorax, with the DIP joint of your left middle finger in the midclavicular line.
3. Begin percussing just below the right nipple. Percuss in the midclavicular line, working inferiorly until the hyperresonant tone of the air filled lungs becomes dull. This line is the superior edge of the liver.
4. Continue percussing inferiorly until the sound again turns tympanitic. This tympani is a result of leaving the dull liver tissue and moving onto the air-filled bowels. This is the inferior border of the liver.

B. **Scratch test**

1. Place the stethoscope on an area that you know to be the liver.
2. Pick an area you know not to be the liver. Use your finger to scratch the skin surface lightly and move toward the stethoscope. When your finger scratches the skin overlying the liver (the liver edge), the scratch sound will be transmitted through both the skin and the liver tissue. This will make the sound louder than the previous scratch. Repeat this from above and below to establish the liver edge.

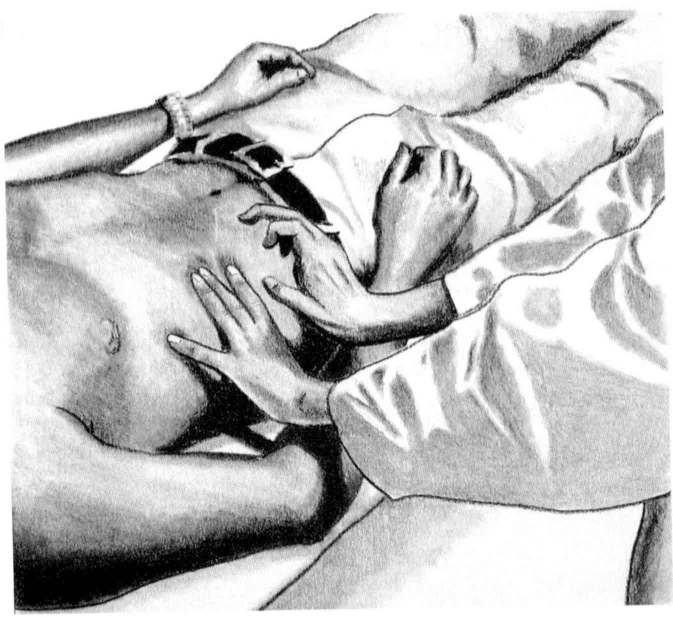

FIGURE 26-3. Percussing to determine liver size.

3. Use caution. As your finger gets closer to the stethoscope, the sound naturally gets louder. To prevent this artifact, make sure the distance between the stethoscope and the scratching finger is the same.

C. Interpretation

1. A larger-than-normal liver (>12 cm from the superior to inferior edge) may be caused by venous congestion (e.g., right-sided heart failure, inferior vena cava obstruction), infiltration (e.g., tumor, fat deposits, parasites), or acute inflammation (e.g., from alcohol or toxins).
2. A smaller-than-normal liver (<8 cm from the superior to inferior edge) may be caused by long-standing inflammation (e.g., hepatitis, alcohol), resulting in fibrosis that has contracted the liver. Normal liver tissue has been replaced by fibrotic nonfunctional tissue (i.e., cirrhosis).

D. The size of other organs is evaluated using the Tier II examination (see Chapter 32).

27. The Tier I Extremity Examination

I THE BIG PICTURE

The Tier I extremity examination identifies abnormalities of the skin overlying the extremities and blood flow to and from the extremities (Table 27-1).

II STEP 1: LOOK FOR SKIN ABNORMALITIES

Start from the top of the scalp and work down. Begin by examining the hair and scalp, progressing to the face, mucous membranes, trunk, upper extremities, fingernails, lower extremities, and toenails. Anything that you have not seen on your own skin is worth careful investigation. If you find an abnormality, use Figure 27-1 to guide your description. Then proceed to your Tier II examination (see Chapter 33, Figures 33-1 and 33-2) to make the diagnosis.

III STEP 2: LOOK FOR NAIL ABNORMALITIES

The fingernails are a valuable clue to systemic disease (Table 27-2).

A. **Clubbing** of the nails results from any chronic hypoxic condition. The exception is emphysema, which does not induce clubbing unless a lung cancer is present. There are three phases to clubbing (Figure 27-2).
   1. Stage 1: **Spongy nail bed.** Early clubbing is characterized by increased blood flow to the nail matrix (the area of the finger just proximal to the nail). The usually firm nail matrix has the spongy feel of the flexor side of the finger.
   2. Stage 2: **Obliteration of the angle.** Ask the patient to hold the left and right nails of corresponding fingers against each other. There should be a small diamond of space between the two where the nail base meets the matrix. Obliteration of this angle is stage 2 clubbing.
   3. Stage 3: **Nails that look like little clubs** (like the South American tree frog).
   4. Clubbing pearls.
      a. Many patients (especially African-Americans) will have a large middle part of the nail with a curvature to the end of the finger. The angle from the nail to the matrix is not involved. This is **terminal beaking,** not clubbing; it has no clinical significance (see Figure 27-2).
      b. Clubbing since birth is congenital clubbing; it has no clinical significance.
      c. Painful clubbing is almost always cancer (usually lung cancer).

TABLE 27-1. Interpretation of the Tier I Extremity Examination

Finding	Interpretation	Tier II Follow-up
Step 1: look for skin abnormalities	See Figure 27-1	Tier II skin examination
Step 2: look for nail abnormalities	See Table 27–2	See Table 27–2
Step 3: assess blood flow to the extremities		
Medial leg ulcers	Venous insufficiency	Tier II heart examination
Lateral leg ulcers	Arterial Insufficiency	Assess pulses
Decubitus ulcers	Chronic bed rest	Assess for signs of infection (Chapter 33)
Cyanosis	Inadequate delivery of oxygen to the tissues	Tier II heart and lung examinations
Poor capillary refill	Inadequate circulation	Tier II heart examination
Lack of normal hair growth	Inadequate circulation	Assess pulses Tier II heart examination
Weak pulses	Inadequate circulation	Tier II heart examination
Asymmetric pulses	Focal arterial obstruction	Angiogram
Step 4: assess blood flow from the extremities		
Edema	Increased venous or lymphatic pressure	Tier II extremity and heart examination
Hyperpigmentation of the skin	Chronic venous stasis	Tier II heart examination
Step 4: feel for warmth or tenderness of the joints	Inflammation Degeneration Infection	Tier II Extremity examination
Step 6: palpate the lymph nodes	Trauma Infection Malignancy	Tier II Extremity lymph node examination

Describe	**A**ll	**T**he	**S**kin	**M**anifestations
		by approaching the		
Distribution	**A**rrangement	**T**ype	**S**hape	**M**argin

FIGURE 27-1. Describing a skin abnormality.

TABLE 27-2. Interpretation of the Tier I Nail Examination.

Finding	Interpretation	Tier II Follow-up
Clubbing	Chronic hypoxia	Tier II pulmonary examination Look for malignancy
Surface changes: signs of internal disease		
Nail pitting	Psoriasis	Look for other skin manifestations of psoriasis
Terry's nails	Alcoholic liver disease	Tier II liver examination
Lindsay's nails	Chronic renal failure	Laboratory testing
Thickening of nails	Fungal infection	None
Onycholysis	Hyperthyroidism	Tier II thyroid palpation
Longitudinal pigmented streaks	Melanoma	Biopsy
Surface changes: signs of incidental trauma		
Splinter hemorrhages	Incidental trauma Endocarditis	None Tier II heart examination (murmurs)
Subungal hematoma	Trauma	None
Partial leukonychia	Incidental trauma	None
Surface changes: signs of malnutrition		
Koilonychia	Iron deficiency	Laboratory testing
Brittle nails, Beau's lines, Muehrcke lines	Malnutrition	Laboratory testing

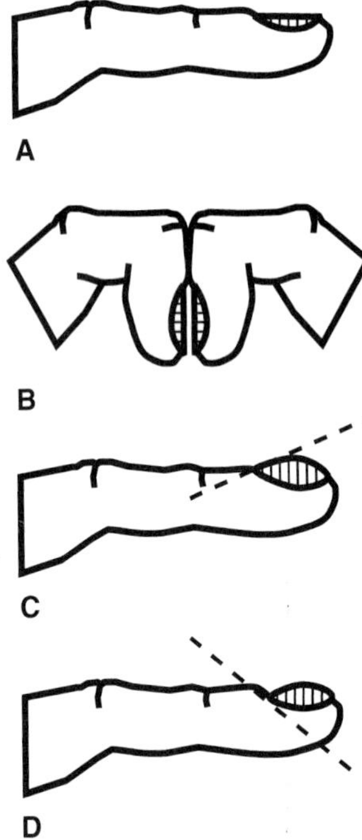

FIGURE 27-2. Three phases of clubbing.

   d. Unilateral clubbing is obstruction of blood flow to that extremity (thoracic outlet syndrome).
   e. Clubbing can develop quickly (within a week) in inflammatory diseases involving the lungs (endocarditis).

B. Surface changes due to systemic disease

1. **Pitting of the nails** (>11 pits/nail) is psoriasis (<11 is random trauma).
2. **Terry's nails**. The normal nail has a white lunate (half moon) at its base; the remainder of the nail is pink. Terry's nails is complete whitening of the nail bed with the exception of a 2-mm strip at the distal nail. It is seen in patients with alcoholic liver disease; congenital Terry's nails is of no clinical significance.
3. **Lindsay's nails** are half and half nails. The proximal half is white, and the distal half is red. This suggests renal failure.
4. **Thickening** of the nails (onychauxis) suggests a fungal infection of the nail.

5. Separation of the nail from the nail bed **(onycholysis)** suggests hyperthyroidism.
6. **Longitudinal pigmented streaks** suggest melanoma of the matrix, extending into the nail.
7. **Nailfold capillaries** (see Chapter 33)

C. Surface changes due to incidental trauma

1. **Splinter hemorrhages** are linear red lines that appear as splinters under the nails. They result from small trauma to the nails (80% of dishwashers will have them) or, rarely, small vessels being occluded with vasculitic material that is in the blood stream (i.e., due to endocarditis).
2. **Subungal hematoma.** Trauma to the nail may induce a hematoma under the nail bed. In the acute setting, the pain may be reduced by heating the tip of a paperclip, and then applying the tip to the nail until it bores a hole through the nail bed. This will reduce the pressure under the nail.
3. **Partial leukonychia** are white spots on the nail due to incidental trauma to the matrix. The spots become visible as the nail grows; they are of no clinical significance.

D. Surface changes due to malnutrition

1. **Koilonychia** is spooning of the nails. There is a cuplike depression in the center of the nail that will hold a drop of water if placed upon it. It is a sign of iron deficiency.
2. **Brittle nails (onychorrhexis)** occur after periods of severe malnutrition or hypocalcemia.
3. **Beau's lines** are linear horizontal depressions corresponding to nail growth arrest during severe illness. The nail grows at 0.1 mm per day; thus, you can estimate the date of the illness from the distance from the depression to the nail matrix. Linear ridges are of no clinical significance.
4. **Muehrcke lines.** These are alternating white and red bands that are not actually in the nail, but instead in the nail bed. They occur during periods of low albumin and resolve when nutrition improves.

IV Step 3: Assess Blood Flow TO the Extremities

A. Observation. The skin, hair, and nails all depend on adequate blood flow to the extremities.

1. Ulcers
   a. Venous insufficiency ulcers occur on the medial leg, because the venous drainage twists from medial to lateral on return to the body.
   b. Arterial insufficiency ulcers (sickle cell anemia, atherosclerosis) occur on the lateral leg. Check the pulses (see below).
   c. Decubitus ulcers occur in places of sustained rest, because the body weight pinches shut the small skin vessels (Table

TABLE 27-3. Staging Decubitus Ulcers.

Grade	Description
Grade 1	Erythema, denuded skin
Grade 2	Extension to the dermis
Grade 3	Extension to soft tissues (muscles)
Grade 4	Exposure of bone

27-3). It is very important to observe the posterior surface of all bed- or wheelchair-bound patients. Decubitus ulcers are common, and they frequently serve as a portal for infection.

HOT 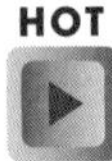 KEY

ALS is the only paralytic disease that does not induce decubitus ulcers, because the arterial walls hypertrophy, preventing closure under the body's weight.

2. **Cyanosis.** Inadequate circulation will result in a blue color of the skin due to deoxygenated blood.
3. **Capillary refill.** Press on one of the patient's nails; this will turn the nail bed white. When you release pressure, the nail bed should return to a pink color within 1 second. Delayed response suggests poor circulation.
4. **Lack of normal hair growth.**

B. **Palpation. Feel for pulses.** The patient's pulses should resemble the strength of your own. Feel both radial pulses and the posterior tibial and dorsalis pedis pulses. If these are adequate, you can assume that more proximal pulses (e.g., femoral, popliteal, brachial) are also adequate.

C. Compare each pulse to the corresponding pulse on the other limb. Asymmetric pulse strength suggests that one limb is receiving less blood than the other.
1. **Finding the dorsalis pedis pulse.** Ask the patient to lift his big toe. Note the tendon that becomes prominent on the top of the foot. Place the tips of your fingers on this tendon; let them roll medially into the groove.
2. **Finding the posterior tibial pulse.** Form your right hand into a "U," as if you were holding a can. Place the web of your thumb on the anterior part of the patient's right ankle so that your fingertips roll into the groove just behind the medial malleolus.
3. **Finding the radial pulse.** Place your fingers parallel to and on the radius bone; let your fingers roll medially into the groove.

D. **Interpretation.** Pulses assess the caliber of the large arteries that might be impaired by atherosclerosis. Even if strong, they do not ensure that circulation is normal. Small capillaries that perfuse the skin, muscles, nerves, and vessels themselves (together referred to as microcirculation) might still be obstructed in diseases such as diabetes mellitus or a paraneoplastic syndrome.

V Step 4: Assess Blood Flow FROM the Extremities

A. Edema. The fluid that leaves the vascular space to the interstitial space is returned to the heart via the lymphatics and the veins. Edema results from either increased venous or hydrostatic pressure (due to obstruction) or inadequate protein in the venous blood to hold onto the fluid. If you observe swelling (edema) in the extremities, use the Tier II examination in Chapter 33 to diagnose the cause.

B. Hyperpigmentation. Inadequate venous return will result in pooling of blood in the extremities (see below). The hemosiderin from the pooled blood stains the skin a dark brown color.

VI Step 5: Assess the Warmth of the Joints.

Trauma, degeneration, inflammation, or infection of the joint space will result in tenderness, warmth, and swelling of the joint. Quickly survey the joints as you perform the above examination. If you find joint abnormalities or if the patient complains of joint pain, use the Tier II method in Chapter 33 to diagnose the cause.

VII Step 6: Palpating Lymph Nodes.

You may also wish to include palpation of the lymph nodes in your Tier I examination.

A. The lymphatic system collects debris in the interstitial space and concentrates it in focal areas (nodes) for destruction and removal.

B. If you know the drainage patterns of the lymph system, you can use focal lymphadenopathy to direct you to the site of the infection/inflammation (it will be distal to the enlarged lymph node) (Table 27-4).

C. Examine the lymphatic system by region. Palpate for the head and neck nodes after your HEENT examination, the axillary nodes after the breast examination, and the periumbilical and inguinal lymph nodes after the abdominal examination (see Table 27-4).

D. Systemic lymphadenopathy implies inflammation/infection that is throughout the body (Table 27-5).

E. The method of palpation is important. Use the tips of your fingers and massage the area in small circles, feeling for the nodes escaping under your moving fingers.

F. If you find an enlarged node, use the character of the lymph node.

1. Size. Measure the greatest width of the lymph node. Lymph nodes >1 cm are of concern.
2. Tenderness. Tenderness suggests an inflammatory or infectious etiology, because it implies that the node has become acutely

TABLE 27-4. Causes of Lymph Node Enlargement by Location.

Location	Interpretation
Head and neck lymph nodes	
Anterior chain (in front of the sternocleidomastoid) and submental (under the jaw) lymph nodes	Usually imply an infection of the mouth.
Posterior chain lymph nodes (behind the sternocleidomastoid)	Are more cause for concern. They are enlarged with lymphoma and mononucleosis, but the most common cause is dandruff.
Periauricular nodes	Suggest a head/neck cancer or lymphoma.
Delphian nodes	Are small midline lymph nodes anterior to the thyrohyoid membrane. They represent malignant or benign thyroid disease.
Axillary lymph nodes	Suggest an arm infection or a breast cancer. Passively abduct the arm, insert you hand into the axillary fossa, and then abduct the arm over your hand. Pull down with your fingers.
Medial epitrochlear space	An infection of the arm or systemic causes.
Left supraclavicular fossa	Contains nodes from the thoracic duct draining the intra-abdominal space. Lymph containing abdominal tumor cells may track along this duct (Virchow's node). To maximize your examination, have the patient perform a Valsalva maneuver while you palpate the supraclavicular space to raise the node to your fingers.
Periumbilical region	Gastric and pancreatic tumors may track along this path. This is the Sister Mary Joseph node, first described by Sister Mary (at St. Joseph's Hospital), who was the scrub-nurse preparing patients for intra-abdominal exploratory surgery for Dr. Mayo. She correlated the presence of the node with patients who were found to have intra-abdominal malignancy.
Inguinal nodes	See Chapter 37.

TABLE 27-5. Causes of Systemic Lymphadenopathy.
Malignancy (lymphoma, leukemia)
Infection (syphilis, mononucleosis, CMV)
Sarcoidosis
SLE
Toxoplasmosis
AIDS
Rheumatic heart disease
Tuberculosis

swollen. As the infection travels through the lymph ducts to get to that node, it induces inflammation. The presence of erythema or reddish streaks leading to the lymph node suggests infection as the cause.

3. Softness/consistency. Fluctuant (squishy) lymph nodes suggest pus inside the lymph node and suggest a bacterial infection. A rubbery node is noted with lymphoma.
4. Mobility. Chronic inflammation (as with cancer) will lead to fibrosis of the node, tacking it down to adjacent tissue. The node will become fixed and immobile.

28. The Tier I Neurologic Examination

I **The Big Picture** The function of the neuromuscular system is to allow the patient to interact and maneuver within his environment. The Tier I neurologic examination evaluates this function (gait, strength, and sensation) (Table 28-1). The Tier II examinations will reveal the cause of these deficits (e.g., weakness, gait abnormalities, sensory loss) (Table 28-2).

II **Step I: Observe the Patient's Gait** Gait is a complex event that requires sensory input, muscle strength, joint integrity, and cerebellar function. As such, it is an excellent screening examination for neuromuscular function, so much so that, depending upon your patient population, you may elect to make gait assessment your sole Tier I neurologic examination. Abnormalities in gait should prompt a detailed Tier II examination (Chapter 34).

HOT

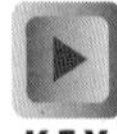

KEY

If a patient with no musculoskeletal complaints has a normal gait, you may assume that the musculoskeletal system is normal.

A. **Abnormal motor nerves**

1. **Parkinsonian gait: *march a petite pas*** ("gait with little steps"). Parkinson disease is characterized by a state of constantly increased muscle tone. The struggle to overcome this hypertonicity to initiate movement is the hallmark of the disease. The first step is slow and short, because the conscious effort to move the foot must overcome the chronic muscle contraction of the leg **(festination).** The next few steps will be small for the same reason. Once the patient starts moving, however, he cannot stop. The result is **propulsion** forward, akin to what you might experience when running down a steep hill. Changing directions (e.g., turning around) re-creates the initial problem of overcoming muscle hypertonicity; turns will be very slow, with frequent small steps in navigating the turn.
2. **Magnetic gait: normal pressure hydrocephalus (NPH).** NPH is a triad of (in order of appearance of the symptom) dementia, ataxia, and urinary incontinence. The arachnoid granula-

TABLE 28-1. Tier I Neurologic Examination.

Step	Action
1	Observe the patient's gait.
2	Observe the muscles for atrophy or fasciculations.
3	Palpate the muscles for tenderness.
4	Assess muscle strength.
5	Assess sensation to light touch.
6	Assess reflexes.

tions that normally reabsorb CSF become plugged, and this puts back-pressure on the ventricles within the brain, which in turn compresses the brain. The patient walks as if her legs were magnetically stuck to the floor (ataxia).

3. **Scissor gait: spastic paraplegia.** This is due to upper motor neuron damage (neurons in the brain or spine) that normally suppresses the reflex arc at the anterior horn of the spinal cord. This causes the leg muscles to be constantly stimulated by the sensory input from the extremities, creating a state of spastic contracture. The scissor gait is characterized by short steps with the toes never leaving the floor. The knees cross and rub against each other, creating the image of a pair of scissors. This gait is classic of **cerebral palsy.**
4. **Steppage gait: foot drop**. **Peroneal nerve damage** results in weakness of dorsiflexion of the foot, making it difficult to lift the toes out of the way when the patient moves the foot forward during gait. To compensate, the hip flexors must lift the whole leg higher than usual. The steppage gait resembles the walk of a clown in big floppy shoes.

B. Weak muscles. Waddling or circumduction (swinging the leg to the side during gait) is due to gluteal muscle weakness. In normal gait, the gluteal muscles lift the right hip upward so the right foot can move forward without catching on the ground. Weakness of the gluteal muscle or hip causes the foot to catch on the ground. To avoid this, patients learn to swing the leg around to the side (circumduction) to move forward.

C. Damaged joints result in limping. The patient puts maximum and prolonged pressure on the good limb, touching the bad limb to the floor just long enough to facilitate "jumping" to the next step on the good limb.

D. Damaged sensory nerves

1. **Wide-based gait.** Dorsal column or cerebellar disease decreases balance because the body no longer knows its spatial position. To compensate, the patient will widen her stance or gait to lower the center of gravity.

TABLE 28-2. Interpretation of the Tier I Neurology Examination.

Finding	Interpretation	Tier II Follow-up
Step 1: Observe the patient's gait		
Festination and propulsion	Parkinsonian gait	
Magnetic gait	Normal pressure hydrocephalus	
Scissor gait	Spastic paraplegia	
Steppage gait	Peroneal nerve damage	
Waddling or circumduction	Weak gluteal muscles or hip injury	
Limping	Damaged joints	Tier II orthopedic examination
Wide-based gait	Dorsal column or cerebellar disease	Tier II sensory and balance examinations
	Cerebellar or vestibular dysfunction	Tier II balance examination
Hyperesthesia gait	Peripheral neuropathy	Tier II sensation examination Tier II weakness examination
Step 2: Assess the health of muscles	Nerve damage	
	Myositis	Drug history Electrolytes Thyroid testing
Step 3: Assess limb strength against resistance		Tier II weakness examination
Step 5: Assess sensation		Tier II sensory examination
Step 6: Assess reflexes		
Increased reflexes	Upper motor neuron disease	Tier II weakness examination
Decreased reflexes	Lower motor neuron disease	Tier II weakness examination

a. **Sensory dysfunction or dorsal column disease.** The cerebellum is normal but receives no input from the limbs. To compensate for this lack of sensory input, the patient **slaps the feet down** to obtain increased sensory input. This is much worse with the eyes closed, because the patient can no longer use visual input to compensate for a lack of proprioceptive input.

b. **Cerebellar or vestibular dysfunction.** The gait is the same as with sensory/dorsal column disease, except that the gait is equally bad with the eyes open or closed (increased visual input does not help if the cerebellum cannot process the information).

2. **Hyperesthesia gait** is the gait of sensory neuropathy. The soles of the feet are so painful that the patient acts as if he or she were walking on hot coals or broken glass. See Chapter 34 for the causes of sensory neuropathy.

E. **Psychiatric disease.** The hysterical gait is characterized by wide swings alternating from left to right. A patient who walks down a hallway alternately hits both sides of the wall. In contrast, a patient with cerebellar damage will consistently deviate to one side of the hall (i.e., to the same side as the lesion).

> **HOT KEY** The patient who is malingering tends to lurch from the hips, maintaining enough control so that he does not fall until he means to. In contrast, the patient with a cerebellar abnormality lurches from the knees.

III STEP 2: ASSESS THE HEALTH OF THE MUSCLES

A. **Observation.** The Tier I examination ensures that the muscles are healthy. Any loss of neural innervation of a muscle will result in muscle fasciculations (wormlike movements of the muscle) and atrophy. Examine all muscles for atrophy and fasciculations.

B. **Palpation.** Myositis is inflammation of the muscles (e.g., viral infection, drug reactions, polymyositis); myopathy is abnormal function of the muscles not due to inflammation (e.g., electrolyte abnormalities, thyroid disease). Look at the patient's face as you palpate: grimacing in response to palpation suggests a tender muscle. Tender muscles suggest myositis; weak muscles without tenderness suggest myopathy.

IV STEP 3: ASSESS LIMB STRENGTH AGAINST RESISTANCE

A. Ask the patient to have a seat on the examination table. If the patient is already on a gurney, ask him to sit with his legs to the side of the bed. Inability to sit will give you an idea of his axial strength.

The examination can be completed with the patient lying in bed, but it will be less sensitive.

B. Always allow the patient to get the muscle in maximum contraction (flexion or extension) before testing strength. Overcoming resistance at rest may be impossible for even a normal muscle because the resting muscle is at a disadvantageous angle.

C. Assess the upper extremity.

1. Biceps strength. Ask the patient to "make a muscle" (flex the elbow). Once flexed, support the back of the patient's humerus with your left hand, and pull down on the distal forearm with your right (just like pulling a lever).
2. Triceps strength. Hold the back of the patient's humerus with your left hand; place your right hand on his distal forearm. Ask the patient to flex his elbow to 90 degrees and then try to extend the elbow while you oppose this movement.
3. Hand grip. Place two fingers in the patient's hand and ask him to squeeze as tight as he can. Using two fingers is important; if you insert one or three, you will get hurt. Also watch for the patient wearing rings; these hurt too.

D. Assess the lower extremity.

1. Quadriceps strength. If the patient is sitting, ask her to lift her knee off the bed or chair and hold it there. Push down on the distal femur toward the bed or chair and ask the patient to resist your pressure.
2. Hip flexors. If the patient is sitting, ask her to again raise her knee off the bed and hold it there. With both hands, reach under the distal femur and support the leg. Ask the patient to push down while you oppose this push.

E. Use the 5-point scale in Table 28-3 to grade strength.

TABLE 28-3. Grading Muscle Strength.

Grade	Muscle Action
0	No movement at all
1	Muscle flickering, but no limb movement
2	Can overcome gravity (i.e., move the extremity) but not much else
3	Good function, but examiner resistance easily overcomes movement
4	Equal strength between movement and examiner resistance
5 (Normal)	Overcomes examiner resistance

A + or − is sometimes added before the grade to designate slightly more or less than the stated grade.

> **HOT KEY** Break-away weakness (good strength suddenly followed by no strength) is always factitious.
> Subjective weakness not confirmed by objective weakness is not always malingering. Polymyalgia rheumatica and Giant Cell Arteritis are diseases of the elderly characterized by this pattern.

V STEP 4: ASSESS SENSATION

A. The Tier I sensory examination is very brief, assessing only light touch. If you notice a deficit, or if the patient complains of loss of or abnormal sensation, perform the full Tier II sensory examination (see Chapter 34).

B. Start at the feet and work superiorly. Stand so that the patient cannot see your touch. Press lightly, asking him if he feels your touch. If you detect a deficit, perform the Tier II examination in Chapter 34.

C. **Expanded Tier I Examination: Pain and Temperature Assessment.** To assess pain and temperature fibers, use a safety pin (always a different safety pin for each patient) or a broken tongue-depressor to touch the skin. With your body, block the patient's view of the pin, so he cannot anticipate the prick. Lightly touch the sharp point of the safety pin to the skin, and ask the patient if he feels it. Then act as if you are touching the skin but do not. Again, ask the patient if he feels anything. Repeat this several times, mixing up the sequence of prick–no prick. Do not press too hard, because this stimulates proprioceptive input as well as pain and temperature.

D. **Expanded Tier I Examination: Proprioceptive.** Explain to the patient what you are planning to do. Raise the toe superiorly and tell the patient that this is "up." Push the toe inferiorly and tell the patient this is "down." Position yourself so that the patient cannot see your movements. Alternately raise or lower the toe, asking the patient each time which direction you are moving the toe.

E. Diabetic patients should have regular assessment of proprioception to detect early peripheral neuropathy (see Chapter 34).

VI STEP 5: ASSESS REFLEXES

A. The key to eliciting reflexes is to find the tendon for that muscle. For example, ask the patient to maximally flex her elbow and feel for the biceps tendon. Keep your thumb on it; tell her to relax her arm. Tap your reflex hammer (or the head of your stethoscope) on your thumb. On larger tendons (such as the knee or Achilles), tap the stethoscope directly upon the tendon.

B. Start at the foot and work up. Use the 1-2, 3-4, 5-6, 7-8 rule to survey the reflexes (Table 28-4).

C. Use the scale in Table 28-5 to grade reflexes.

TABLE 28-4. Key Reflexes and Their Associated Nerve Roots.

Spinal Root	Reflex	How to Perform the Exam
S1/S2	Ankle reflex	Ask the patient to "press down on the gas" with his foot slightly. Tap on the Achilles tendon.
L3/L4	Knee reflex	Let the lower leg dangle off of the table. If the patient is in bed, lift the upper leg so that the knee is at 45-degree flexion. Tap on the lower patellar tendon.
C5/C6	Biceps reflex	Ask the patient to maximally flex his elbow and feel for the biceps tendon. Keep your thumb on it. Tap your reflex hammer on your thumb.
C7/C8	Triceps reflex	Ask the patient to stand with his arms like a scarecrow (humerus straight out; elbows at 90 degrees so that the forearms point to the floor).

D. Important rules about reflexes:

1. If the patient anticipates your strike, the reflex will be blunted. Tell her you are going to count to three, and then tap. Tap on two.
2. You cannot call an absence of reflexes until you have evoked the Jurdasic maneuver. Ask the patient to clench her fists or jaw. This tension will heighten all reflexes in the body.

E. Interpreting reflexes.

TABLE 28-5. Grading Reflexes.

Grade	Muscle Action
0	There is no movement at all.
1	The muscle twitches. The limb does not move.
2	The limb moves.
3	The limb moves. Other muscles not involved in the reflex arc also move as the energy from the reflex arc spills over into neighboring anterior horn cells.
4	Clonus. The limb moves and keeps moving.

A + or − is sometimes added before the grade to designate slightly more or less than the stated grade.

1. Increased reflexes are due to an upper motor neuron lesion (from the brain to the anterior horn of the spinal cord). Inhibitory neurons run along upper motor neurons, dampening the reflex arc. When destroyed, the inhibition is lost. Stroke, multiple sclerosis, spinal cord trauma, and spinal cord mass are the most common etiologies.
2. Decreased reflexes are due to either anterior horn disease (polio) or peripheral neuropathy (see Chapter 34).
3. Assessing reflexes are predominately used to assess the cause of weakness (see Chapter 34).

PART IV

Tier II Physical Examination

29. The Tier II Head and Neck Examination

I THE BIG PICTURE

A Tier II head and neck examination should be performed on patients who have specific head and neck–related complaints.

The 10 common complaints of the head and neck include the following:

A. Facial trauma and epistaxis
B. Headache
C. Hearing loss
D. Ear pain
E. Diplopia
F. Eye pain
G. Abnormal vision
H. Rhinitis
I. Mouth pain
J. Mass in the neck or jaw

II FACIAL TRAUMA AND EPISTAXIS

A. All head and neck trauma should begin with an assessment of a possible cervical neck fracture. When there is very low suspicion for a fracture, a cervical spine fracture can be excluded by the absence of spinal tenderness with palpation. If there is moderate suspicion, however, cervical neck radiographs should supersede the examination. All of the maneuvers in this chapter require manipulation of the head, which can displace a neck fracture, leading to paralysis.

B. Facial trauma. Make sure that no vital structures have been broken.

1. **Ask the patient to close her jaw tightly.** The teeth should align. If not, the jaw may be broken or dislocated. Radiographic films will confirm the diagnosis.
2. **Look in the nose.** Make sure the septum is not deviated so that it obstructs one of the nares. Ask the patient if she can breathe

out of the nose while occluding one nostril at a time. If the septum is not obstructing the nare, a broken nose is of cosmetic importance only. Surgical correction can be performed electively. Cerebrospinal fluid draining from the nose or the external ear suggests a basilar skull fracture. This fluid is clear and, unlike nasal drainage, is high in glucose (it tests positive for glucose on a urine dipstick).

3. **Carefully examine the extraocular muscles.** An orbital floor fracture (as might occur with a blow to maxilla) can trap the inferior rectus muscle. If not surgically released, the eye will be permanently damaged. Stabilize the patient's head by grasping her chin with your left hand. Ask her to follow your right index finger as you slowly move it to all four quadrants. Pay attention to the patient's chin in your left hand. If she is having difficulty following your finger with her extraocular muscles, you will feel her head move against your hand. Watch for inattention. If the patient's attention wanes, bring her back to task by snapping your fingers as you move your hand.
4. **Evaluate visual acuity.** Damage to the eye, including posterior vitreous or anterior chamber bleeding, may not be apparent on the first presentation. Both types of bleeding affect visual acuity, however, which is the key to making the timely diagnosis (see VIII below).
5. **Examine the zygomatic arches.** These bridges along the lateral face are highly susceptible to injury. A fracture will result in tenderness along the bone and jaw malalignment. Surgical correction is required.
6. **Look in the external auditory canals.** Sufficient forward force can dislodge the jaw into the external auditory canal. Blood will be apparent in the canal if this has occurred.
7. **Look for loose or dislocated teeth,** which pose a risk for aspiration.
8. **Know what to expect.** Swelling of the eye and subconjunctival hemorrhage (homogenous redness of the white of the eye) are expected findings following trauma to the face. Black eyes (raccoon eyes) or Battle's sign (blood behind the ear) usually occurs 24 to 48 hours after the injury. If either sign is apparent in acute trauma, suspect that the trauma has occurred at least once previously. Be highly suspicious of domestic abuse in all patients with facial trauma. Examine the patient in the absence of the partner.

C. **Epistaxis.** There are two types of nosebleeds. Anterior nosebleeds can be imminently treated; posterior nosebleeds require otolaryngology consultation.

1. **Anterior nosebleeds** are due to trauma of the turbinates; nosepicking is the most common etiology. Bleeding is primarily

through the nares, not into the pharynx; it is possible to touch the source of the bleeding with a cotton-tipped swab. Thus, the nosebleed is amenable to anterior packing. To treat an anterior nosebleed, tell the patient to blow her nose. The residual clot continues to irritate the lesion, perpetuating the bleeding. Then tape two tongue depressors together to form a pincher. Maximally extend the patient's head, and place the pincher on the nose.

2. **Posterior nosebleeds** are usually due to medical diseases such as hypertension or a bleeding diathesis. Call otolaryngology immediately; because the lesion is out of reach of direct compression, posterior packing will be required.

III HEADACHE

Because the etiologies of headache have similar and nondescript presentations, the best method is to consider each cause of headache by considering each layer of tissue, from the brain to the skin. Start with the vessels in the brain and work outward: consider the subarachnoid space, the meninges, the subdural space, the epidural space, the skull, the muscles, and finally the skin. The brain does not have sensory fibers of its own. Headache from the brain occurs only when it is forced against the skull wall or when the sensory fibers around intracerebral vessels are distended.

A. **Migraine headaches.** These headaches result from abnormal constriction of a vessel, followed by hyperdilation that distends pain fibers. They usually occur on the side of the head corresponding to the side of the distended vessel (hence the name, "hemi-cranium," or "mi-cranium"). Onset is sudden (minutes to hours), and duration may range from hours to days. Triggers include stress or substances that cause vasoconstriction (e.g., caffeine, chocolate). The first onset of migraines usually occurs before 21 years of age; there is a close association with motion sickness as a child. Headaches that begin after the age of 21 are more likely to be nonmigraine types of headache. Vasoconstrictive medications (e.g., ergotamine, sumatriptan) are used to treat migraine.

1. The classic migraine is preceded by an aura that corresponds to the location of the constricted vessel. Common auras include flashing lights, abnormal sensation, or motor deficits.
2. The common migraine has no aura, only pain.
3. The complicated migraine is associated with neurologic deficits (e.g., Bell's palsy) that resolve as the headache resolves.
4. Catamenial migraines are associated with menses.
5. The "ice cream" headache is similar to a migraine in that it results from cerebral vasoconstriction followed by vasodilation due to excessive cold stimulation of the carotid receptors in the back of the throat.

B. Cluster headaches. These headaches occur in clusters; a patient may have several headaches in a 2-week period and then no headaches for several months. Affected patients usually are 30- to 50-year-old men. Retro-orbital pain associated with unilateral tearing is characteristic. Oxygen often helps.

C. Tumor headaches. These headaches are caused by increased cerebral pressure from the tumor in the brain. Onset is insidious, occurring over months as the tumor enlarges. The headaches are worse in the morning (lying down at night increases pressure in the head) and with increased intracerebral pressure (e.g., coughing, sneezing). They are associated with nausea and vomiting and occasionally focal neurologic deficits.

D. Headaches due to brain hemorrhage

1. **Subarachnoid hemorrhage** is due to a rupture of an intracerebral arterial aneurysm into the subarachnoid space. Patients will describe the headache as "the worst headache of my life." The headache is sudden; the pressure from the bleed may cause herniation of the brain and neurologic deficits.
2. **Subdural hemorrhage** is due to shearing of veins overlying the brain following head trauma. Alcoholics and the elderly are particularly at risk because cerebral atrophy allows the brain to bounce within the skull with even minor head trauma, shearing surface veins on the brain. Reduced cognition is common and may be the only presenting complaint. Neurologic deficits are rare, because there is a limit to brain compression: intracerebral pressure tamponades the low-pressure venous bleeding.
3. **Epidural hemorrhage** is due to rupture of the middle meningeal artery as it is displaced from its groove in the temporal bone. The diagnosis is usually obvious: temporal bone trauma will be described in the history, and there will be a displaced skull fracture along the temporal bone. Characteristically, the patient loses consciousness as a result of the acute concussion, then regains consciousness (the lucid interval), and then gradually loses consciousness again as the arterial bleed gradually compresses the brain. The diagnosis must be made during the lucid interval, because brain herniation and death will result during the arterial compression of the brain. A patient with a concussion who begins to lose consciousness must be immediately reevaluated.

E. Meningeal headaches. There are four types of meningitis: bacterial, aseptic drug, aseptic viral, and cancer. Ask the patient to touch the chin to the chest. This stretches the meningeal lining of the brain, worsening the pain. The inability to touch the chin to the chest suggests meningitis (meningismus).

1. **Kernig's sign.** Have the patient lie flat on the bed and flex the hip. This stretches the meninges; a patient with meningitis will raises his head off the bed to reduce this stretch.

2. **Brudzinski's sign.** With the patient lying flat on the bed, have her flex her neck. This stretches the meninges; a patient with meningitis will flex her hips to reduce the meningeal stretch.
3. **Jolt-acceleration.** Facing the patient, rapidly turn his head side to side (make sure you have excluded spinal trauma) for 30 seconds. Progressively increasing pain indicates meningitis.

HOT

KEY

Meningitis with cranial nerve abnormalities should prompt suspicion for either tuberculous meningitis or carcinomatous meningitis (meningeal carcinoma), because both diseases favor the base of the brain, where cranial nerves exit.

F. Headaches originating in the skull and neck

1. **Sinus headaches.** These headaches are often associated with upper respiratory tract infections. They may be accompanied by purulent nasal discharge, sinusoidal tenderness to palpation, and maxillary toothache.
2. **Mastoiditis.** This condition is infection (sinusitis) of the mastoid sinuses. As with frontal sinusitis, the danger is extension via venous drainage to the brain. The mastoids may be tender to palpation.
3. **Posttraumatic headache.** See II A.

HOT

KEY

Never flex the patient's neck if a neck fracture is suspected.

G. Headaches originating in the muscles, subdermal vessels, and skin

1. **Tension headaches.** These headaches occur in response to neck strain or stress, usually at the end of the day when stress has been maximal. The neck muscles begin at the posterior neck and insert over the top of the head. The pattern of pain follows this course, radiating from the neck over the top of the head. The neck muscles may be tender to palpation.
2. **Inflammatory headaches.** Temporal arteritis is also known as giant cell arteritis and is often associated with polymyalgia rheumatica; it is predominately a disease of the elderly. This vasculitis of the temporal artery is characterized by headache and a dull jaw pain with chewing (jaw claudication). Without immediate treatment, the vasculitis will limit blood flow to the anterior ophthalmic artery, and vision will be lost. A new-onset headache in an elderly patient should raise suspicion for giant cell arteritis. This is one of the few diagnoses in which a sedimentation rate

is useful, because it will be elevated in temporal arteritis and meningitis, but not in other causes of headache.

3. **Herpetic headache.** Herpes zoster/shingles is due to varicella virus that is reactivated in the dermatomal nerve root. Pain begins as the virus migrates along the sensory nerve root. The headache may precede the appearance of vesicles by a day or two. If cranial nerve V (ophthalmic branch) is affected (e.g., vesicles on or around the eyes or the tip of the nose), the patient must receive intravenous acyclovir to prevent involvement of the cornea. Ramsay-Hunt syndrome is involvement of cranial nerve VII, resulting in pain around the external ear and facial paralysis. In both cases, the headache is one-sided (only one nerve is involved) and the skin is exquisitely sensitive to light palpation.

Hearing Loss

The ear receives sound vibrations through the external auditory canal. Sound is received by the tympanic membrane and amplified by the bones of the middle ear (conduction system), and passed to the cochlea, which converts the vibration to a nueral impulse, and then to CN VIII and the brain (nervous system). To determine the type of hearing loss, follow sound from its source and work inward.

A. **External ear.** Look in the external ear for cerumen impaction or foreign bodies. Start with the good ear if possible, because this will establish the appearance of normal for this patient. When examining the left ear, hold the otoscope with the left hand and pull the pinna posteriorly with the right hand to straighten the external auditory canal. Reverse the roles of your hands when examining the right ear.

HOT
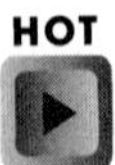
KEY

If cerumen is obstructing the ear canal, remove the needle from an IV catheter and attach the needleless-catheter to a 10-ml syringe. Insert the catheter into the ear (no farther than one third of the way into the external canal) and repeatedly flush with a mixture of hydrogen peroxide and normal saline until the cerumen is removed. Do not try to remove the cerumen with a cotton swab; this will only pack the cerumen deeper in the ear.

HOT

KEY

The most common foreign body found in the ear is an insect (e.g., small cockroach). If discovered, flood the ear with viscous lidocaine and then rinse. The lidocaine will paralyze the insect.

B. **Findings on examination of the tympanic membrane (TM).** The normal TM resembles a transparent sail; pressure variations (e.g., from sound waves) cause it to move back and forth. The pressure behind the TM causes the center to bulge slightly toward the examiner, forming a subtle cone. The light from the otoscope bounces to all sides of the cone, creating a slight light reflex.

1. Perforation appears as a visible hole in the TM.
2. Vesicles on the TM indicate bullous myringitis, which is due to a mycoplasma infection.
3. Erythema of the TM suggests otitis media, an infection of the middle ear (behind the TM). Obstruction of the eustachian tubes traps oral anaerobic bacteria in this enclosed space, leading to infection. This is common in children because their eustachian tubes are floppy, having not fully developed, leading to obstruction. The crying child is an important confounder, because this will increase blood flow to the TM, creating the appearance of erythema. In this case, use an insufflation device (a bulb attached to the otoscope) to pulse air into the external auditory canal. The TM will move freely if the erythema is due to crying; the pressure behind the TM (in otitis media) will prevent the TM from moving with insufflation. In most cases of otitis media, decongestants and antibiotics are indicated.
4. A completely white TM is caused by pus behind the TM. This condition is indicative of purulent otitis media, and antibiotics and decongestants are indicated.
5. Noninfected fluid trapped behind the TM indicates serous otitis. Decongestants open the eustachian tube and drain the fluid; antibiotics are not required.

C. **Middle ear bones to the cochlea.** The two components of hearing are **conduction** from the external auditory canal to the cochlea and **nerve transmission** from the cochlea to the brainstem.

1. **Weber test.** This test is useful if the patient describes *one* ear with decreased hearing. Ask the patient to identify which ear has the hearing deficit. This test distinguishes a conduction deficit from a neural deficit. Strike a tuning fork and place it on the center of the top of the head. Ask the patient in which ear he feels the vibration the greatest.
   a. If the bad ear feels the vibration greater than the good ear, the hearing deficit is due to a conduction deficit. In this case, the conduction failure (e.g., a plugged external auditory canal, a damaged TM, damaged ear bones) reduces external sound; the ear focuses entirely on the bone vibration. (You can try this on yourself; plug one ear with your finger and then hum. The plugged ear will feel the vibration from the hum greater than the open ear).
   b. If the good ear feels the vibration greater than the bad ear, the hearing loss is due to a nerve defect: the bad ear cannot detect the vibration.
2. **Rinne test.** This test is reserved for patients who have a hearing deficit in <u>both</u> ears. Strike the tuning fork and place the single end on the mastoid process (behind the ear). The vibration will

bypass the conduction system and go straight to the cochlea. Place the forked part of the tuning fork next to the external ear. Ask the patient which sounds stronger. Although solids conduct vibration better than air, the amplification system of the normal ear (middle ear bones) makes air conduction (AC) greater than bone conduction (BC). This pattern (AC > BC) is preserved unless the amplification system is damaged, in which case the pattern is reverse (BC > AC).

   a. If the problem is due to a conduction deficit, bone conduction will be greater than air conduction (BC > AC). The tuning fork on the mastoid will be felt greater than the tuning fork next to the external ear.

   b. If the problem is due to a nerve deficit, the normal pattern is preserved, but at a lower level of volume (AC > BC).

3. **Patient speech.** The other clue to the cause of the hearing loss is listening to the patient talk. If the patient has a conduction deficit, she will still sense the volume of her voice through bone conduction as she speaks. Her voice volume will be normal. If she has a nerve deficit, however, she cannot determine the loudness of his voice and will usually speak very loudly.

 V EAR PAIN

Begin with the external ear and work inward.

A. Pinna. Erythema of the external ear is due to one of three conditions:

1. **Cauliflower ear.** Trauma to the ear (e.g., from wrestling) causes a hematoma between the cartilage and the skin. There is little to be done for chronic cauliflower ear, but an acute hematoma should be drained to avoid damage to the cartilage.
2. **Malignant external otitis.** This rare and dangerous bacterial infection can be seen in patients with diabetes mellitus because of impaired immune function. The patient will present with pain involving the external ear (as in external otitis [swimmer's ear; see later discussion]), with tenderness to palpation of the mastoid process. It can progress to the brain and possibly result in death.
3. **Relapsing polychondritis.** In this rare autoimmune disease, the body destroys its own cartilage. The key finding is involvement of other cartilaginous structures, such as a saddle nose (a dip in the upper bridge of the nose) and softening of the larynx (soft voice, choking following swallowing of food). Early steroid therapy is important to prevent tracheomalacia (softening of the trachea) and respiratory obstruction.

B. External otitis (swimmer's ear) causes erythema and tenderness in the external auditory canal. Topical antibiotics and steroids are the therapy.

C. Tympanic membrane (see the discussion in IV B).

D. Middle ear (see the discussion in IV C).

E. Inner ear (cochlea) infections are usually viral and painless. The usual symptom is vertigo (the room spinning) (see Chapter 34).

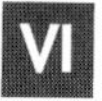

DIPLOPIA (DOUBLE VISION) Eye examination involves the inspection of the extraocular muscles. Diplopia, a disorder of the extraocular muscles, is caused by neuromuscular disease, a mass behind the eye (fungus, tumor), or swelling of the extraocular muscles as occurs in Graves' disease.

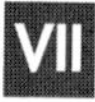

EYE PAIN Eye pain originates from the periocular structures or the eye itself.

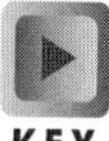

Always have a low threshold for ophthalmology consultation for vision loss or eye pain. Vision loss is a devastating problem with long-term effects on quality of life.

A. **Exclude periocular causes of eye pain or redness.**
   1. **Blepharitis** is inflammation of the eyelids. Most cases can be treated with gentle scrubs with a baby shampoo. Pubic lice can also affect the eyelids, because the hair caliber is the same as that of pubic hair. Look carefully at the lashes for pubic lice.
   2. **Hordeolum** (sty) is a plugged eyelash follicle. This is treated with warm compresses; drainage is usually not required.
   3. **Preseptal or orbital cellulitis** is infection of the skin and structures surrounding the eye, causing pain with eye movement. In addition to intravenous antibiotics, emergency consultation with an ophthalmologist is required.

B. **Approach the eye layer by layer.**
   1. **Conjunctivitis** causes dilatation of the conjunctival vessels (i.e., the bloodshot eye). See Chapter 23 for how to distinguish the causes.
   2. **Subconjunctival hemorrhages** cause homogeneous, painless redness of the eyes (see Chapter 23).
   3. **Corneal abrasions** are common with contact lenses, trauma, or foreign bodies in the eye. The patient will present with redness of the eye, pain, and a sensation of a retained foreign body. The foreign body is frequently absent; the sensation comes from the abrasion. Nevertheless, evert the eyelid with a cotton-tipped swab to make sure that no foreign body is present.
      a. Place the swab just above small cartilage strip at the edge of the eyelid, and grasp the eyelashes and pull up. The eyelid will roll over the swab. Ask the patient to look down during the procedure to prevent counterproductive eyelid contractions.
      b. Fluorescein reveals any abrasions. Touch the strip of fluorescein (orange strip) on the inner surface of the lower eyelid. Ask the patient to blink a few times. Darken the room and look at the eye with a Wood's lamp (black light). An abrasion

holds the fluorescein and reveals itself as a yellow line. Abrasions on the front of the cornea or stellate abrasions (starlike, suggesting herpes) require immediate ophthalmologic evaluation, because improper healing can lead to corneal scarring and blindness. Other abrasions can be treated conservatively with antibiotic ointment and an eye patch. Do not give the patient anesthetic eye drops, because this will mask worsening eye pain that warrants immediate reevaluation.

   c. Consult an ophthalmologist immediately for all welding injuries. The heat of the particles and the speed of impact can penetrate the front of the eye, depositing the metal fragment in the posterior chamber.

4. **Pingueculum** and **pterygium** are fibrotic streaks on the eye surface resulting from previous trauma or exposure to ultraviolet light. Surgical removal is possible if vision is affected.
5. **Chemosis** (see Chapter 23)
6. **Iritis** is inflammation of the iris. Shining a light in the patient's eye causes pupillary constriction and increased pain.
   a. Iritis is inflammation of the iris that usually results from antibody-antigen complexes becoming trapped in the anterior chamber of the eye (i.e., the anterior chamber is a filter). Chronic infections that cause an antibody-antigen complex (e.g., syphilis, tuberculosis, certain viruses) or rheumatologic disease may lead to iritis.
   b. If the inflammation is long-standing, fibrosis may lock the pupil in position (nonreactive) and form an irregular appearance.
7. **Anterior uveititis** is inflammation of the anterior chamber due to accumulation of antibodies in this space. On slit-lamp examination, the inflammatory material will make the anterior chamber appear opaque (known as "cell and flare").
8. **Hyphema** is pooled blood in the anterior chamber, usually following trauma to the eye.
9. **Hypopyon** is similar to hyphema, but it is pus that causes a milky-white layer of fluid in front of the iris.
10. **Glaucoma** is increased pressure in the eye. The increased pressure in the eye opposes the vascular blood pressure that is supplying the eye structures, leading to ischemia and blindness.

HOT
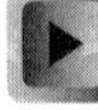
KEY

Make it a practice to screen for glaucoma. Refer anyone with a family history of glaucoma to an ophthalmologist.

   a. Narrow-angle glaucoma
      (1) The anterior chamber fluid is created behind the iris and then travels in front of the lens, through the pupil, to the

anterior segment, where it is reabsorbed. The iris separates the anterior from the posterior chambers; narrow-angle glaucoma is narrowing of the passage between these two chambers.

(2) When the angle acutely closes, pressure in the posterior chamber builds quickly, causing pain, erythema, and, due to a vagal response, abdominal pain and vomiting. This angle closure also holds the pupil in a fixed midposition. This is an ophthalmologic emergency; consult an ophthalmologist immediately.

b. **Open-angle glaucoma**

(1) Pressure builds because drainage of anterior fluid is obstructed. Over time, the increased pressure on the retina obliterates vascular flow, leading to retinal ischemia and blindness.

(2) The smallest vessels furthest away from the cup/disc (where vascular flow originates) are squeezed shut first. Visual loss, therefore, begins at the periphery of the retina and works inward, leading to tunnel vision. Open-angle glaucoma is painless, and unless you screen for it, you are unlikely to make the diagnosis until the eye is beyond recovery.

VIII ABNORMAL VISION

Consider this as a process by which light travels through the layers of the eye, one layer at a time.

A. **Assess the patient's visual acuity.** This is the most important part of the examination.

1. Visual acuity is expressed in terms of OD, OS, or OU. OD refers to the right eye, OS refers to the left eye, and OU refers to both eyes. A score is given for each eye or, if the score is the same for both eyes, one score is given.
2. The patient should stand 20 feet from the vision chart.
3. The top number (e.g., "20" from a score of 20/100) is the distance at which the patient can read the top letter on the chart; the bottom number (e.g., "100" in the example above) is the distance at which a patient with normal visual acuity can read the same letter.

B. **Inspect the cornea.** Corneal scarring or damage refracts light, but allows it to pass, resulting in blurry vision.

C. **Inspect the anterior chamber.** Anterior uveitis. Light passes but is refracted as it passes (blurry vision) (see VII B 7).

D. **Inspect the vitreous chamber.** Few diseases affect the posterior chamber. The most common are:

1. **Bleeding in the vitreous chamber** from a detached retina. Severely myopic patients are at risk for this, because the oval eyeball puts tension on the retina. A sudden scintillating flash of light with visual loss suggests the diagnosis.

2. **Floaters** are tiny pieces of retinal tissue that have broken free and float in the vitreous fluid. Patients complain of "a spot" in their vision that persists even with eye movement.

E. **Inspect the retina.** A vision of scintillating light (similar to what you "see" when you close your eye and rub it repeatedly) suggests sudden retinal disease. To perform a retinal examination, always dilate both eyes. An undilated examination has poor sensitivity.

1. **Using a standard ophthalmoscope**
   - **a.** Darken the room.
   - **b.** Place an "X" on the wall about 7 feet from the floor so the patient gazes slightly superiorly.
   - **c.** Look through the ophthalmoscope and focus (at 6 inches away) on the wrinkles of your palm. Turn the dial on the scope until the lines are clear. Note the number at the bottom of the scope. This will be your number for all eye examinations.
   - **d.** Place the ophthalmoscope so the top of it rests flush against your eyebrow. When it is fixed to your eyebrow, it should not move at all, allowing you to make very fine adjustments while looking at the retina by moving your head slightly.
   - **e.** On the ophthalmoscope, turn down the dial for the light to its lowest level. The back of the eye is dark. You will not need much light, because it causes pupillary constriction to oppose your efforts.
   - **f.** Stand in front and a few feet from the patient at a 30-degree angle. Look through the ophthalmoscope with your *medial* eye (i.e., your left eye if you are looking at the patient's left eye) until you see a red reflex from the retina. Looking through your medial eye will keep your from "kissing" the patient when you get close. When you have the red reflex in sight, you are at the proper angle. Follow that angle all the way to the patient's eye.
   - **g.** Before you move in with the ophthalmoscope, place your lateral hand on the patient's forehead with your thumb pointing downward. Place your thumb on the eyelid and lift up. Your hand on the patient's head prevents bumping the scope in her eye, and your thumb prevents blinking.
   - **h.** Move in with the scope. Get very close (a centimeter or less away from the eye). Close the medial part of your mouth and breathe out the lateral side to avoid breathing in the patient's face.

HOT

KEY

You are not going to see the complete view of the retina depicted in the textbooks. Instead, you will only see one circle's worth of the retina. Make fine movements with your head to move around the retina, mentally putting the circle pieces together until you have a total picture of the retina.

2. **Using a panoptic scope**
   a. Darken the room.
   b. Look through the panoptic scope with your medial eye and focus on something 10 feet away. Do not make any further adjustments to the scope. Turn down the light to its lowest level.
   c. Perform all the preceding steps above (VIII E 1 d to h). With the panoptic scope, place the soft rubber cup over the patient's eye.
3. **What to look for:**
   a. Find the blood vessels and follow the direction of their branch points; like little arrows, they point toward the optic cup and optic disc. The optic cup is a small depression of the retina that contains the optic disc, which is the end of the optic nerve. The two appear as yellow circles—one on top of the other. The cup should be three times the size of the disk.
      (1) **Papilledema.** If there is only one circle, the optic nerve has been pushed through the cup toward you by elevated pressure in the brain (cerebral edema).
      (2) **Optic neuritis.** If the disk is enlarged (i.e., the cup-to-disk ratio is less than 3:1), the optic nerve is inflamed and partially moved forward, occupying more space in the optic cup.
      (3) **Glaucoma.** Pressure inside the eye pushes the optic nerve head (the disk) back toward the brain and makes the cup deeper. Some of the veins and arteries originate inside the cup. Normally, these vessels approach the cup and gradually disappear into it. If the cup is deep, the vessels approach the lip of the cup and suddenly disappear. A sharp demarcation of the vessels as they approach the cup suggests glaucoma.
   b. Inspect the retinal veins and arteries.
      (1) A **retinal vein occlusion** causes all the veins to dilate. The retinal veins look like a cluster of worms. "Thunder and lightening" is used to describe a retinal vein occlusion because of its dramatic appearance.
      (2) A **retinal artery occlusion** causes pallor of the retina. The vessels are not apparent. A cherry-red spot represents the artery just to the point of occlusion. The surrounding pallor is a function of the decreased blood flow to the retina.
      (3) Look at the color of the retinal veins and arteries. Normal vessels appear red because the vessel is one tenth vessel wall (white) and nine tenths blood (red). When the vessel wall hypertrophies, there is more white than red. The copper wire appearance of the vessel is due to the hybrid of the white and red. If vessel wall hypertrophy continues,

the vessel becomes mostly white ("silver wire" appearance).

(4) Look for new vessels. The sticky, sugar-coated proteins of diabetes occlude the retinal vessels. This stimulates the retina to grow new vessels (neovascularization).

(5) Look for other abnormalities:

(a) **Flame hemorrhages** are ruptured vessels resulting from hypertension or diabetes mellitus.

(b) **Cotton wool spots** look like little patches of cotton. They represent embolic material (e.g., from endocarditis) that has occluded the vessel.

c. **Macular degeneration** is the most common cause of blindness in the United States. It is difficult to diagnose without benefit of the ophthalmologist's indirect ophthalmoscope. Be aware of it, but do not expect to see in on your direct retinal examination.

F. Inspect the optic nerve. Inflammation of the optic nerve is almost always due to multiple sclerosis (see Chapter 34).

G. Check for visual field defects.

1. Sit 2 feet in front of the patient and ask him to stare at your nose; you stare at his nose.
2. With your arms straight out to your sides and your hands behind your head where you cannot see them, hold up one finger in your left hand and two fingers in your right. Slowly move your hands forward. Ask the patient to tell you when he can first see your fingers and to tell you how many total fingers you have up (right plus left hand).
   a. If the answer is three, the visual fields are normal.
   b. If the answer is four, the right lateral visual field is defective. The patient sees two fingers from your right hand and assumes that your left hand also has two fingers extended.
   c. If the answer is two, the left visual field is defective. The patient sees one finger from your left hand and assumes that your right hand also has one finger extended.
   d. If the answer is zero, both lateral fields are defective.
3. The standard nomenclature for drawing a deficit (i.e., in your admission note) is to black out the part of the circle that the patient does not see. For example, a blacked-out marking of the lateral left circle means that the patient cannot see the lateral world with his left eye. Because light crosses as it enters the eye (i.e., a lateral image is detected on the medial part of the retina), the damaged part of the retina or nerve is *opposite* to what the patient does not see (e.g., in this example, the medial retina of the left eye is damaged). Figure 29-1 will help you localize the deficit.

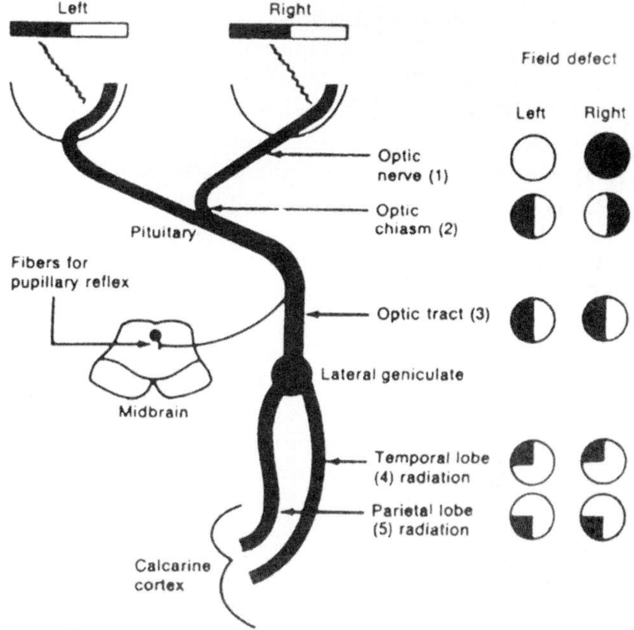

FIGURE 29-1. Visual pathways. (From Weiner HL, Levitt LP, Rae-Grant A: *Neurology*, 6th ed. Philadelphia: Lippincott Williams & Wilkins, 1999.)

IX **RHINITIS** Look in the nose with the nasal speculum. The nose goes straight back into the head, parallel to the floor. Lift the tip of the nose with your finger and insert the nasal scope directly back.

A. Allergic rhinitis. The mucosa of the nose will be pale white.

B. Viral rhinitis. The nasal mucosa is inflamed and red.

C. Bacterial rhinitis or sinusitis. Pus in the nose is suggestive of bacterial sinusitis.

D. Deviated septum. Always look for this condition before inserting nasogastric tubes. Surgical correction is necessary only if it causes chronic sinusitis or airway obstruction (e.g., the patient cannot breath through that nare with the opposite nare occluded).

E. Perforated septum. This condition is commonly seen in cocaine users.

F. Nasal polyps. These appear as fleshy, nontender masses in the nose. They are part of an important triad: asthma, aspirin hypersensitivity, and nasal polyps.

X MOUTH PAIN (see Chapter 23)

A. Oral ulcers
B. Gingivitis
C. Oral cancer

XI MASS IN THE NECK/JAW (see Chapter 23)

A. Lymph nodes
B. Thyroid
C. Mouth cancer

30. The Tier II Lung Examination

I The Big Picture of Consolidation of Lung Tissue

A. The alveoli in the lungs are normally held open by the surfactant on their interior surface. When foreign matter disrupts the surfactant, as occurs with bacterial pneumonia, the normally air-filled alveoli consolidate into a solid mass. For the most part, **consolidation implies pneumonia** (Table 30-1).

B. Alveoli are also kept open by the constant flow of air in and out of these pockets. If this flow stops, as might happen with bronchial obstruction, the alveoli may collapse and consolidate. **Nonpneumonia causes of consolidation are collectively referred to as atelectasis.** The examination findings are the same as pneumonia (including fever), except the elevated white blood cell count and positive blood and sputum cultures of pneumonia will be absent with atelectasis.

C. The cornerstone of the diagnosis of consolidation is that **sound travels best in solids, moderately well through air, and poorly through liquids.** Sound and vibration from the larynx conduct through consolidated alveoli (solid) better than air-filled alveoli. In contrast, fluid in the pleural space buffers sound and vibration, resulting in diminished palpable and ausculatory findings (Figure 30-1).

II Suspected Consolidation

A. Symptoms that should prompt this Tier II examination. Any symptom of pneumonia (e.g., fever, productive cough, dyspnea) or unexplained hypoxemia should prompt a search for signs of lung consolidation.

B. Tier I findings that should prompt this Tier II examination

1. **Absence of breath sounds.** This can result from a **dense consolidation, pleural effusion,** or **pneumothorax.** The presence of bronchophony, egophony, or whisper pectoriloquy suggest consolidation (see below). The presence of hyperresonance on percussion suggests pneumothorax. The absence of all of these signs suggests effusion.
2. **Bronchophony** is radiation of bronchial (tubular) breath sounds from the bronchi through a consolidation to the periphery of the lung (see Chapter 24).
3. **Crackles** (see Chapter 24). Crackles are due to alveoli "popping open."
   a. **A very dense consolidation may *not* have crackles,** because the density of the consolidation prevents the alveoli from pop-

TABLE 30-1. Diagnosing pneumonia.

- If the vital signs are normal, the probability of pneumonia is very low. The elderly are the exception, because they may not be able to mount the expected fever and tachycardia.
- In diagnosing pneumonia, examination abnormalities usually precede chest radiographic findings by 1 to 2 days.
- It may take 4 weeks for radiographic findings to resolve. Confirm resolution of pneumonia with a physical examination.
- Symptoms of pneumonia (fever, cough, dyspnea) without signs of consolidation on examination make atypical pneumonia (due to *Mycoplasma* or *Chlamydia* infection) more likely, especially if the radiograph is also normal.

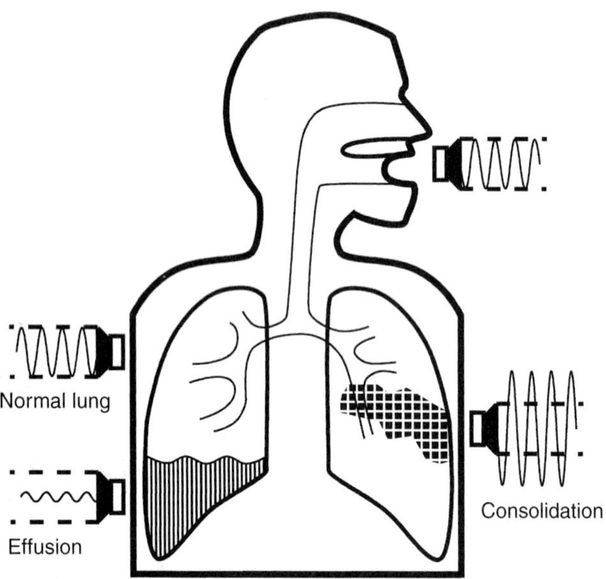

FIGURE 30-1. Sound through consolidation, air, and pleural effusions.

ping open during inspiration to cause the "crackly" sound. The same is true of consolidation distal to an obstructed bronchus (e.g., distal to a cancer).

b. **A less dense consolidation will have crackles,** because bacteria in the alveoli cause the alveolar walls to stick together by disrupting surfactant. The alveoli pop open during inspiration.

c. **Causes of crackles other than consolidation.**
   (1) **Pulmonary edema** (heart failure, fluid overload). Look for other associated signs of heart failure (e.g., S_3, elevated JVP, displaced PMI) (see Chapter 31).
   (2) **Chronic bronchitis.** Look for other signs of chronic obstructive pulmonary disease (COPD) (see IV).
   (3) **Pulmonary fibrosis** (see III). As opposed to other causes of crackles, the crackles of pulmonary fibrosis are **dry-sounding,** like the sound of Velcro being ripped open.

B. Egophony ("E to A changes")

1. Place the diaphragm of the stethoscope over the area where you suspect consolidation. Have the patient say "beee" for 3 seconds. Compare this to a part of the lung you suspect to be normal (Figure 30-2).
2. The "beee" sound created at the larynx is composed of two frequencies: the low-frequency parent tone (sounding like "baaaa")

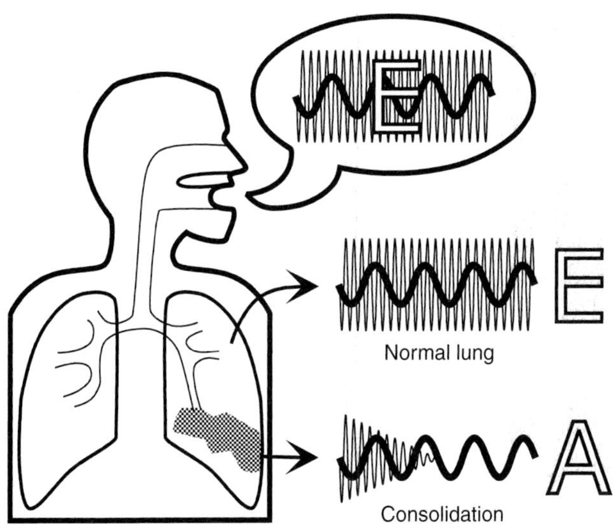

FIGURE 30-2. Egophony.

and high-frequency tones that overlie the parent tone. The combination of the two tones sound like "beee." Through normal lung, both frequencies are transmitted undisturbed, sounding like "beee" at your stethoscope. Consolidated lung tissue absorbs the high-frequency sounds of the "beee," allowing only the low-frequency parent tone ("baaaa") to be transmitted to your stethoscope.

C. Whisper pectoriloquy

1. Place the diaphragm of the stethoscope over the suspected consolidation. Have the patient whisper "sixty-six whiskies please." Compare this to a part of the lung suspected to be normal (Figure 30-3).
2. Normal lung allows transmission of the high-frequency tones that make the words spoken at the larynx sound fuzzy ("sisisis whissies pleze"). Consolidated lung absorbs the high frequencies, resulting in a crisp "sixty-six whiskies please" at your stethoscope. **The consolidation makes the sound *crisper,* not louder.**
3. Whisper pectoriloquy occurs only in dense consolidations. Although it is a good confirmatory test, its **sensitivity is less than 50%.**

D. Fremitus

1. Stand behind the patient and place both of your hands on the chest so that the heels of your hands are in the midclavicular line and your fingers extend around the sides. Ask the patient to say

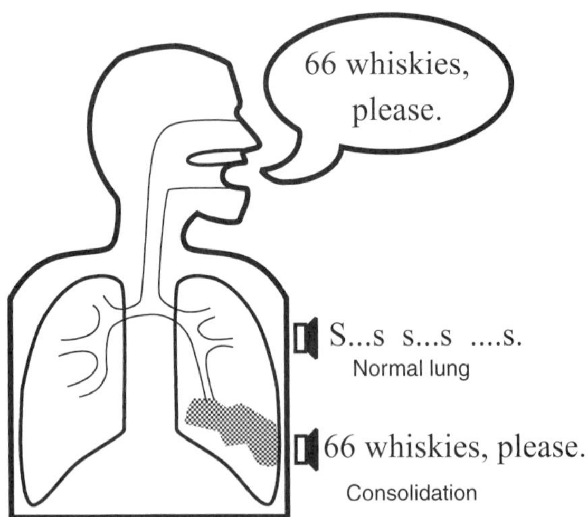

FIGURE 30-3. Whisper pectoriloquy.

"toy boat" or a similar phrase that has multiple vowels. Vowel sounds are phonated in the chest; constants are phonated in the pharynx. The greater the number of vowel sounds in the words you ask the patient to say (e.g., toy boat, Scooby Doo, blue balloons), the greater the vibration in the chest, and the more sensitive the fremitus sign will be.

2. Remember that **consolidated lung tissue** acts like a solid; it **transmits the vibration of the "toy boat" better than normal, air-filled lung tissue.** You feel (**f**remitus is a **f**eel) a stronger vibration over the consolidation.
3. **Compared to egophony and whisper pectoriloquy, fremitus is the least specific finding of consolidation;** the solid mass of the liver, spleen, and heart can cause false positive results. For this reason, **use fremitus only when distinguishing a suspected effusion versus a suspected consolidation** (i.e., when you have found dullness to percussion on your Tier I examination). It is very useful in this setting because effusion (liquid) and consolidation (solid) are on opposite ends of the spectrum with respect to transmitting vibration (see Figure 30-1).

E. All signs of consolidation (crackles, bronchophony, egophony, whisper pectoriloquy, and fremitus) depend on an open bronchus. **If dense consolidation is visible on a radiograph but there are no findings of consolidation, suspect segmental bronchial obstruction due to cancer or a foreign body.**

HOT
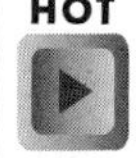
KEY

To best elicit fremitus, ask the patient to say words that have multiple vowels in them, such as "blue balloons." The German phrase "n**eu**n und n**eu**nzig" is also a good example; the English translation "ninety-nine" is not.

II SUSPECTED PLEURAL EFFUSION

Pleural effusion is accumulation of fluid in the pleural space, between the lung parenchyma and the chest wall. Do not confuse pleural effusion with pulmonary edema, which is accumulation of fluid in the interstitial space between the alveoli and the pulmonary capillaries.

A. Sound generated by the larynx is generated in an air medium. **If you listen over a pleural effusion, you do not hear sound,** because the sound generated at the larynx does not penetrate the effusion but rather bounces off the air–fluid interface. This applies to all sounds, including egophony, bronchophony, and whisper pectoriloquy.

B. There is no fremitus over a pleural effusion for the same reason. The vibration from the larynx bounces off and does not penetrate the effusion; you feel no vibration. In fact, the normal side of the lung has a *greater* vibration than the effusion.

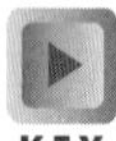

HOT KEY: Consolidation amplifies vibration, and effusion suppresses vibration. Fremitus is therefore very useful in distinguishing effusion from consolidation.

C. Physical findings in pleural effusion

1. Dullness to percussion
2. No breath sounds
3. No egophony, bronchophony, or whisper pectoriloquy
4. No fremitus (no vibration)

D. Skodaic resonance. A very large pleural effusion may compress the portion of the lung just above the effusion. Be aware of this; this 2-inch strip of compressed lung may exhibit all the findings of consolidation (e.g., crackles). The diagnosis is made by finding signs of effusion below the consolidation (see II C).

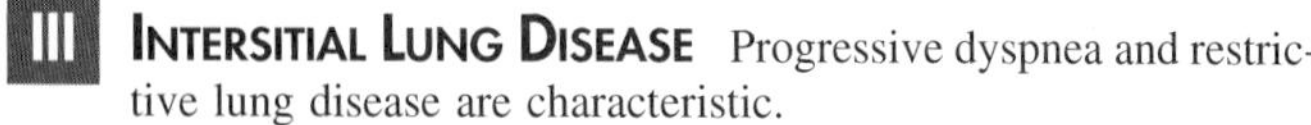

III INTERSITIAL LUNG DISEASE Progressive dyspnea and restrictive lung disease are characteristic.

A. The fibrosis between the alveoli and capillaries may compress the alveoli during exhalation. During inspiration, these alveoli may pop open, creating a **dry crackle** (see Figure 24-4).

B. Although the interstitial fibers do not represent a consolidation, thousands of these fibers act like fiberoptic cables, transmitting sound vibrations to the periphery of the lung as if it were a consolidation.

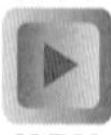

HOT KEY: Egophony heard at all areas of the lung suggests interstitial pulmonary fibrosis.

IV GENERAL FEATURES OF OBSTRUCTIVE LUNG DISEASE Healthy terminal bronchioles normally remain open during exhalation so alveolar air (rich in CO_2) can empty. As the chest wall contracts, positive pressure is put on the alveoli, pushing the air out of the lungs. There are four ways that this can be impaired:

A. Terminal bronchioles are damaged and become floppy. The increased thoracic pressure pinches them closed, trapping air in the alveoli (emphysema).

B. Terminal bronchioles become plugged with secretions (chronic bronchitis).

C. Musculature of these bronchioles is hyperactive, causing them to spasm and close the bronchiole (asthma).

D. Interstitial pressure compresses the terminal bronchioles (congestive heart failure; see Chapter 31).

V SUSPECTED AIRFLOW OBSTRUCTION

A. **The wheeze.** The most diagnostic finding in obstructive lung disease is the wheeze, which results from the floppy bronchiolar walls vibrating as expiratory air passes (see Chapter 24). Common causes of wheezing include:

1. **Emphysema and chronic bronchitis.** Long-term smoking destroys the terminal bronchial walls, making them floppy. High intrathoracic pressure during expiration pinches the bronchioles closed, causing them to vibrate like an oboe reed as expiratory volume passes.
2. **Asthma.** Bronchiole muscle hyperreactivity narrows the bronchioles; the bronchioles vibrate as expiratory flow passes. If severe, the bronchioles may vibrate during inspiration as well, giving inspiratory wheezes. Very severe attacks will allow little to no airflow; there will be no sounds.
3. **CHF.** Left-sided heart failure increases pulmonary venous pressure, pushing fluid into the interstitial space between the capillaries and the alveoli (see Chapter 31). This fluid compresses the terminal bronchioles from the outside-in; the bronchioles vibrate as expiratory air passes.
4. **Upper-airway obstruction.** The hallmark examination finding in upper-airway obstruction is **stridor (inspiratory wheezing).** Stridor is usually due to obstruction in the airway that occurs outside of the thorax (e.g., the larynx). For all other causes of wheezing, the negative intrathoracic pressure pulls apart the terminal bronchioles during inspiration, relieving the obstruction. This prevents inspiratory wheezes. An obstruction outside of the thorax is not pulled open by the negative intrathoracic pressure of the chest because it is outside of the chest; for this reason, inspiratory wheezes suggest an upper-airway obstruction.

B. **Assessing the severity and chronicity of obstruction. Spirometry testing is ideal, but in the acute care of the patient, spirometry measurements are rarely available.** The essential part of the Tier II examination is to assess the severity and chronicity of the exacerbation by providing estimates of spirometry values.

1. The severity of bronchial obstruction is usually measured by the FEV_1/FVC ratio (the FEV_1 %). The FVC is the total volume of air the patient can expel from the lungs; the FEV_1 is the volume of air the patient can expel in the first second. The FVC and the FEV_1 are reduced in both obstructive and restrictive disease, but the FEV_1 is reduced out of proportion to the FVC in obstructive lung disease. The harder the patient with emphysema tries to push air out of the lungs, the greater the pressure on the outside of the floppy bronchioles and the greater the impediment to the first second of flow.

2. The greater the obstruction, the lower the $FEV_1\%$ (FEV_1/FVC). Normal is 80% to 100%; severe obstruction is less than 50%.

C. Assessing the severity of obstructive lung disease

1. **Listen to the patient speak.** The ability to speak full sentences is the most sensitive measure of assessing severity of obstruction. Speaking full sentences requires maintaining a prolonged exhalation. It also requires that the patient is not "air hungry." **If the patient is speaking in one- or two-word sentences, the obstruction is usually severe (acute $FEV_1\%$ <50%).**
2. **Observe the patient's breathing.**
   a. **Accessory muscle use.** Observe the abdomen and neck. The abdomen should move outward with inspiration as the diaphragm descends; the chest wall should move out as the intercostal muscles expand the chest wall. The neck muscles should not move, because the diaphragm and intercostal movements should be sufficient to maintain inspiration. If the diaphragm and intercostal muscles fatigue as part of the exacerbation, the patient will compensate by using the sternocleidomastoid muscles to expand the chest. If you note accessory muscle movement, be prepared to intubate the patient soon, because these muscles will also soon tire.
   b. **Pursed-lip breathing.** Pursed-lip breathing is a way of increasing back-pressure on the collapsed bronchioles. This method keeps the bronchioles open long enough during exhalation to allow the air trapped in the alveoli to escape.
   c. **Panting with shallow, rapid breaths.** This suggests that so much air is trapped in the lungs that it is opposing inspiration. To compensate for this lack of tidal volume, the respiratory rate increases, but with a shallow volume per breath.
   d. **Orthopnea** is the state of breathing better while upright (ortho = straight) or difficulty breathing while flat. It primarily occurs in three diseases.
      (1) **COPD.** When the patient lies flat, more blood is shunted to the top of the lungs. The V/Q mismatch is greatest in this part of the lung because the high alveolar pressure found in COPD has an even greater effect on compressing the pulmonary arteries when the pulmonary artery pressure is lower.
      (2) **Heart failure.** When the patient lies flat, extra volume from the legs is returned to the chest, increasing pulmonary congestion.
      (3) **Apical lung disease.** When the patient lies flat, more blood is shunted to the affected part of the lungs (apex), causing inadequate oxygenation and dyspnea.
3. **Perform the 6-second breath test.**
   a. Ask the patient to take as big a breath as possible and hold it. Then ask her to blow it out as fast as she can, not stopping

until all the air is out of the lungs. Measure how long this takes.

b. The harder the patient tries, the greater the pressure is on the outside of the bronchioles. If the patient has floppy terminal bronchioles (i.e., obstructive lung disease), the air immediately becomes trapped, requiring longer than 6 seconds to be expelled from the lungs. The FEV_1 is less than 50%.

4. Determine the pulsus paradoxus. Use the method in Table 30-2 to assess the pulsus paradoxus.

a. When a patient inspires, the chest wall expands, creating a negative pressure in the thorax. This sucks blood into the right ventricle. The right ventricle has three ways of accommodating this increased volume:

(1) Expansion of the RV free wall

(2) Expansion of the septum

(3) Expansion of pressure into the pulmonary artery

b. When the septum expands, it bulges into the LV outflow tract. This decreases the cardiac output of the left ventricle, temporarily decreasing the blood pressure (see Figure 31-7). This decrease in the blood pressure corresponds with the decrease you find with the blood pressure cuff (i.e., pressure B) (see Table 30-2). Pressure A is the pressure when the septum is

TABLE 30-2. Procedure for Determining Pulsus Paradoxus.

Step	Action
Step 1	Tell the patient to breathe normally. Take his pulse (e.g., 90 beats/min).
Step 2	Place a blood pressure cuff around the patient's arm and inflate it until you hear no sounds. Auscultate over the brachial area just as if you were taking his blood pressure.
Step 3	Slowly lower the pressure. At some point you will begin to hear sounds, but the sounds will not correspond to every heart beat; (e.g., you will hear 55 beats/min instead of the patient's 90 beats/min). Note the blood pressure at this point (pressure A).
Step 4	Continue to lower the pressure until you hear every sound (90 beats/min). Note this pressure (blood pressure B).
Step 5	Subtract pressure A from pressure B to determine the pulsus paradoxus. (A normal pulsus paradoxus is 12 mm Hg or less.)

not bulging into the left ventricle, that is, when the patient is not inspiring.

c. The normal pulsus paradoxus is 12 mm Hg or less. It is so named because Kussmaul found it paradoxical that the blood pressure should decrease instead of increase when blood return to the heart was maximal (during inspiration).

d. **Pulsus paradoxus in COPD and asthma:** The pulsus paradoxus increases anytime the accommodation by the RV free wall or the pulmonary artery is impaired. Tamponade increases the pulsus paradoxus by impairing the RV free wall (see Chapter 31); asthma and COPD increase the pulsus paradoxus by increasing pulmonary artery pressure (due to hypoxia and volume retention).

D. Assessing chronicity of obstructive lung disease

1. Sternocleidomastoid hypertrophy

a. Ask the patient to hold her thumb next to the sternocleidomastoid.

b. **If the patient's sternocleidomastoid is larger in diameter than her thumb, her chronic FEV_1 is likely to be <50%.** Chronic use of accessory muscles leads to hypertrophy of the muscles.

2. **Dahl's sign** (hyperpigmentation of the distal thighs)

a. In chronic COPD, the air trapped in the lungs flattens the diaphragms. When a flat diaphragm contracts during an inspiratory effort, it pulls the sides of the chest inward, opposing inspiration. Patients with a chronic COPD will compensate by chronically leaning forward with their elbows on their knees while sitting. This pushes the abdominal contents into the chest, recreating the normal curvature of the diaphragm. When the diaphragm contracts, it now pistons down like a normal diaphragm, allowing for an effective inspiration.

b. **Chronically sitting in this "tripod" position causes chronic erythema of the skin proximal to the knees** (Figure 30-4). The hemosiderin from the red cells trapped in the skin stains the skin brown.

VI Pulmonary Hypertension

A. Primary pulmonary hypertension is rare. More common is secondary pulmonary hypertension due to either chronic hypoxemia or severe left-sided heart failure. If the patient has no signs of left-sided heart failure, but a loud S_2 to the left of the sternum, you can be confident that he has been subject to chronic and severe hypoxemia.

B. **Loudness of S_2.** The pressure downstream from a valve is responsible for how loudly the valve closes. Because aortic pressure is usually much higher than pulmonary arterial pressure, the aortic space has the louder S_2 (i.e., A_2 is usually louder than P_2). An S_2 that is louder

TABLE 30-3. Interpretation of the Tier II Lung Examination.

	Consolidation	Pleural Effusion	Pulmonary Edema	Pulmonary Fibrosis	COPD	Pneumothorax
Breath sounds	Yes or no	No	Yes	Yes	Yes	No
Crackles	Wet or absent	None	Wet	Dry	Wet or absent	No
Percussion	Dull	Dull	Normal	Normal	Like a drum	Like a drum
Tactile fremitus	Increased	Decreased	Normal	Normal	Normal	Decreased
Whispered pectoriloquy	Yes	No	No	No	No	No
Bronchophony	Yes	No	No	No	No	No
Egophony	Baaa	None	Beee	Baaa	Beee	None

COPD, Chronic obstructive pulmonary disease.

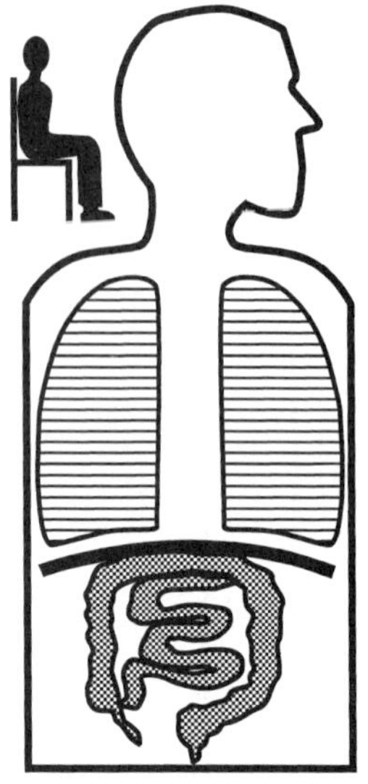

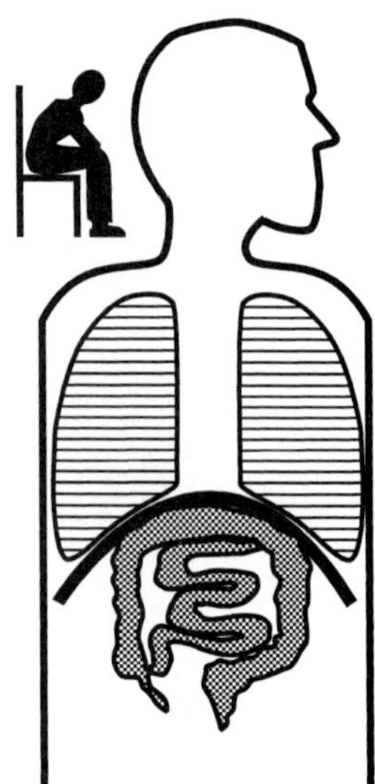

FIGURE 30-4. Tripoding.

in the left second intercostal space (overlying the pulmonic valve) than the right suggests pulmonary hypertension.

VII Other Pulmonary Findings

A. **Friction rubs** are caused by inflammation between the visceral and parietal pleura. The most common cause is bacterial infection that has extended to involve the pleural space. Other causes are tuberculosis, cancer, and asbestosis.
   1. The friction rub sounds like **creaking leather.**
   2. Pericardial friction rubs are due to similar inflammation within the pericardial sac and also sounds like creaking leather. You can differentiate the two by asking the patient to hold his breath. If the rub continues, it is pericardial.

B. **Signs of pneumothorax.** The additional air in the pleural space makes that area of the lung hyperresonant to percussion. A pneumothorax occurs in four types of patients; if you suspect a pneumothorax, repeat your percussion of the thorax carefully.
   1. Lung hyperinflation leading to a popped bleb (patients with end-stage COPD)
   2. Trauma (including central line and thoracentesis needles)
   3. Young men with sudden dyspnea (spontaneous pneumothorax)
   4. Patients with heterogeneous lung disease who are placed on a ventilator. Patients with lung disease such as *Pneumocystis cari-*

nii pneumonia or severe asthma who are placed on a ventilator are at great risk for a pneumothorax. The high pressure used to open the stiff parts of the lungs is diverted to the nonrestricted normal portions, resulting in rupture of these alveoli.

VIII **ABNORMAL BREATHING PATTERNS** The respiratory pattern should oscillate evenly. Note the following patterns:

A. **Cheynes-Stokes breathing.** The patient takes deep, rapid breaths, followed by absence of breathing for a time, then deep, rapid breaths again. This usually indicates **congestive heart failure.** The failing heart cannot pump enough blood to the brain; the brain becomes acidotic as a result, and this stimulates the lungs to breathe rapidly to make up for the lack of oxygen delivery and CO_2 retention. The deep breathing suddenly increases oxygen delivery to the brain and causes a decline in CO_2. This shuts off the breathing.

B. **Biot breathing.** The patient breaths very fast with equal intensity. This is usually due to a **midbrain infarction or bleed.** The prognosis is usually quite poor.

C. **Apneustic breathing.** The patient breaths in irregularly irregular gasping breaths. This is **a sign of brain death** and a harbinger of death.

D. **Kussmaul's respirations.** These are deep, fast breaths. This usually indicates metabolic acidosis (the patient is trying to expel CO_2 to normalize his pH), but can also indicate hypoxemia (the patient is trying to get more oxygen into his lungs). You have likely experienced Kussmaul's breathing after vigorous exercise (the CO_2 produced during muscle contraction is being expelled).

E. **Panting.** Fast shallow breathing is either hypoxemia or pain. It may also be seen in obstructive airway disease when the chest is so full of trapped air that it cannot take in additional volume.

31. The Tier II Heart and Vascular Examination

I THE BIG PICTURE OF THE TIER II HEART EXAMINATION

The Tier II heart and vascular examination consists of diagnosing four problems:

A. Diagnosing the cause of a heart murmur
B. Confirming the diagnosis of heart failure
C. Confirming pericardial disease
D. Assessing adequacy of peripheral blood flow

II HEART MURMURS

Murmurs are due to turbulence created by either **increased flow** across a valve or **decreased valve area.**

A. Increased flow occurs from one of three etiologies.

1. **Increased total blood volume.** An excessive amount of volume returning to the heart causes increased **flow** across the valves. Examples include renal failure (i.e., fluid retention due to the failure to urinate) and normal pregnancy.
2. **High-output failure.** An excessive amount of volume returning to the heart as a result of low systemic vascular resistance (SVR) causes increased **flow** across the valves. The low resistance allows more arterial volume to be directly delivered to the venous volume and thus to the heart. Any condition that requires more blood flow to the tissues to meet the tissues' metabolic needs (e.g., fever, sepsis, thryotoxicosis, anemia) will reduce the SVR.
3. **Mitral/tricuspid insufficiency.** Because the atria are low-pressure chambers, mitral or tricuspid insufficiency will result in high flow from the ventricles (contracting chambers) into the atria (holding chambers).

B. Decreased valve area occurs from pulmonic stenosis, aortic stenosis, or idiopathic hypertrophic subaortic stenosis (IHSS).

III DIAGNOSING MURMURS

If you hear a murmur on your Tier I examination, use the following approach to diagnose the cause (Figure 31-1).

A. Determine whether the murmur is systolic or diastolic. Systolic murmurs occur between S_1 and S_2; they are heard at the same time you feel the carotid pulse. If the murmur is systolic, proceed to III B. Diastolic murmurs occur between S_2 and S_1. If the murmur is diastolic, proceed to III E.

B. If the murmur is systolic, determine whether it is a "front-door" or "back-door" murmur. The ventricles receive blood from the

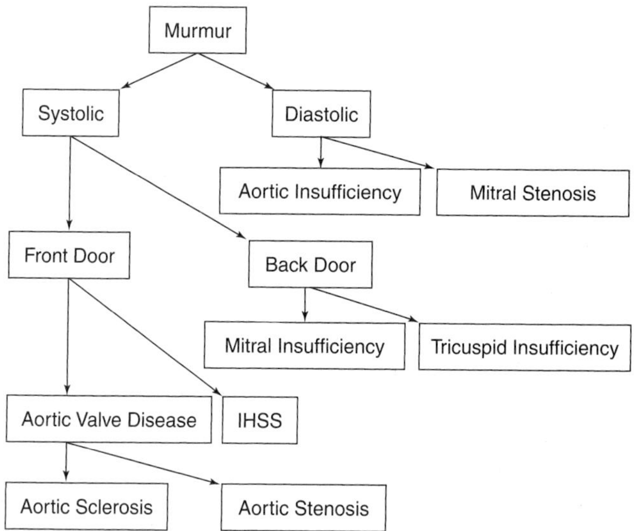

FIGURE 31-1. Determining the cause of heart murmurs.

"back doors" (i.e., the mitral and tricuspid valves) and sends it out the "front doors" (i.e., the aortic and pulmonic valves).

1. **"Front-door" murmurs** are caused by turbulence created as blood flows in the correct direction over an **aortic or pulmonic valve with decreased area.** Although these murmurs are **best heard at the base** (second intercostal spaces), they can be heard elsewhere in the chest. They have the following characteristics.
   a. **Crescendo-decrescendo shape.** The obstructing valve initially impairs blood flow during early systole, and because there is no flow, there is no murmur (Figure 31-2B). In midsystole, the pressure overcomes the obstruction, allowing flow to occur. The combination of high flow with a decreased area causes a loud murmur. During late systole, the ventricle begins to relax. Flow decreases and the obstruction again impairs flow. The murmur diminishes.

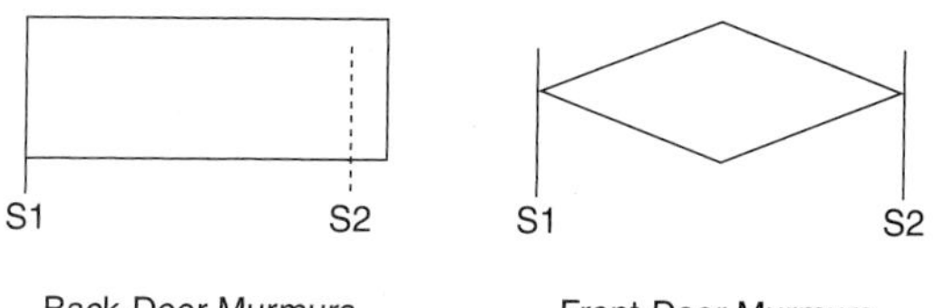

FIGURE 31-2. Murmur shapes.

b. **S_2 at the end.** By definition, the second heart sound (S_2) is closure of the aortic and pulmonic valves. When closed, there can no longer be flow over these valves, and thus there cannot be a murmur. Thus, the S_2 is not obscured in front door murmurs.

HOT
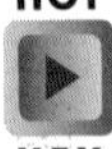
KEY

A systolic murmur with a clearly heard S_2 is a front-door murmur.

2. **"Back-door" murmurs** are caused by turbulence created as blood flows in the wrong direction (i.e., back into the atria through a leaky valve). The pressure in the atria is usually less than 10 mm Hg, and the pressure in the ventricles during systole is as high as 600 mm Hg. If the valve is incompetent, you can count on high flow in a backward direction. The high-pressure gradient between the atria and ventricles produces the following two characteristics. Back-door murmurs are **best heard at the apex** but can be heard elsewhere.
   a. **Rectangular shape.** The high-pressure gradient between the ventricle and the atria causes the murmur to begin at full force immediately on initiation of systole. It remains at that rate throughout systole, leading to a holosystolic, or rectangular, shape (Figure 31-2A).
   b. **Obscured S_2.** The aortic valve closes when the aortic pressure is greater than the LV pressure. If the diastolic aortic pressure is 80 mm Hg at the time of the aortic valve closure, the LV pressure at the precise moment of S_2 must be 79 mm Hg (i.e., just a shade smaller than the closing pressure in the aortic root). This is what has closed the aortic valve. Because the pressure in the left atrium is less than 10 mm Hg, there is still a large pressure gradient (79 mm Hg to 10 mm Hg) from the ventricle to the atria at the precise moment of S_2. Flow therefore continues, and thus so does the murmur. The back-door murmur tends to obscure the second heart sound (S_2).

HOT
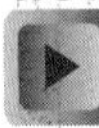
KEY

Systolic murmurs that obscure S_2 are back-door murmurs.

C. **"Front-door" murmurs** are due to one of three abnormalities: pulmonic stenosis, aortic stenosis/sclerosis, or idiopathic hypertrophic subaortic stenosis (IHSS).
   1. Pulmonic stenosis is rare. Unless the history directs you otherwise (Table 31-1), consider a front-door murmur as due to either aortic valve disease or IHSS.

TABLE 31-1. Causes of Systolic Heart Murmurs.

Types of Murmurs	Etiologies
Back-Door Murmurs	
Tricuspid insufficiency (regurgitation)	**Endocarditis** (valve is destroyed by bacteria) **Dilated cardiomyopathy** (the valve is pulled apart by the dilated ventricle)
Mitral insufficiency (regurgitation)	**Myocardial infarction** of the papillary muscles **Endocarditis** **Dilated cardiomyopathy** (pulling the valve apart) **Rheumatic heart disease** **Degeneration**
Front-Door Murmurs	
Aortic stenosis **Aortic sclerosis**	**Calcification** of the valves **Congenital bicuspid valve** **Rheumatic heart disease**
IHSS	
Pulmonic stenosis (rare)	**Congenital heart disease** (tetralogy of Fallot) **Rheumatic heart disease** **Medications** (phen-phen diet drugs)

2. Aortic stenosis or sclerosis can be distinguished from IHSS by having the patient squat, which squeezes blood from the legs back to the heart. This initially increases blood flow to the right ventricle, and then after three or four beats, increases volume to the left ventricle. The increased volume increases flow over the aortic valve, thereby increasing the murmur if it is aortic stenosis or sclerosis (note that the increased volume did not change the aortic valve's area) (Figure 31-3).
3. To distinguish aortic stenosis from aortic sclerosis, determine whether the obstruction of aortic stenosis decreases aortic blood flow. Feel the carotid pulse while you listen to the murmur.
   a. **Aortic sclerosis** is a calcification of the aortic valve, but it does not limit blood flow. The carotid pulse will be synchronous with the murmur.
   b. **Aortic stenosis limits blood flow over the aortic valve.** The carotid pulse will come slightly after the murmur. It will also be weaker than expected, because flow to the carotids is limited (pulsus parvus et tardus).

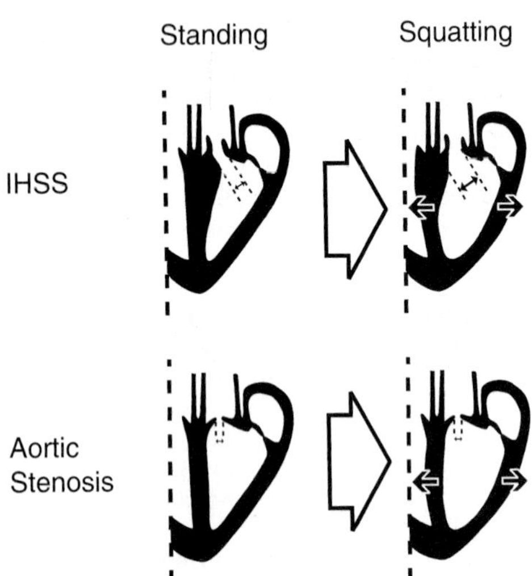

FIGURE 31-3. Idiopathic hypertrophic subaortic stenosis versus aortic stenosis.

4. The septal hypertrophy of IHSS causes a murmur by decreasing the area of the left ventricle outflow tract (Figure 31-3). When the patient squats, increased volume is returned to the left ventricle. This stretches the left ventricle walls, pulling the ventricular walls apart. Although the increased volume increases flow (as it did with aortic stenosis), the increased volume also increases the area of the outflow tract due to ventricular stretch. The increased flow is outweighed by the increase in valve area. **The murmur of IHSS decreases with squatting.**

HOT 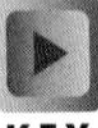 KEY

IHSS is the most common congenital heart abnormality. Because the abnormal septum puts the patient at risk for arrhythmias, its detection is a prominent part of preparticipation sports physicals. The most common murmurs in young athletes are flow murmurs (due to increased circulating blood volume) and IHSS. Flow (benign) murmurs increase in intensity with squatting as volume to the heart increases; IHSS murmurs decrease in intensity as the increased volume to the heart relieves the obstruction.

D. Back-door murmurs are due to tricuspid or mitral insufficiency (regurgitation).

1. Tricuspid insufficiency can be distinguished from mitral insufficiency by increasing blood flow to the right ventricle. If the murmur is due to tricuspid insufficiency, the increased volume in the

right ventricle will increase flow over the tricuspid valve during systole, thereby intensifying the murmur. See Table 31-2 for maneuvers you can use to increase blood volume to the right ventricle.

2. **Maneuvers that increase blood flow to the left side of the heart.** If the murmur is due to mitral regurgitation, an increased pressure in the left ventricle will intensify the murmur.
   a. **Have the patient perform the Valsalva maneuver.** Ask her to bear down as if having a bowel movement or to forcibly blow out against a closed airway. This increases intrathoracic pressure and squeezes blood from the pulmonary veins into the left ventricle. The increased left ventricle volume will result in more flow over a regurgitant mitral valve during systole. **A back-door murmur that increases with Valsalva is mitral regurgitation.**

TABLE 31-2. Maneuvers Used to Diagnose the Cause of Murmurs.

Maneuvers That Increase Blood Flow to the Right Side of the Heart (Increase Preload)*	Maneuvers That Increase Pressure in the Left Ventricle (Decreasing Preload)
1. **Raise the legs** (venous flow returns to the right ventricle). 2. Have the patient **inspire** (negative intrathoracic pressure pulls blood into the chest). 3. Have the patient **squat** (squeezing blood back to the right ventricle). 4. **Push on the abdomen** (the abdominal pressure squeezes blood from the abdomen back to the heart).	1. **Valsalva maneuver.** Have the patient bear down as if having a bowel movement, or ask him to forcibly blow out against a closed airway. This increases intrathoracic pressure and squeezes blood from the pulmonary veins into the left ventricle. The increase in intrathoracic pressure also decreases blood flow to the right ventricle (the opposite of taking a deep inspiration). 2. **Hand grip.** Have the patient tightly **grip both hands.** This will increase systemic vascular resistance, thus increasing back-pressure in the left ventricle. This will increase the gradient between the ventricle and the atria, thus increasing mitral regurgitation murmurs.

* The increase in blood flow to the right side of the heart is transitory (perhaps three or four heart beats). This volume is ultimately transferred to the left ventricle.

b. **Have the patient clench both fists tightly.** This increases systemic vascular resistance and increases back-pressure on the left ventricle. The increased left ventricular pressure required to overcome this resistance will result in more flow over a regurgitant mitral valve. **A back-door murmur that increases with hand-grip is mitral regurgitation.**

E. **If the murmur is diastolic, use your physical examination to determine its cause** (Table 31-3).

1. **Aortic insufficiency** occurs when blood leaks back into the left ventricle from the aorta.
   a. Have the patient lean forward to bring the aortic valve as close to the chest wall as possible.
   b. Position your stethoscope to the left of the sternum, in the third intercostal space. The turbulence of aortic insufficiency, and thus the associated murmur, occurs along the LV outflow tract.
   c. Know what the murmur of aortic insufficiency sounds like.

> **HOT KEY**
>
> Perform this simple maneuver to train your ears to recognize the frequency of the murmur of aortic insufficiency. Place the diaphragm of the stethoscope next to the larynx of your throat. Softly say the word, "parrrr." The "p" represents the S_2; the "arrrr" is the murmur of aortic insufficiency.

TABLE 31-3. Causes of Diastolic Heart Murmurs.

Types of Murmurs	Etiologies
Tricuspid stenosis (rare)	Rheumatic heart disease. It is rare; when it occurs, it usually involves the aortic and mitral valves first.
Pulmonic insufficiency (rare)	Endocarditis Severe biventricular dilated cardiomyopathy
Mitral stenosis	Rheumatic heart disease
Aortic insufficiency	Endocarditis Valvular stenosis (valves calcify in an open position) Valvular degeneration Any cause of aortic root dilatation (syphilis, Marfan's syndrome) as the dilatation pulls the valves apart

d. Ask the patient to hold his breath. The murmur of aortic insufficiency has the same frequency as normal breath sounds; it will be obscured unless the patient holds her breath.

e. Look for peripheral signs of aortic insufficiency. All of these findings are due to the rapidly declining diastolic pressure caused by the incompetent aortic valve's inability to seal the diastolic chamber, and the increased systolic pressure resulting from augmented LV stroke volume from the additional preload the aorta adds to the normal volume from the atria. The high systolic blood pressure and the low diastolic blood pressure lead to **a wide pulse pressure,** manifest in many different pulses (Table 31-4).

> **HOT KEY**
>
> The pulse abnormalities seen with aortic insufficiency only occur if the ventricle has had **time to dilate** to accommodate the increase blood volume and the left ventricular **contractility is preserved.** Aortic insufficiency without pulse abnormalities is due to either acute aortic insufficiency (e.g., endocarditis), or chronic aortic insufficiency with a damaged left ventricle (one that will not tolerate the high resistance of a surgically placed new valve).

2. **Mitral stenosis** occurs because of thickening of the mitral valve due to rheumatic heart disease. Flow over the mitral valve occurs

TABLE 31-4. Peripheral Signs of Aortic Insufficiency.

Sign	Description
Water-hammer pulse	Strong radial pulse felt when patient's wrist is held above the head. Normally, a faint or absent pulse is felt.
Quincke's pulse	Alternation of nail bed like a flashlight between pink (systolic pulsation) and white (rapid diastolic collapse).
Corrigan's pulse	Bobbing of head with each systolic pulsation.
Rappaport's pulse	Bobbing of ear lobes with each systolic pulsation.
Hill's pulse	Pistol-shot femoral pulses.
Derioze's pulse	To-and-fro murmur heard when stethoscope is applied over the femoral artery at 30-degree angle (pointing toward the feet).

during diastole, and the murmur of mitral stenosis is a low-frequency diastolic rumble. The sound has the characteristic pattern "did-hee baar ruup."

a. The "did-hee" sound is due to the S_2 ("did") followed by the opening snap ("hee") of the thickened mitral valve.

b. The "baaar" sound is due to the atrial volume rumbling across the mitral valve (i.e., the diastolic rumble).

c. The "ruup" sound is due to the loud S_1 caused by the closure of a thickened mitral valve.

HOT

KEY

The murmur of mitral stenosis sounds like a bowling ball rolling down a lane. The "did-hee" is the sound of the ball hitting the wood and making a small bounce; the "baar" is the ball barreling down the lane toward the pins. The "ruup" is the ball crashing into the pins.

The greater the distance between the "did" and the "hee," the greater the degree of stenosis, because severe stenosis will delay opening of the mitral valve (i.e., the opening snap comes late).

F. Determine the severity of the murmur (Table 31-5).

1. Grades 1 and 2 murmurs are sometimes pathologic (i.e., valve is abnormal) but can also be due to increased flow over a normal valve (i.e., a flow murmur). Murmurs caused by increased flow over a normal valve are called flow murmurs. See II A above

TABLE 31-5. Grading Heart Murmurs.

Grade	Description
1	**The valves do not close as crisply as expected.** The S_1 and S_2 should be sharp; if they are not, it is a grade 1 murmur.
2	The murmur is appreciated with ease, but it is **not the most prominent sound in the chest** (i.e., S_1 and S_2 are most notable).
3	The murmur is the **most prominent sound on auscultation.** It is the first thing you hear upon initiating auscultation.
4	A thrill. The murmur is felt as well as heard.
5	The murmur is heard with the stethoscope tangential to the skin.
6	The murmur is heard with the stethoscope off the skin or without a stethoscope.

for causes of increased flow over the valves. The difference between a grade 1 and 2 murmur is clinically unimportant.

2. **Grade 3 murmurs always imply an abnormal valve.** Although high-flow states (see II A above) may still be contributing to the murmur, a decrease in valve area is ensured when a grade 3 murmur is heard. This rule applies only to front-door murmurs; all back-door murmurs are abnormal regardless of grade, because there should be no flow over a normal mitral or tricuspid valve.
3. **Other clues as to the cause of a murmur:**
   a. **Location of radiation.** The radiation of a murmur is a clue as to the responsible valve. Use caution, however; a vibration in one part of the heart may vibrate the rest of the heart, causing the murmur to travel to unpredictable locations (Table 31-6).
   b. **Location of auscultation.** The location at which you hear a murmur can also be a clue as to the murmurs cause (see Chapter 25). Again, this is a clue, not a rule; the same caveat for radiation of murmurs applies here.

HOT
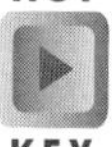
KEY

If you are listening for a left-sided murmur, have the patient lean forward. This brings the heart as close to the chest wall as possible. If you suspect a mitral murmur, roll the patient onto her left side.

IV Congestive Heart Failure

A. General considerations

1. Congestive heart failure manifests in one of two ways:
   a. Symptoms of inadequate blood flow to the tissues (i.e., **forward failure,** leading to prerenal renal failure; weakness; syncope).
   b. Symptoms of backup of blood behind the heart (i.e., **backward failure,** leading to shortness of breath resulting from pulmonary edema, crackles, elevated JVP, peripheral edema).
2. Do not rely solely on radiographs and echocardiograms; radiographs may lag behind the clinical condition and may not give

TABLE 31-6. Classic Radiation Patterns of Murmurs.

Murmur	Radiation Pattern
Aortic stenosis	To the carotids
Aortic sclerosis	To the carotids
IHSS	To the carotids
Mitral stenosis	To the axilla or the back
Mitral insufficiency	To the axilla or the back
Tricuspid insufficiency	No radiation (stays at the apex)

you a timely assessment of the patient's condition and response to therapy. Echocardiograms are often not available when you need them to make clinical decisions, and echocardiograms cannot be ordered each morning to assess response to therapy. Use your physical examination to make day-to-day assessments of the patient's condition.

B. Etiology

1. **Systolic heart failure** occurs when the ventricle loses contractility and cannot squeeze blood forward.
2. **Diastolic heart failure** occurs when the blood in the atria does not have enough time during diastole to flow into the left ventricle to be pumped forward. This occurs when the ventricle wall is very stiff and opposes filling from the left atrium (as might occur from long-standing hypertension; see Appendix A, Equation 10 for a clue as to why).
3. **High-output heart failure.** When the tissues' metabolic demands increase (e.g., hyperthyroidism, sepsis, thiamine deficiency) or when delivery of oxygen is low (e.g., anemia; see Appendix A, Equations 3 and 7 as to why), the arterioles will dilate to allow more blood flow to the tissues. This increases blood volume in the veins, eventually "piling up" at the heart. When the excess volume is too much for heart to keep up with, the volume floods the lungs causing **high-output heart failure.**

HOT
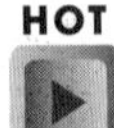
KEY

The physical examination is critical to distinguishing between systolic and diastolic heart failure.

C. Understanding heart failure. To understand systolic heart failure, think of the sequence of events that lead to its pathogenesis. Use the equations in Appendix A as you proceed.

1. First, there is an insult to the myocardium (e.g., ischemia, toxins) that decreases contractility.
2. This leads to decreased stroke volume (Equation 4), decreased cardiac output (Equation 5), and decreased mean arterial pressure (Equation 6), thus decreasing blood flow to the kidneys. This is termed **forward heart failure**.
3. The decrease in renal blood flow prompts the kidney to produce more renin, increasing angiotensin II and thus aldosterone. Aldosterone prompts the kidney to retain more salt and therefore more volume. The increased venous volume increases left ventricle preload, which compensates for the poor contractility (Equation 4); the stroke volume is returned to normal.
4. The price to be paid is that the increased preload also increases pressure in the pulmonary veins, pushing fluid into the pulmonary

interstitium. The physical findings of crackles, increased JVP, ascites, and edema are a result of retaining more preload. This is termed **backward heart failure.**

5. The management of heart failure is like walking a tightrope. There should be enough preload to maintain an optimal cardiac output (forward function), but not so much that the patient has dyspnea and edema (backward dysfunction). The physical examination will help you determine which side of the tightrope the patient is on (i.e., whether preload is excessive or inadequate).

> **HOT KEY**
> The brain natriuretic peptide (BNP) level is a useful test for distinguishing CHF from COPD, because it increases as the volume in the heart increases. Use caution, however; the BNP will be elevated in even well-compensated heart failure patients, because these patients rely on increased preload to survive. Use your physical examination and the patient's symptomatic response to guide your therapy, not the BNP level alone.

D. **Signs of inadequate forward function** (forward failure)
   1. **Hypotension**
   2. **Weak peripheral pulses**
   3. **Pulsus alternans,** a phenomenon of beat-to-beat alternation in the strength of the pulse. Feel the radial pulse for the alternate weak pulse and a strong pulse.
      a. The weak pulse results from the poor forward pumping function of the heart. During this weak contraction, only a small percentage of the preload is pumped forward (e.g., 20%); the remaining 80% remains in the ventricle.
      b. The strong pulse occurs with the next systolic contraction, when the volume from the atrium is joined by the 80% of residual volume from the previous beat. The ventricle now has a supernormal preload, which increases the left ventricular stretch, causing the next beat to be much stronger. As with all measures of LV failure, the finding may be prominent during acute failure, but absent when the patient has received diuresis.
   4. **Soft S_1.** The LV contraction closes the mitral valve. When contractility is strong, valve closure is brisk. S_1 is loud when the ventricle is strong but weak when it is not.

E. **Signs of excessive preload** (backward failure)
   1. **Dyspnea**
   2. **Crackles.** The increased pressure in the pulmonary capillaries pushes fluid into the interstitium.
   3. **Edema.** Increased venous pressure pushes fluid into the interstitium of the legs.
   4. **JVP** (see Chapter 25)

5. **The third heart sound (S_3).** The S_3 is caused by a large bolus of blood falling from the left atrium into a large residual volume in the left ventricle (much like a very large man falling into a swimming pool). The result is a low-frequency "bluub" that immediately follows S_2; thus, it is termed the third heart sound, or S_3.
   - **a.** Immediately following S_2, the mitral valve opens and volume from the left atrium falls into the left ventricle. The normal heart ejects most of its diastolic volume (ejection fraction >60%), leaving very little LV volume at the beginning of diastole. Thus, the extra sound is not heard in normal hearts.
   - **b.** The failing heart, however, ejects only a small fraction of its diastolic volume (ejection fraction <30%), leaving a large amount of volume in the ventricle. When the mitral valve opens, the atrial bolus of fluid falls into the residual LV volume creating a low-frequency "bluub."
   - **c.** The best place to listen for an S_3 is directly over the PMI. Listen for S_1 and S_2 for several cycles and then concentrate on hearing what happens just after S_2. S_3 is not crisp like S_2; the S_2-S_3 combination will sound like a "dub-blub." Like pulsus alternans, the S_3 will disappear when the patient has had the excess preload volume removed by way of diuresis.
   - **d.** Because S_3 is due to excessive volume in the left ventricle at the beginning of diastole, any other cause of excess total blood volume overload can produce these same signs (e.g., renal failure, pregnancy, young athletes). Look for other signs of heart failure to confirm the diagnosis.

> **HOT KEY**
>
> You can recreate the sound of an S_3 in the privacy of your home. Stand above a toilet (fresh bowl), and quickly dump a cup of water into the bowl. The low-frequency sound you hear is the S_3. To recreate the sound you will hear in your patient, hold the stethoscope in your left palm; make a fist with the palm pointing downward. With your right index finger, pull across the MCP knuckles toward you.

IV Other Abnormal Heart Sounds

A. The third heart sound **(S_3)** (see IV E 5).

B. The fourth heart sound **(S_4)** occurs after S_3 and just before the cycle starts over again (S_1). The S_4 occurs only in **noncompliant (i.e., thick) left ventricles,** as might occur after long-standing hypertension (see Appendix A, Equation 10).

1. Normally, the majority of diastolic filling of the ventricles occurs in early diastole, when atrial volume passively falls into the left

ventricle. If the ventricle is very thick, however, this flow is impeded, and the atria must squeeze the residual atrial volume into the ventricle at the end of diastole.

2. The sound is much like the sound you hear when you drop a bowling ball (large atrial bolus) onto a stiff mattress (stiff left ventricle), as opposed to a baseball (normal atrial bolus) onto a featherbed (normal lef ventricle).
3. Like the S_3, the best place to hear an S_4 is at the PMI. Also like an S_3, it is a low-frequency sound, so **use the bell of the stethoscope.**
4. An S_4 is a marker for diastolic heart failure, because the thick left ventricle that causes the sound also impedes diastolic filling of the ventricle (see IV B 2).
5. An S_4 cannot be heard with atrial fibrillation, because the fibrillating atria cannot provide the atrial squeeze that causes the S_4.

HOT
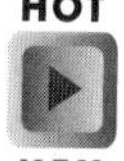
KEY

You can simulate an S_4 by placing the head of your stethoscope in your left hand. Make a fist with the palm pointing downward. With your right index finger, drag across the knuckles away from you.

C. Split heart sounds

1. To understand split heart sounds, remember the following key points:
   - **a.** A ventricle will continue to contract until it has done its job. A valve will close later if the ventricle has a larger blood volume to expel or if it must overcome the resistance of a stenotic valve or downstream pressure (i.e., arterial/pulmonary hypertension).
   - **b.** If the ventricle starts contraction late (i.e., the electrical bundle is blocked), it will close late.
   - **c.** In all people, the pulmonic valve will closer later in inspiration than in expiration. The negative intrathoracic pressure with inspiration delivers more blood to the right ventricle; it will take longer for the right ventricle to finish ejecting this greater blood volume.
2. **Method.** Listen to S_2 at the base of the heart **during exhalation.** S_2 should be a single sound.
   - **a.** If the S_2 is single, stop the investigation; the S_2 is normal. There is no need to listen during inspiration, because **splitting of the second heart sound during inspiration is normal.**
   - **b.** If the S_2 is split during exhalation (you hear two sounds making up the S_2), one of the valves that causes the S_2 (aortic or pulmonic) is closing *later* than the other. **The late valve is the abnormal valve.**
   - **c.** Then listen as the patient takes a deep breath and holds it. You have only a few seconds during the inspiration, so listen

What you hear on auscultation during exhalation:

Exhalation	S1	x2	y2

Listen during inspiration to determine which valve (aortic or pulmonic) is X and Y.

Example 1: The split disappears.

Exhalation	S1	x2	y2
Inspiration	S1		→ x2y2

The X2 has moved into Y2. This means that X2 is the pulmonic valve (since it moved), and the late closing valve (the abnormal valve) had to have been the aortic valve (Y2).

Example 2: The split persists.

Exhalation	S1	x2	y2	
Inspiration	S1	x2	→	y2

In example 2, the Y2 has moved away from the X2. This means that Y2 had to be P2 (the movable valve). P2 is the late valve, and thus the abnormal valve.

FIGURE 31-4. Split heart sounds.

carefully. Remember that with inspiration, the pulmonic valve (P_2) always closes later than normal (see IV C 1 c).

d. **If the S_2 split disappears** during inspiration (i.e., becomes a single S_2 sound), the pulmonic valve was the first of the two split sounds. It has now moved to the right (closing later) to merge with the aortic valve to form a single sound (Figure 31-4). **The aortic valve was the late-closing, abnormal valve.**

e. **If the S_2 split widens with inspiration**, the second sound was the pulmonic valve, because inspiration pushed it farther to the right (closing later), widening the split. **The pulmonic valve was the late-closing, abnormal valve.** This is referred to as **persistent split S_2**; do not confuse this with a fixed split S_2 (see IV C 4).

3. **Etiologies.** When you have diagnosed a split S_2, use the following method to diagnose the cause. First, think of an elevator with a late-closing door. The elevator will close its doors only after it has completed its job (emptying passengers). The four causes of a late-closing elevator door are:

a. Stenotic doors: Aortic or pulmonic stenosis. Listen for murmurs.
b. Many passengers inside the elevator: Left-to-right (late closing pulmonic valve) or right-to-left (late closing aortic valve) ventricular shunt. Listen for murmurs.
c. Many bystanders outside of the elevator opposing the passengers from exiting the elevator: High downstream pressure in the form of aortic or pulmonic hypertension. Listen for a loud S_2 in the pulmonic space to exclude pulmonary hypertension; obtain the diastolic blood pressure to exclude aortic hypertension.
d. Poor electricity: Left or right bundle branch block. Obtain an ECG.

4. **A fixed split S_2 implies an atrial septal defect (ASD).** The pulmonic valve closes a bit later than the aortic because of increased blood flow from the left atrium to the right atrium (the left atrium has a slightly higher pressure). During inspiration, volume increases to the right atrium, causing the pressures between the atria to equilibrate; this shuts off the left-to-right flow through the ASD. The pulmonic valve still closes later than the aortic due to the increased inspiratory volume that has replaced the increased volume from the left atrium.
5. **Split S_1.** A split S_1 has the same causes as a split S_2, although usually it is clinically benign.
6. A word of caution. A split S_2 can be confused with a third (S_3) heart sound. To distinguish an S_3 from a split S_2, remember that the low-frequency S_3 is <u>not</u> heard with the diaphragm, where a split S_2 is.

HOT
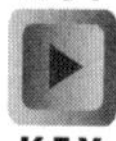
KEY

When a heart sound is split (either S_1 or S_2), the late valve is *always* the abnormal valve.

D. **Midsystolic click.** Mitral valve prolapse is a redundancy of the mitral valve leaflets. This causes the middle of the valve to buckle into the left atrium (Figure 31-5). If the buckling is severe, it may pull the valves apart, resulting in a **mitral regurgitant murmur.** If the buckling is brisk, the middle part of the valve may snap like a sailboat's sail catching the wind. This results in a **midsystolic click.**
E. **Pericardial knock** (see VI)

V RIGHT-SIDED HEART FAILURE

A. **Right-sided heart failure** symptoms include elevated JVP, peripheral edema, and ascites. Causes include left-sided heart failure, pericardial disease, RV infarction, or sudden rupture of the tricuspid

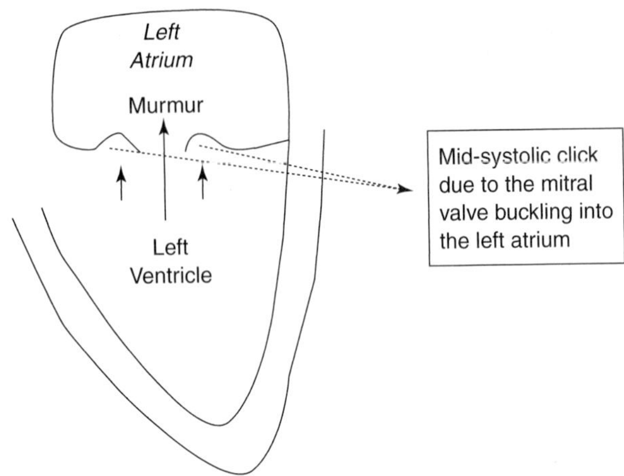

FIGURE 31-5. Mitral valve prolapse.

valve. Follow this method to make the diagnosis:

1. **Evaluate left-sided heart failure.** This is the most common cause of right-sided heart failure. If you hear crackles, the cause of the elevated venous pressure is most likely due to left-sided heart failure.
2. Evaluate **cor pulmonale.** Pulmonary vascular resistance is increased solely by the presence of hypoxia. Assess the probability that your patient has chronic hypoxia by asking about emphysema (Is he a smoker? Are there signs of obstructive lung disease?) and sleep apnea (Is he overweight? Is there a history of snoring?). Listen for a loud S_2 in the pulmonic space. Obtain an echocardiogram to confirm the diagnosis if necessary.
3. **Pericardial disease.** Constrictive pericarditis and tamponade will oppose venous blood flow into the right ventricle. Simple pericarditis will irritate the pericardial wall, but will not cause right-heart failure (see VI).
4. **Evaluate a sudden rupture of the tricuspid valve.** Over time, many patients will develop tricuspid insufficiency. If the valve suddenly ruptures, however, a large portion of the RV output escapes out the "back door" (to the atria and the vena cava) instead of being pumped into the pulmonary artery. This causes right-sided heart failure and an elevated JVP. Recognizing the three waves of the JVP can help determine if the tricuspid valve has suddenly been damaged (Figure 31-6).
   a. **A wave**. The first venous pulsation is from the **atrium contracting** during late diastole. There is no valve between the atrium and the jugular vein; therefore, part of the volume from

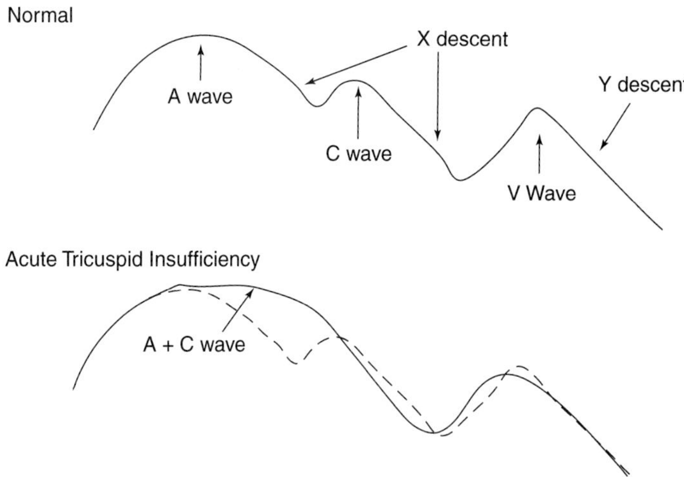

FIGURE 31-6. ACV jugular pulsation waves. **Descents:** *X,* atrial relaxation; *Y,* blood flowing into right ventricle when the tricuspid valve opens. **Waves:** *A,* atrial contraction; *C,* "cusp" of tricuspid bulges back into right atrium during ventricular systole; *V,* blood enters right atrium during ventricular systole with closed tricuspid valve.

this contraction is ejected into the vena cava and into the jugular vein.

b. **C wave**. Following diastole, the right ventricle contracts, **closing** the tricuspid valve. The tricuspid valve bows into the right atrium, sending a reverberation of fluid into the jugular vein. This usually is so small that it is unnoticed except as a small flutter immediately after the A wave.

c. **X descent.** The ventricle continues to contract. As it does, it shortens and pulls down on the floor of the right atrium. The atrium is now slightly larger, and this draws some fluid from the jugular vein into the right atrium. This fluid causes the pulsation to diminish for a millisecond.

d. **V wave.** At the end of systole, the **ventricle relaxes** and the atrium resumes its previous shape. Blood from the extremities is drawn into the right atrium, and some of this volume overshoots the right atrium and goes to the jugular vein. This volume causes another small pulsation in the jugular vein.

e. **Y descent.** The tricuspid valve then opens and blood spills into the right ventricle. This pulls blood from the vena cava and thus from the jugular vein into the right atrium. The jugular pulsation declines.

f. **Duration.** All of this takes place in a second; it is virtually impossible to see each component of the cycle. Do not try to see each step; instead, get a sense of what the entire complex (A wave, C wave, X descent, V wave, Y descent) looks like in a normal person. Then when you see something different, you will know that something is amiss.
   (1) The normal pattern looks like "large blip small."
   (2) To help you visualize this, draw a cursive "m," and make the second hump smaller than the first. Draw it over and over again and watch your hand as your do so. This is the normal pattern of the JVP. Each "m" is the same, and the first hump is always larger than the second.

g. **Sudden rupture of the tricuspid valve.** The C wave is lost (the tricuspid valve cannot close because it is damaged) and replaced by a much bigger wave caused by volume ejected from the right ventricle into the jugular vein. The normal pattern of the complex is replaced by "laaaaarge small." Draw the cursive "m" again, but this time make the first hump much larger than the second. The "ms" are always the same shape, but the first hump is larger than the second. This is called A-C merger (i.e., merging of the **a**trial contraction wave with the **c**losure wave) and suggests the tricuspid valve has been acutely damaged.

h. **Cannon A wave.** This occurs when the atrium and ventricle are not synchronized. In other words, it is complete heart block. In this case, the atrium contracts at a different rate (e.g., 70 bpm) than the ventricle (e.g., 40 bpm). When the atrium contracts while the ventricle is also contracting, the atrium contracts against a closed tricuspid valve. All of energy in the atrial contraction is used to force blood back into the vena cava and into the jugular vein. You see a huge A wave pulsation when this occurs. Draw the normal cursive "m" over and over again, and make an occasional *huge* first hump followed by a very small second hump.

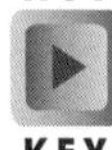

The A wave disappears if the patient is in atrial fibrillation, because there is no atrial contraction.

VI PERICARDIAL DISEASE

A. **Pericarditis** is inflammation occurring between the pericardium and the heart wall. As the heart contracts, it rubs against the inflamed pericardium, and this friction creates pain and a rub.
   1. Characteristically, the pain is less when the patient sits forward; this reduces the friction between the heart and the pericardium.

Pericardial effusions do not cause these symptoms, because fluid insulates the pericardium from the myocardium, thereby preventing the friction responsible for the pain and the rub.

2. The rub sounds like a cowboy climbing into a leather saddle. Said quickly in your lowest voice, "Rubb, bubb, bubb," it simulates the sound of a pericardial rub.
3. Classically, there are three components to a friction rub, though not all components are heard on every patient. The three components are due to the friction caused by atrial systole, ventricular systole, and ventricular diastole.
4. The diffuse ST segment elevation on ECG is due to damage of the epicardial cells from this friction.

HOT KEY

You can simulate the sound of pericarditis. Begin by lightly pinching your ear lobe with your thumb and index finger. Now put your finger in your ear (keep your thumb under your earlobe), and quickly drag it out over the tragus (the cartilage in the ear), the ear lobe, and finally to your thumb while maintaining light pressure between your thumb and finger.

B. Constrictive pericarditis is calcification of the pericardial sack. It occurs from long-standing, chronic pericarditis, as might be seen with tuberculosis, cancer, or end-stage renal disease. The abdominojugular reflux sign is used to assess the presence or absence of constrictive pericarditis.

1. Remember that one way to see the JVP is to push on the patient's abdomen, increasing venous return to the right side of the heart; some of this venous blood overshoots the right atrium, thereby causing the JVP to elevate temporarily (see Chapter 25). This lasted only a few seconds, because normally the normal right ventricle is able to accommodate for the extra volume and pump it through to the left ventricle.
2. The **abdominojugular reflex sign** assesses the right ventricle's ability to accommodate extra venous return. If it cannot accommodate this return, the extra volume remains in the JVP even after 15 seconds. Causes include:
   - **a.** The right ventricle free wall cannot expand. Constrictive pericarditis is a calcified, rigid pericardium that results from chronic inflammation of the pericardium and prevents the right ventricle free wall from expanding.
   - **b.** Pulmonary hypertension opposes the off-loading of pressure into the pulmonary artery.
3. **Method**
   - **a.** Position the patient at an angle so you can see the JVP. You must be able to see the meniscus of the JVP. It should increase by at least 3 cm and remain elevated for longer than 15 seconds.

b. Tell the patient you are going to press on her abdomen. If you surprise the patient with a quick abdominal punch, she will tighten up, and this will force blood out of the chest instead of pushing abdominal blood into the chest.

c. Press in the middle of the abdomen with 35 mm Hg of constant pressure, and hold the pressure for at least 15 seconds.

(1) To press with 35 mm Hg of pressure, unfold a blood pressure cuff and place it over the abdomen. Inflate it to 30 mm Hg of pressure. Press on the abdomen through the cuff until the sphygmomanometer goes to 65 mm Hg (30 + 35 = 65).

(2) Do not press on the liver (hepatojugular reflux sign), because this induces pain in the patient with a swollen liver. The patient will tighten up, negating the sign.

4. **Kussmaul's sign** is a variant of the abdominojugular reflux sign. Normally, inspiration causes intrathoracic pressure to become more negative. This augments venous return to the heart and causes the JVP to decrease. If the right ventricle cannot accommodate this extra volume, the volume is displaced to the jugular vein, where it remains. If the JVP fails to decrease during inspiration, suspect that the right ventricle cannot accommodate the increased volume; causes include constrictive pericarditis, restrictive cardiomyopathy, tricuspid stenosis, or pulmonary hypertension.

C. **Pericardial tamponade.** Tamponade is fluid in the pericardial sack that compresses both the right and left ventricles. The result is **Beck's Triad:**

1. **Venous hypertension:** elevated JVP; venous blood cannot enter the right ventricle.
2. **Arterial hypotension.** The left ventricle receives no preload volume from the compressed right ventricle.
3. **Muffled heart sounds.** The fluid insulates the heart sounds.
4. Note that in patients with tamponade, the lungs are clear (i.e., no crackles), because the pericardial effusion prevents the right ventricle from pumping blood into the lungs to begin with.
5. **Pulsus paradoxus.** The pericardial fluid compresses the right ventricle free wall. As the patient takes a deep breath (bringing more venous volume to the right heart), the right heart must rely upon septal expansion to accommodate this increased volume. With each breath, the septum deviates into the left ventricle outflow track, obstructing LV cardiac output and thus decreasing the strength of the pulse (Figure 31-7). See Chapter 30 V C 4 and Table 30-2 for how to measure pulsus paradoxis.

VII INADEQUATE ARTERIAL PULSES

The Tier I examination addresses the peripheral pulses. If you find abnormalities, perform a Tier II examination to evaluate other pulses. If you find an obstruction, listen for bruits. **A bruit is a murmur of a periph-**

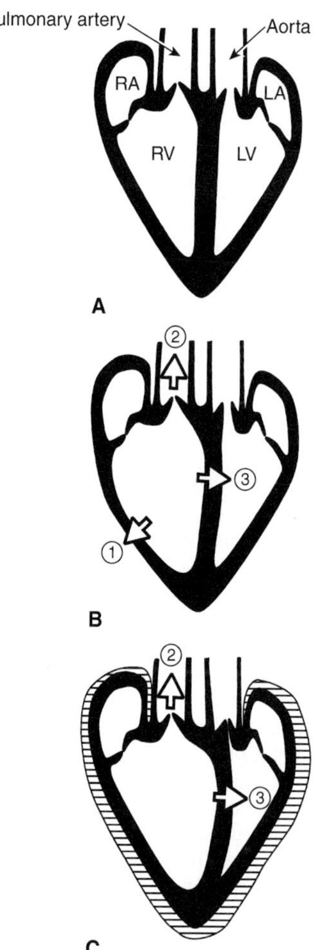

FIGURE 31-7. The physiology of cardiac tamponade. **A,** normal heart during exhalation. **B,** mechanisms of right ventricle expansion to accommodate increased volume returning to the right ventricle with inspiration. ①, RV free wall expansion; ②, pressure off-loaded to the pulmonary artery; ③, septal shift into the left ventricle outflow tract. **C,** tamponade: the inability of the right ventricle free wall to expand causes greater septal shift into the left ventricle outflow tract.

eral artery and, like murmurs, is a function of flow divided by area. The smaller the area (i.e., obstruction), the larger the bruit is, until the obstruction becomes so great that it limits the arterial flow.

A. Carotid bruits. Locate the trachea with your fingers, and let your fingers fall laterally into the grove between the trachea and the sternocleidomastoid muscles. Place the stethoscope there and move it superior to just below the jaw.

C. Renal bruits. The aorta bifurcates into the iliac arteries at the umbilicus. The renal arteries obviously branch laterally from the aorta proximal to this point. Position your stethoscope halfway between the umbilicus and the xiphoid, and move 5 cm laterally. Ask the patient to bend his knees and lie flat to relax the abdominal muscles. Ask the patient to take a deep inspiration followed by a deep exhalation; during the exhalation, depress your stethoscope into the abdomen. Have the patient hold his breath in exhalation while you listen.

D. Allen test. The Allen test ensures that the ulnar artery is capable of supplying blood to the entire hand.

1. Check the ulnar pulse before every arterial blood gas or arterial line procedure. Absent or insufficient ulnar blood flow results in hand ischemia if you cannulate the radial artery.
2. Occlude both the radial and ulnar arteries simultaneously. Ask the patient to open and close a fist until the hand blanches. Then release only the ulnar artery while maintaining pressure on the radial. The entire hand should turn pink as it fills with blood. If it does not, there is ulnar artery insufficiency.

E. The ankle-brachial index. Normally, the blood pressure in the arm is greater than the blood pressure in the leg because it is closer to the heart. The ankle to brachial ratio, therefore, is normally greater than 0.6. To assess the ankle-brachial index (ABI), measure the systolic blood pressure in the arm (see Chapter 25). This is the brachial pressure. Then find a large blood pressure cuff (a thigh cuff) and wrap it around the lower leg. You will need a Doppler stethoscope (the nurses can help you find one). Place the Doppler probe on the dorsalis pedis artery and press lightly. You will hear a swooshing sound. Inflate the cuff until you no longer hear the swoosh. This is the ankle pressure. Divide the systolic pressure in the arm by this pressure. This is the ABI. A ratio of less than 0.5 is an indication that surgery may be needed to revascularize the leg.

32. The Tier II Abdominal Examination

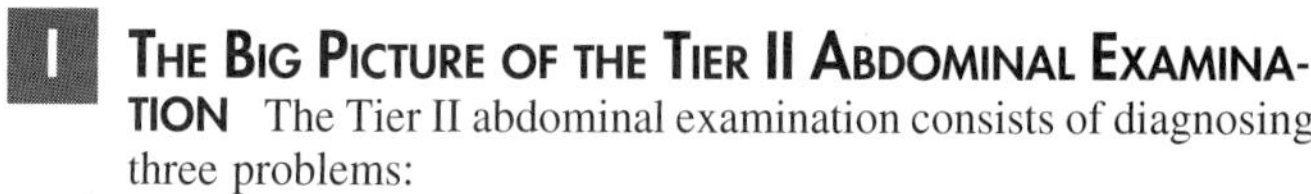

I THE BIG PICTURE OF THE TIER II ABDOMINAL EXAMINATION

The Tier II abdominal examination consists of diagnosing three problems:

A. Diagnosing the cause of abdominal pain
B. Confirming the diagnosis of liver disease
C. Confirming the diagnosis of splenomegaly

II GENERAL APPROACH TO ABDOMINAL PAIN

A. **Step 1:** Before you touch the abdomen, **think of each organ in the abdomen.** Begin with the esophagus, consider the stomach and all associated structures, the small bowel, the large bowel, and the rectum. Do not overlook the organs in the right and left upper quadrant (liver, gallbladder, and spleen), the retroperitoneal organs (pancreas, kidneys, aorta, and paraspinous muscles), and the pelvic organs (uterus, ovaries, vagina, prostate, and bladder). Start with this mental list and narrow it using the following principles.

B. **Step 2: Determine the character of the pain.**
   1. **Colicky pain** comes and goes. This suggests an obstruction of a hollow tube. As the tube squeezes against the obstruction, the patient feels pain. As the squeeze relents, the pain abates. Hollow tubes in the abdomen subject to obstruction (from top down) include the bile ducts, the small bowel, the large bowel, and the ureters.
   2. **Constant pain** suggests a disease of a solid organ or a hollow tube that has now become a solid organ (e.g., appendicitis, diverticulitis).

C. **Step 3: Use the progression of the pain to help make the diagnosis.**
   1. Obstruction (small bowel obstruction, appendicitis) begins with **anorexia** (the body is trying to keep any additional food from entering the body), **nausea** (vagal response to the distention), then **pain.** Other causes of abdominal pain begin with pain followed by these symptoms.
   2. **Early pain** begins at the embryologic origin of the affected organ. Small bowel (the appendix) originates at the umbilicus and large bowel in the suprapubic region.
   3. Next, the pain moves to the location of the organ.
   4. Finally, the pain becomes diffuse as the organ bursts.

D. Step 4: Use color clues (Table 32-1).

E. Step 5: Look for fever. Fever implies one of the following:

1. A hollow tube has burst, releasing its bacterial contents into the abdomen. Fever and an elevated WBC are evidence the infection has extended into the bloodstream. Do not wait for these signs to begin treatment.
2. There is a localized pocket of infection. Fever is a common feature of systemic infections, but it is not typically a feature of viral or bacterial infections localized within the gastrointestinal tract (e.g., gastroenteritis or bacterial colitis).

F. Step 6: Consider extra-abdominal causes of pain. A few diseases can cause referred pain to the abdomen. They are rare but worth considering before your abdominal examination. Think of the mnemonic "PM BAD LUNCH."

Systemic causes of abdominal pain **(PM BAD LUNCH):**

Porphyria

Mediterranean fever (familial Mediterranean fever): Armenian heritage; family history; 72-hour history of paroxysms of fever and abdominal pain

Black widow spider bite: history of a black widow spider bite

Addison's disease: associated hypotension; history of steroid use, autoimmune disease or tuberculosis (most common causes of Addison's disease)

Diabetic ketoacidosis

TABLE 32-1. Color Clues in Diagnosis of Abdominal Pain.

- **Green** anywhere suggests bile duct or gallbladder rupture.
- **Purple** ecchymosis (blood) in the flanks or around the umbilicus suggests a ruptured vessel in the abdomen.
- **Blue,** cold, pulseless extremities suggest involvement of the intra-abdominal aorta.
- **Yellow** skin, eyes, or dark urine suggests bile duct obstruction or liver injury.
- **Black** tarry stool (melena) suggests an upper gastrointestinal bleed. The black color is a product of bile mixing with blood. The tarry component only occurs when gastric acid is mixed with the blood.
- **Red** blood in the stool suggests lower gastrointestinal bleeding (colon) or brisk upper gastrointestinal bleeding (peptic ulcer). Dark blood suggests involvement of the right colon and bright blood involvement of the left colon or hemorrhoids.
- **Silver** stools are due to melena without the bile (i.e., a tumor obstructing the bile duct that is bleeding into the duodenum).

Lead poisoning (especially in children, painters, and welders)
Uremia
Narrow-angle glaucoma: red, painful eye (see Chapter 29)
Calcium: hypercalcemia causes chronic constipation due to chronic bowel contraction
Herpes zoster: vesicular rash may occur a day or so later than the dermatomal pain

G. Step 7: Consider the location of the pain. Use the "around-the-clock method" to use the location of the pain to guide your differential diagnosis (Figure 32-1).

H. Step 8: Exclude diagnoses that may be fatal. For example, in **peritonitis,** or inflammation of the abdominal lining, **death is imminent unless there is immediate surgical intervention.** Signs of peritonitis include guarding, tenderness on cross palpation, and a completely still body position.

1. **Shallow palpation: guarding**. The peritoneum lines the abdominal cavity and is heavily innervated with sensory fibers. Depressing the peritoneal lining sends a reflex arc to constrict the abdominal muscles; the muscle constriction creates a rigid, boardlike protection from outside stimuli (Figure 32-2). When the peritoneal lining is inflamed, this reflex arc is heightened. Even small depressions by palpation cause boardlike tightening of the abdominal wall (guarding).
   - **a.** Each of the three phases of guarding represents an increasing level of peritoneal irritation. Begin by testing for the most severe phase and then work backward.
     - **(1)** Phase III guarding (most severe): splinting. Observe the abdomen as the patient takes a deep breath, and look for one area of the abdomen that fails to rise. In severe peritonitis, even movement with breathing is sufficient to cause the abdominal muscles to constrict and limit motion.
     - **(2)** Phase II guarding: laying of hands. Lightly lay the palm of your hand on the abdomen. Feel the muscles constrict under your hand. This implies moderate peritoneal inflammation; only light touch stimulates the abdominal muscles to constrict.
     - **(3)** Phase I guarding: making a dent. With four fingertips, indent the abdomen 1 to 2 inches. If the peritoneum is mildly inflamed, this will cause the abdominal muscles to constrict. Tenderness may be elicited, but it is guarding only if you feel the abdominal muscles involuntarily constrict.
   - **b.** Tenderness or voluntary guarding (conscious constriction of the abdominal muscles) can occur in patients without peritonitis.
2. **Cross palpation.** Rebound tenderness refers to pressing deeply into the abdominal wall and then quickly releasing to see if pain

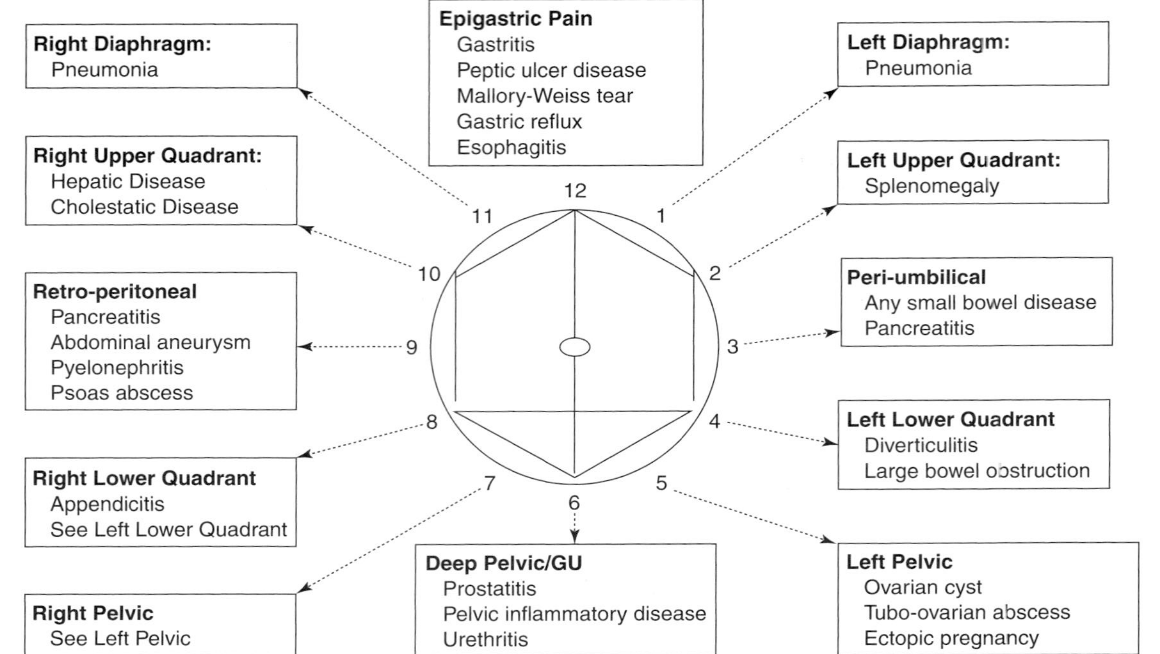

FIGURE 32-1. The clock method: generating a differential diagnosis for abdominal pain.

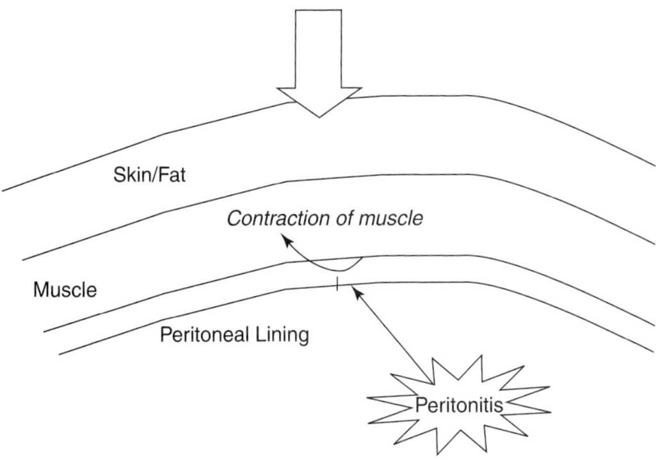

FIGURE 32-2. Diagram of the peritoneal reflex arc.

results. The quick release vibrates the peritoneum and induces pain if the peritoneum is inflamed. It is cruel to do this; if it is painful when going down (i.e., the patient has guarding), it will be painful when coming up. The exception to this is cross palpation. Press on a *nontender* area of the abdomen and then quickly let go. This makes all parts of the abdominal lining vibrate, and if peritonitis is present in another part of the abdomen, the pain will be localized to that area (i.e., not to the area at which pressure was applied and released).

3. **Completely still body position.** In later stages of peritonitis, the patient lies completely still so she does not shake the peritoneum and worsen the inflammation. Even subtle movements that shake the peritoneum (tapping the heel of the foot or bumping the side of the bed) are enough to exacerbate peritoneal pain.

HOT 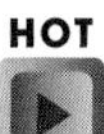 KEY

The presence of peritonitis should prompt an immediate call to surgery.

Every case of peritonitis begins with a distended organ that has not yet burst. Patients without signs of peritonitis may develop them later.

III OTHER COMPONENTS OF THE TIER II ABDOMINAL EXAMINATION

A. Exclude a gastrointestinal bleed.

1. **Perform a rectal examination.** It is possible to palpate most of the abdomen, but the pelvis is beyond reach. Peritonitis in the

pelvis is inaccessible except by rectal examination, which allows probing of the inside of the pelvis with the finger. The rectal examination also allows you to obtain stool and look for blood.

2. **Perform a guaiac test.**
   a. In general, ruptured peptic ulcers do not bleed; the blood is going into the peritoneum, not the bowel.
   b. In general, bleeding peptic ulcers do not rupture; the erosion is toward the bowel wall, not away from it.
3. **Obtain a hematocrit immediately.** This is the baseline by which subsequent hematocrits are measured. Order coagulation studies and a platelet count early.
4. **Prepare for the worst.** While evaluating for a gastrointestinal bleed, make sure there is adequate venous access (e.g., two large-bore peripheral IV lines) in case the patient suddenly needs volume resuscitation.

B. **Exclude a bowel obstruction.**
   1. Large bowel obstructions are characterized by **distention.**
   2. **Borborygmus**
      a. This is the sound of **"tinkles and rushes"** on auscultation of the abdomen. The "tinkles" are high-pitched sounds that result from a strong peristaltic attempt at pushing bowel contents through a small bowel obstruction. The "rushes" are the result of the peristaltic wave overcoming the obstruction and pushing bowel contents through. (a "rush" is the sound made when a person blows out a candle).
      b. This finding is **intermittent;** it occurs only with peristaltic waves. When the peristaltic wave hits the obstruction, the patient has pain; when there is no wave, there is no pain. As you obtain the history from the patient, place your stethoscope on the patient's abdomen with the earpieces out of your ears (so you can continue with the history). When the paroxysm of pain hits, quickly drop the earpieces in your ears and listen for the "tinkles and rushes."

C. **Exclude abdominal distention.** Percuss throughout the abdomen to determine the cause.
   1. **Solid.** Constipation due to a bowel obstruction or bowel ileus (the bowel is temporarily asleep) causing retained fecal matter. Percussion will be dull, reflecting the hard stool that is absorbing the percussion note.
   2. **Gas.** Ileus or bowel obstruction may also trap air within the colon or small bowel, thereby distending the abdomen. In this case, the percussion note will be hyperresonant like a drum.
   3. **Liquid.** Use the methods in section IV.D below to determine if ascites is present.

D. **Palpate for deeper structures.**
   1. It is possible the patient has a distended organ that has not yet burst. Moderate palpation will detect such tenderness.

2. Ask the patient where the pain is greatest. Palpate this area last. Palpate with the fingertips. Start with slow circles, extending 3 to 5 cm into the abdomen.
   a. Do not watch the abdomen as you palpate. Instead, keep your eyes on the patient's face. Watch for facial grimaces or a snarl (raising of the upper lip). Further distention of an already inflamed or distended organ elicits a vagal response that prompts nausea. The nausea reflex raises the upper lip in preparation for vomiting.
   b. If you see the upper lip rise, you know you have just palpated a distended or inflamed organ. You should be careful, because the patient may vomit.

HOT 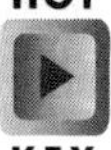 KEY

Do not be deterred by fear that your gentle palpation may rupture an organ. If it is that close to rupturing, its rupture is imminent. It is better to know of it before it ruptures.

3. **Liver and spleen.** See sections IV and V for an approach to examining the size of the liver and spleen.
4. **Gallbladder.** Look for **Murphy's sign** to assess for **cholecystitis.** Face the patient. Place your left hand on the patient's right costal margin, so your index finger is parallel to and along the lower costal margin. Your finger should point toward the xiphoid process. As the patient *exhales,* rotate your thumb into the patient's abdomen about 3 cm. Then ask the patient to take a deep breath. Murphy's sign is the *cessation of breathing* (not the presence of pain) as the diaphragm pushes the gallbladder against your thumb.
5. **Aortic aneurysm.** To palpate for this, place both hands flat on the patient's abdomen so that the MCP knuckle of the index finger of both hands is on the umbilicus. Open your hands so that the ulnar surface of both hands rests on the abdomen. Ask the patient to take a deep breath in, then out. During exhalation, press down 6 cm with both hands and move them toward each other. Hold your hands in that position and feel for a pulsating mass.
6. **Kidneys.** Palpating the kidneys is possible in very thin patients but is a futile exercise for the most part. The key is to make sure the kidneys are not swollen from obstruction or infection. Form your hand into a fist and lightly tap on the costovertebral border of the back. Exquisite tenderness suggests pyelonephritis.
7. **Pancreas.** Although is impossible to palpate the pancreas, ecchymosis in the flanks (Grey Turner's sign) and around the umbilicus (Cullen's sign) suggests hemorrhagic pancreatitis.
8. **Psoas and obturator muscles.** The psoas and obturator muscles, which form the posterior wall of the abdomen, are responsible for flexion of the hip. Infections may seed these muscles, creating

an abscess. Moving the muscle moves the abscess, and this increases the pain. With the patient lying supine, flex the hip by lifting the leg while keeping the knee straight. This will stretch the psoas muscle. With the hip flexed, flex the knee to 90 degrees and rotate the foot medially. This stretches the obturator muscle.

IV Liver Problems

A. **Liver enlargement.** Assessing the size of the liver is a Tier I examination (see Chapter 26). If the liver is enlarged, palpate the lower margin for consistency.

1. Stand at the right side of the patient's thorax, facing toward her left foot. Place your hands side by side with the palms down, so all fingers are pointing toward her feet. Find the lower costal margin. Place your hands so your palms are against the thorax and the fingers extend over the costal margin onto the abdomen. Keep your fingers touching the abdomen but raise your palms off the body.
2. When the patient exhales, the abdomen should go down. Now insert your fingers into the abdominal wall.
3. Flex your DIP joints (this requires slightly flexing the PIP joints as well). Your fingers should look as if you are holding onto the ledge of a cliff.
4. Push in 2 cm, flex the DIP joints, and pull back 1 cm. This creates a ledge across which the liver edge passes (Figure 32-3). As the patient takes a deep breath (the abdomen should rise), the diaphragm will move the liver across your fingers. Watch the patient's face as you do this. If the liver is acutely swollen, the patient will grimace as the liver edge moves across your fingers.
5. Liver enlargement resulting from tumor invasion feels nodular. All other causes of liver enlargement have a smooth edge.

B. **Portal hypertension.** The swelling of an enlarged liver or the contraction of the cirrhotic liver constricts the venous flow within the organ, causing an increase in portal vein pressure and swelling of the spleen and the bowel wall.

1. Ascites is the accumulation of serous fluid in the peritoneal space. The increased venous pressure increases fluid flow across the bowel and spleen membranes, dripping fluid into the abdominal cavity.
2. Opening of venous anastomosis. The elevated portal vein pressure will open old anastomoses, returning venous volume to the heart via hemorrhoids and distended veins on the abdominal surface (caput medusae and caput "Wiese"; see Chapter 26).

C. **Systemic signs of liver failure.** The signs of liver disease correspond to the functions of the liver.

1. **Inadequate progesterone metabolism.** Progesterone has two important functions.

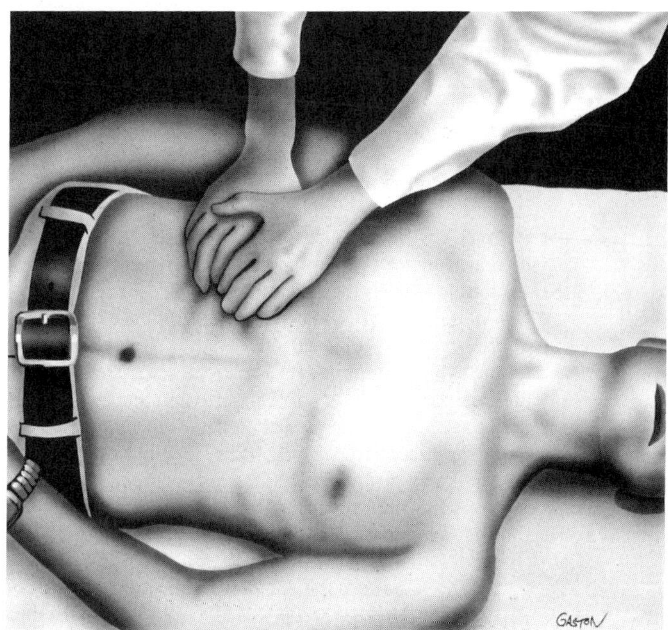

FIGURE 32-3. Liver palpation.

a. Stimulates respiration at the medulla

b. Decreases systemic vascular resistance by dilating arteriovenous connections. The examination may reveal signs of these arteriovenous shunts, including:

   (1) Spider angiomata (telangiectasias). These look like **small red spiders.** The body of the spider is the arterioles heading toward the skin, and the legs are small arteriole tributaries. The spider is apparent because it is opening up into a venule that sits just below the skin. If you push on the body of the spider, its legs disappear. Spider angiomata resulting from liver disease occur only on the parts of the body that are superior to the liver. Diffuse spiders suggest Osler-Weber-Rendu disease.

   (2) "Gin blossoms." These are small spiders that occur on the face, so named for their association with excessive gin consumption. Do not confuse gin blossoms with dilated small veins on the face and nose; these may occur in alcoholism but are seen in association with other causes of frequent vomiting. To be a spider, the mark must have the body and legs of a spider.

(3) **Hepatopulmonary syndrome.** Small arteriovenous malformations may also open within the lung arterioles, shunting blood from the right side of the heart to the left side. This manifests in hypoxia, which in turn increases pulmonary hypertension. The hypertension loudly slams the pulmonic valve closed at the end of systole, creating an S_2 sound that is louder in the pulmonic space (left of sternum; 2nd intercostal space) than in the aortic space.

(4) **Palmar erythema.** The loss of end-arteriolar resistance increases blood flow to the palmar surface.

(5) **Low blood pressure and narrow pulse pressure.** The loss of systemic vascular resistance decreases the mean arterial pressure, which decreases the afterload pressure the heart must pump against. Patients with liver disease appear to gain cardiac protection from this; they almost never have coexisting cardiac disease. Patients with alcoholic cardiomyopathy rarely have liver disease.

2. **Decreased estrogen clearance.** Excess estrogens, especially for men, result in gynecomastia and testicular atrophy.
   a. The normal testicle is 3 to 4 cm in length. The testes are atrophic if less than 2 cm.
   b. Gynecomastia requires augmentation of glandular tissue, not just excess fat around the areola. To identify true gynecomastia, feel for glandular tissue superior to the areola.
   c. The excess estrogen opposes testosterone's effect at the hair follicle, leaving a full, rich head of hair. Most men begin to have a receding hairline by 35 to 40 years of age, except for those who have liver disease.
   d. **Dupuytren's contractures** are contractures of the palmar flexor tendon that are associated with liver disease. They may also be found in persons with other diseases (e.g., epilepsy, vascular insufficiency), as well as in otherwise healthy people of Scandinavian and Celtic descent.

3. **Fetor hepaticus.** Ammonia is normally cleared by the liver. When it accumulates, NH_3 gas is expelled by the lungs, generating the odor of rotten shrimp. NH_3 is a soluble gas that penetrates into the cerebrospinal fluid, where it is locked in the form of NH_4^+. Its presence creates toxic metabolic encephalopathy.
   a. **Asterixis** (loss of postural tone)
      (1) Ask the patient to hold his hands with the wrists fully extended, as if he was stopping traffic. The patient tries to maintain this tone, but the motor neurons momentarily fade and the patient lowers his hands. The patient quickly realizes this, and a compensatory extensor movement occurs at the wrist. This gives the wrist a **flapping appearance.**

(2) Alternatively, ask the patient to squeeze two of your fingers and hold the squeeze. Momentary loss in tone results in relaxation followed by resumption of the squeeze, as if the patient was milking a cow.

HOT
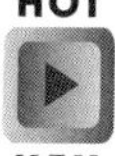
KEY

Tremor in the hand does not constitute asterixis.

b. **Encephalopathy** (see Chapter 34)
c. **Spatial apraxia.** Ask the patient to complete a dot-to-dot puzzle or sign his name; both tasks require spatial skills (with minimal cognitive skills) to complete.
d. **Day-night reversal.** Patients with liver disease awaken at night and sleep during the day. Be wary of ascribing daytime somnolence to hepatic encephalopathy; the patient simply may be tired from being up all night.

4. **Decreased albumin production** resulting in ascites and peripheral edema (see Chapter 33).
5. **Hyperbilirubinemia.** Bilirubin derives from biliverdin, the breakdown product of hemoglobin. The liver passively (no ATP energy is required) conjugates the bilirubin to be excreted as bile. The hyperbilirubinemia of liver disease is conjugated bilirubin, and even a few damaged cells can cause it. The increase in bilirubin is due to the obstruction of intrahepatic bile ducts from liver swelling or cirrhosis. The bilirubin deposits in all membranes, especially the eyes, mouth, ears, and skin.

D. **Ascites.** Physical examination is not reliable in detecting small collections of serous fluid in the abdominal cavity ascites, so use this examination with caution. The following techniques can be useful in detecting larger amounts of ascites:

1. **Ascites as fluid.** Fluid goes to the most dependent location, causing the flanks to bulge as the patient reclines. This test is sensitive, but because fat drops to the sides as well, it is not specific.
2. **Shifting dullness.** The air-filled bowels float on top of the fluid, forming a meniscus of air at the apex of the patient's abdomen. Have the patient lie flat and begin percussing at the umbilicus. There should be a tympanic sound. Continue percussing as you move laterally (to the patient's left) from this point. At some point, the percussion note will become dull. This is the point where you have moved off the air bubble. Mark this point of dullness. Now roll the patient one fourth of the way to his right (toward you). Begin percussing at the umbilicus, again moving toward the left. If ascites is present, the air bubble will float to the highest elevation in the abdomen. The line of dullness should have shifted to the patient's left.

3. **Fluid wave.** Place one hand (the patient's or an assistant's) in the middle of the patient's abdomen. Place your right hand on the patient's left lateral abdomen (toward the flank). With your left hand, give the patient's right flank a vigorous tap. The assistant's hand in the middle should prevent the fat jiggle from mimicking thc fluid wave vibrating your other hand. If there is ascites in the abdomen, your right hand should feel the wave of fluid (caused by your left hand) hitting the right abdominal wall.
4. **Distinguishing the cause of the ascites**
   a. **Increased hydrostatic pressure.** Swelling or fibrosis of the liver causes constriction of the hepatic veins, increasing portal vein pressure. The increased venous pressure expands the spleen and bowels, and fluid leaks from both. This also swells the bowels, resulting in constipation and distention. If bacteria leak from the bowels, spontaneous bacterial peritonitis can result.
   b. **Increased oncotic pressure** in the abdomen results from **cancer** that has seeded the abdominal wall or from **tuberculosis.** The liver is more likely to be large, because the cancer has infiltrated it, and the spleen will not be palpable. Because the spleen and bowels are not distended (portal pressure is normal), the signs of caput medusae, caput "Wiese," and hemorrhoids are absent. For the same reason, there is no risk of spontaneous bacterial peritonitis.

V Spleen: Splenomegaly

A. The spleen is a retroabdominal organ. The causes of splenomegaly have two features in common: **chronic inflammation** and **infiltrative diseases.**

Causes of **SPLENOMEGALY**
Sarcoidosis
Portal hypertension
Leukemia
Endocarditis
Neoplasia
Opportunistic infections
Malaria
Epstein-Barr virus (mononucleosis)
Gaucher's disease
Autoimmune disease (Felty's disease, lupus)
Lymphoma

B. To palpate the spleen, use the method for palpating the liver, except now stand on the patient's left side. The spleen is a very mobile organ; it floats like apples in a bobbing apple tank. **Do not push too hard,** or you will push the spleen away from you. Let the spleen come to you (via the diaphragm pushing down during inspiration). In addition, remember that the spleen moves toward the umbilicus during its initial expansion (not toward the feet, as with liver enlargement). Position your hands accordingly.

HOT
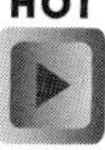
KEY

A palpable spleen is always abnormal.

33. The Tier II Extremity Examination

I THE BIG PICTURE OF SKIN ABNORMALITIES A detailed Tier II extremity examination should be performed if you identify one of the problems listed below as part of your history or Tier I examination.

A. Rash
B. Suspected skin cancer
C. Leg ulcers
D. Nail abnormalities
E. Peripheral edema
F. Lymph nodes
G. Hand pain
H. Wrist pain
I. Loss of hand function
J. Abnormal skin over the hand and wrist
K. Infected joints
L. Elbow pain
M. Shoulder pain
N. Back pain
O. Hip pain
P. Knee pain
Q. Ankle pain
R. Suspected compartment syndrome

II SKIN LESIONS/RASHES Your primary task is to describe the skin lesion and then use a dermatology atlas to diagnose the cause. Get close—skin lesions should be evaluated from a distance of less than 20 cm. Use Figure 27-1 to guide your description.

A. Distribution

1. **Isolated lesions** suggest contact dermatitis or infection. **Symmetric lesions** suggest a diffuse infection or a systemic disease.
2. **Photosensitivity rashes** occur in sun-exposed areas (face, arms). The erythematous rash (occasionally with vesicles) is due to inflammation from a foreign substance (porphyrins in the case of porphyria; Ag-Ab complexes in the case of lupus, dermatomyositis, and drugs) that when exposed to ultraviolet light creates oxygen free-radicals that damage the tissue.
3. **Intertriginous lesions** (between the toes or in the groin) are due to fungus (because it requires the moist environment to survive)

or scabies. If cellulitis is present, look for concomitant fungal infections. The bacteria and fungus rely on each other, so the cellulitis will not respond to antibiotics unless the fungus is treated. Scabies is a skin mite that creates linear burrows between the fingers. These are highly pruritic (scab = to itch).

4. **Follicular lesions** imply damage to the hair follicle occurring with infection or scurvy (twisted hairs within the follicle).
5. **Groin lesions** suggest fungus, erythrasma (*Corynebacterium* infection), or sexually transmitted diseases (see Chapter 36).
6. **Hands** have the greatest exposure to the environment; contact dermatitis or atopic dermatitis are the most common.

B. Arrangement

1. **Linear and serpiginous** (snakelike) imply a histamine-mediated urticarial lesion or a type IV reaction (poison ivy).
2. **Reticulated lesions** (spider web appearance) follow the pattern of the reticulated vessels beneath the skin. This implies vasculitis.
3. **Dermatomal lesions** imply herpes zoster (reactivation of the varicella virus along the infected dermatome).
4. **Primary lesions with smaller satellite lesions** suggest *Candida* infection.
5. **Grouped and annular lesions** are likely to be a primary dermatologic lesion or fungal infection (tinea corporis). You will have to use other clues to make the diagnosis.

C. Type of eruption. If the distribution and arrangement of lesions has not made the diagnosis, use the type of lesion to narrow the differential. There are three important questions: Can you feel the lesion? What is its size? What does it contain? (Figures 33-1 and 33-2).

1. **Flat lesions (Figure 33-2)**
   a. **Macule.** A colored or depigmented area that cannot be palpated. Erythematous macules are usually drug reactions, especially if they blanch (see below for nonblanching lesions) (Table 33-1). **Depigmented macules are due to vitiligo** or tinea veriscolor (antibodies to melanin destroy the pigment).
   b. **Patch.** A greater than 1-cm macule. The most common cause is coalescing macules.
2. **Raised lesions**
   a. **Papule.** A raised, punctate lesion. This may be due to dilatation of a vessel or a burst vessel (vasculitis; see below) (Table 33-2).
   b. **Plaque.** A flat-topped area elevated above the skin surface. This implies infiltration of the dermis that is raising the epidermis (see Table 33-2).
   c. **Nodule.** A dome-shaped mass elevated above the skin surface (Table 33-3).
   d. **Tumor.** A nodule greater than 2 cm. The etiologies are the same as for nodules (see Table 33-3).

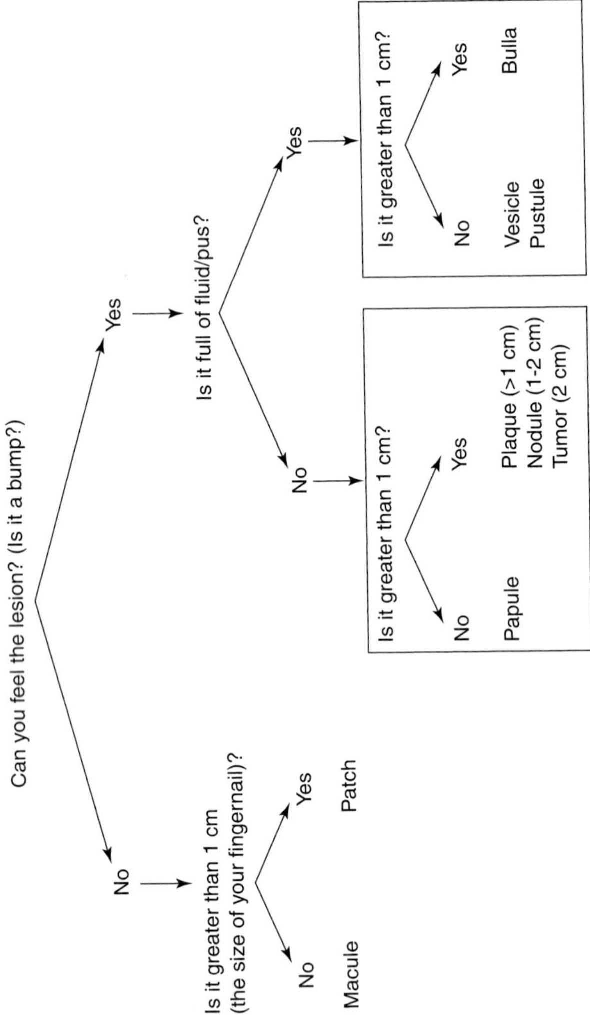

FIGURE 33-1. An approach to determining the type of lesion.

Primary lesions

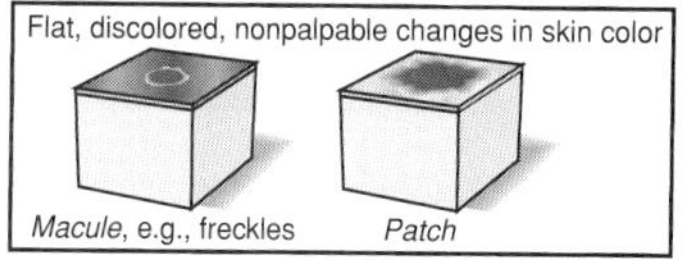

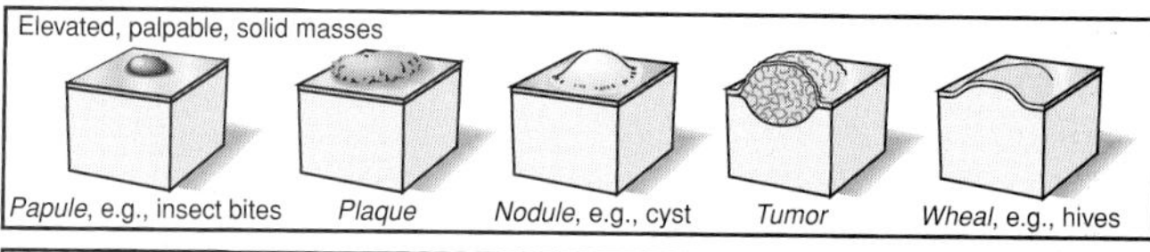

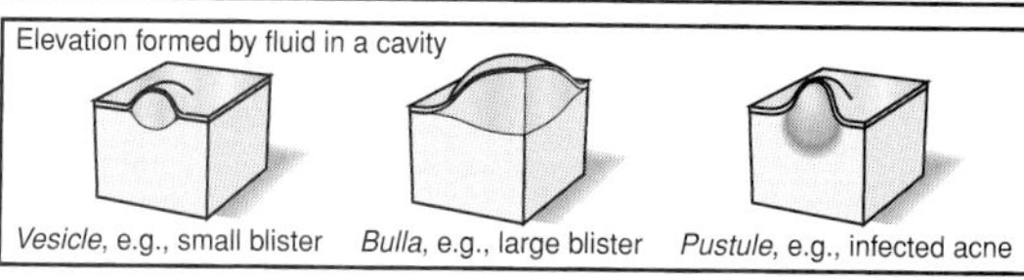

Secondary lesions

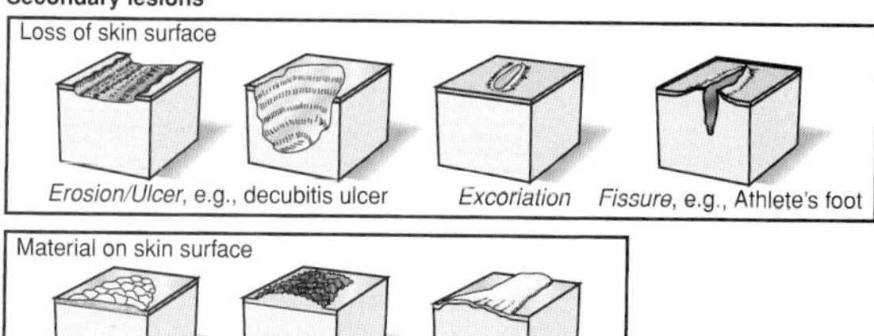

Vascular lesions

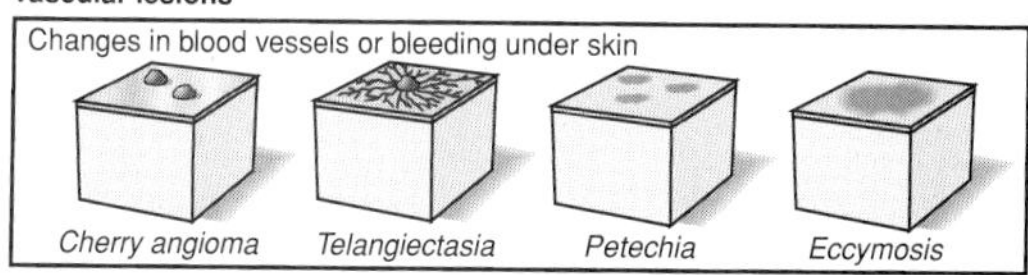

FIGURE 33-2. Types of skin lesions. (From *Stedman's Medical Dictionary*, 27th ed. Baltimore: Lippincott Williams & Wilkins, 2000.)

3. **Fluid-filled lesions**
   a. **Vesicle.** A transparent fluid-filled elevation. Vesicles form when inflammation resulting from an infection or autoimmune disease splits the layers of the skin. Tense vesicles are due to a split between the dermis and epidermis; flaccid vesicles are a split within the dermis (Table 33-4).

TABLE 33-1. Causes of Macules and Patches

Lesion	Location	Special Features
Erythematous Lesions		
Erythema multiforme	Anywhere; palms especially	Usually due to a drug reaction or herpes or *Mycoplasma* infection. Target lesions and lesions of multiple shapes.
Lupus erythematosus	Sun-exposed areas	
Pityriasis rosea	Back/trunk	Christmas tree pattern on the back.
Seborrheic dermatitis	Scalp, face, skinfolds, groin	Suspect immunocompromised condition.
Secondary syphilis	Anywhere; does involve the palms and soles	May be macular or papular; nonblanching (vasculitis).
Rocky Mountain spotted fever	Extremities; does involve the palms and soles	May be macular or papular; nonblanching (vasculitis).
Drug eruption	Anywhere	Erythematous or pigmented. Drug reactions can occur at any time.
Tinea corporis	Trunk	Erythematous; pruritic.
Pigmented Lesions		
Junctional melanocytic nevi		
Melanoma	Anywhere, but especially sun-exposed areas.	See text for the ABCD criteria for melanoma.
Lentigines (freckles)	Sun-exposed areas	Benign.
Peutz-Jegher's	Face/lips	Associated with GI complaints, especially GI bleeding.

(Continued)

TABLE 33-1. Continued

Lesion	Location	Special Features
Melasma	Face	Hyperpigmented areas of the face; associated with pregnancy or estrogens.
Café-au-lait lesions	Anywhere	Neurofibromatosis.
Urticaria pigmentosa	Trunk	
Drug reactions	Anywhere	
Depigmented Lesions		
Vitiligo	Face/trunk	Depigmented.
Tinea versicolor	Trunk	Under the breasts. Fungal infection. Usually pruritic.
Tinea corporis	Trunk	Trunk. Fungal infection. Usually pruritic.
Erythrasma	Groin	Due to *Corynebacterium* infection. Coalesces blue under Wood's lamp.
Tinia cruris	Groin	Groin. Fungal infection. Usually puritic, scaling.

   b. **Bulla.** A lesions greater than 1 cm. The causes are the same as for vesicles.
   c. **Pustule.** A vesicle filled with pus. (See Table 33-5.)
4. **Excavated lesions**
   a. **Erosion.** Loss of all or part of the epidermis.
   b. **Ulcer.** An erosion that has extended into the dermis. This usually implies focal ischemia to the tissue resulting from vascular plugging or damage. The ulcer is the result of the necrosis (Table 33-6).
5. **Purpuric lesions.** The purple color is due to extravasation of blood cells into the skin.
   a. **Petechia.** Pinpoint purpura. This is due to rupture of small capillaries as a result of trauma or vasculitis. Normal platelets

TABLE 33-2. Causes of Papules and Plaques.

Lesion	Location	Special Features
Erythematous		
Acne	Scalp/face;	
Actinic keratosis	sun-exposed areas	Premalignant lesion. Flaky surface.
Basal cell carcinoma	Scalp/face	Nodule with heaped-up, pearly borders.
Chronic eczema	Scalp/face/trunk	
Cryoglobulinemia	Extremities, ears (cold areas)	
Dermatomyositis	Anywhere	
Dermatitis herpetiformis	Dorsal trunk and extremities, knees	Iodides or gluten sensitivity induces IgA deposition that causes the rash.
Erysipelas	Face	Localized cellulitis of the face.
Erythema migrans (Lyme disease)	Trunk/extremities	Erythematous lesion with central clearing at the site of the tick bite.
Granuloma annulare	Dorsal extremities	Annular lesions that may appear similar to tinea corporis (ringworm). Self-limiting.
Hypersensitivity vasculitis (palpable purpura).	Extremities	Inflammation of venules due to antigens from drugs, infections, or IgA (Henoch-Shönlein purpura).
Lichen planus	Trunk, extremities	

(Continued)

TABLE 33–2. Continued

Lesion	Location	Special Features
Lupus erythematosus	Anywhere, but especially on sun-exposed areas	Butterfly rash.
Morphea	Anywhere	"Carnauba wax" central area surrounded by lilac border. May be associated with scleroderma.
Mycoses fungoides	Trunk	Cutaneous T-cell lymphoma. Erythematous, serpiginous.
Papular uritcaria	Trunk	
Pityriasis rosea	Trunk/back	Preceded by a herald patch. Christmas tree pattern. Remits spontaneously.
Psoriasis	Scalp, ears, elbows, soles, genitalia, hands, lower back, and rectal crease	
Pyogenic granuloma	Face	Rapidly developing hemangioma at the site of previous trauma; bleeds spontaneously.
Rosacea	Face	See above.
Sarcoid	Face	Lupus pernio.
Syphilis	Face/trunk	
Urticaria pigmentosa	Face/trunk	
Skin Colored		
Squamous cell carcioma	Face/scalp	
Molluscum contagiosum	Face/trunk	
Verruca (planuua or vulgaris)	Anywhere	
Neurofibromatosis	Trunk	

(Continued)

TABLE 33–2. Continued

Lesion	Location	Special Features
Pigmented		
Melanocytic nevi (mole)	Scalp/face	
Melanoma		
Seborrheic keratosis	Scalp/face, trunk	Stuck-on, waxy appearance.
Angiofibroma	Scalp	
Hereditary hemorrhagic telangiectasia		

will prevent petechia resulting from trauma unless the platelet count is less than 50 (see above).

b. Ecchymosis. Extensive in size. Bruising, draining blood, or necrotizing fasciitis (see below).

c. Hematoma. Massive in size.

6. Scaling lesions are due to psoriasis (see below), seborrheic dermatitis (around the head, face, and groin), lupus, or actinic keratosis (Table 33-7).

D. Shapes. Oval, annular (ringlike), serpiginous, angular, or linear (see II B).

E. Margins. Defined or ill-defined. Look for satellite lesions.

F. Blanching. Press on the lesion with a clear glass slide (or your glasses). Assess whether the lesion blanches (goes away) or does not blanch. Blanching lesions are due to dilation of vessels, usually in response to histamine (i.e., drug or food reactions). Because the vessel is still intact, pressure will push the blood out either side of the vessel tube, eliminating the lesion's color. Nonblanching lesions are due to inflammation (vasculitis) that has breeched the vessel wall or the body's inability to repair incidental damage to the vessel (see petechia above). Blood makes its way into the interstitium, forming a small hematoma that cannot be squeezed back into the vessel with pressure. The lesion's color remains with pressure. Syphilis (and other spirochetes), Rocky Mountain spotted fever, primary vasculitis, and emboli (endocarditis, cholesterol emboli) are examples.

III SKIN CANCER

The four varieties of skin cancer are all most common on sun-exposed areas. Look for these carefully; skin cancer is the most common cancer.

A. Actinic keratosis (AK) is a scaling, premalignant lesion.

B. Squamous cell cancer appears as a crusted plaque. It is usually a progression from an AK.

TABLE 33-3. Causes of Nodules or Tumors.

Lesion	Location	Special Features
Erythematous		
Amyloidosis	Anywhere	
Granuloma annulare	Trunk/extremities	
Pyogenic granuloma	Face	
Sarcoid	Face	Lupus pernio.
Erythema nodosum	Trunk/extremities	Sarcoid, post-*Streptococcus* infections, TB, fungus, sulfa drugs, estrogens.
Pretibial myxedema	Extremities	Graves' disease.
Skin Colored		
Benign neoplasms	Anywhere	
Lipoma	Anywhere	A benign collection of fat.
Malignant neoplasms	Anywhere	Squamous and basal cell carcinomas.
Melanocytic nevi	Anywhere	
Metastatic tumors	Scalp/face/trunk	Breast, renal cell, melanoma.
Neurofibromatosis	Trunk	
Nevus sebaceous	Scalp/face	
Pigmented		
Basal cell carcinoma	Face	
Blue nevus	Face	
Kaposi's sarcoma	Face/trunk/extremities	
Melanocytic nevus	Face/trunk	
Melanoma	Face/trunk	
Seborrheic keratosis	Face/trunk	

C. Basal cell cancer is a nodule with heaped-up pearly borders.

D. Melanoma. Melanomas elicit an immune response that destroys some but not all of the tumor. This creates the classic appearance. The ABCDEs: **A**symmetric, irregular **B**orders, mottled **C**olor, **D**iameter greater than 6 mm and **E**levation/**E**nlargement over time. Obtain a biopsy of all suspicious lesions, especially if they change over time.

TABLE 33-4. Causes of Vesicles.

Lesion	Location	Special Features
Bullous impetigo	Face/trunk	
Bullous pemphigoid	Trunk	
Contact dermatitis	Scalp/face	
Dermatitis herpetiformis	Scalp/face/trunk	
Drug reactions	Scalp/face/trunk	
Dyshidrotic eczemae	Hands/feet	Tapioca-like vesicles; pruritic.
Eczematous dermatitis	Scalp/trunk	
Herpes simplex	Face	
Herpes zoster	Scalp/face/trunk	
Pemphigus vulgaris	Scalp/face/trunk	
Porphyria cutanea tarda	Sun-exposed areas	Especially seen in alcoholics.
Scabies	Trunk	
Varicella	Trunk	

TABLE 33-5. Causes of Pustules.

Lesion	Location	Special Features
Acne	Scalp/face/trunk	
Drug reactions	Face/trunk	
Fungal infections	Anywhere	Systemic *Candida* infection.
Hidradenitis suppurativa	Axilla	
Hot tub folliculitis		*Pseudomonas* infection.
Impetigo	Face/trunk	
Staphylococcus folliculitis	Scalp/face/trunk	
Rosacea	Face	Untreated, it may cause blindness.
Scabies	Trunk	
Tine corporis	Trunk	

TABLE 33-6. Causes of Ulcers.

Lesion	Location	Special Features
Carcinoma	Scalp/face	
Ecthyma gangrenosum	Extremities	*Pseudomonas*-induced. Deep ulcer on an erythematous base.
Factitial/neurotic excoriations	Scalp/face	
Melanoma	Scalp/face	
Arterial insufficiency	Extremities	Lateral/ventral extremities.
Venous insufficiency	Extremities	Medial extremities.
Decubitus ulcers	Dependent areas	
Pyoderma gangreosum		Crohn's, ulcerative colitis.

IV Leg Ulcers

See Chapter 27, IV.

V Nail Abnormalities

A. See Chapter 23 for an approach to nail abnormalities.

B. Nailfold capillaries. This underutilized test consists of placing a drop of immersion oil on the nail matrix (the skin that abuts the nail base). Look at it under a dissecting microscope (10×) or even an ophthalmoscope. The capillaries should come to the end of the matrix, make a "U" turn and return the body, forming a capillary loop. Vasculitic diseases such as lupus, scleroderma, and CREST syndrome obliterate these capillaries.

VI Peripheral Edema

Use Equation 9 (Appendix A) to diagnose the cause of the edema. The causes of edema include:

A. High hydrostatic venous pressure. Start with the aortic root and work backward to the edema. Remember that a stenotic or incompetent valve will put back-pressure all the way to the effusion. Use the physical examination to evaluate each possibility (Table 33-8).

B. Low oncotic pressure. Picture a rib eye steak on a plate. Follow its path as the protein makes its way from the plate to the liver. Then exclude cause of protein loss (Table 33-9).

TABLE 33-7. Causes of Scales, Lichenification, and Crusts.

Lesion	Location	Special Features
Atopic dermatitis	Scalp/trunk	
Basal cell carcinoma	Scalp	
Contact dermatitis		
Eczematous dermatitis	Anywhere	
Lichen simplex chronicus	Posterior neck, groin, thighs, scrotum, lateral shins, Achilles	Long-term consequence of repeated scratching of atopic dermatitis.
Lichen planus	Sun-exposed areas. Also occurs in the mouth.	Shiny, flat-topped, pruritic lesions.
Lupus erythematosus	Scalp	Chronic.
Nummular eczema	Lower legs	Older males; round patches of eczema.
Psoriasis	Scalp/face/trunk	
Pyogenic infections	Scalp	SSSS, impetigo, TEN.
Seborrheic dermatitis	Scalp	
Tinea capitis	Scalp	
Tinea corporis	Trunk	
Zinc deficiency	Scalp/face	

C. High permeability.

1. Sepsis. Look for other signs of infection.
2. Hypothyroidism. Obtain a TSH value.
3. Anaphylaxis. Review the medication history.
4. Drugs. Calcium channel blockers, clonidine, minoxidil, hydralazine, corticosteroids, estrogen, testosterone, and progesterone may increase vessel permeability.
5. Pit viper bites. The venom inhibits degradation of bradykinin in the lungs, increasing vessel permeability.

D. The location of the edema is an additional clue in diagnosing the cause.

1. Focal edema suggests a hydrostatic cause just proximal to that area. The left leg is almost always the first extremity to be involved because the left ileac vein must cross under the aorta to get to the IVC; this compression increases the pressure. The right ileac vein drains directly into the IVC.

TABLE 33-8. Causes of Edema: High Hydrostatic Pressure.

1. Aortic stenosis/insufficiency. Listen for murmurs.*
2. Cardiomyopathy. Look for an S_3, diffuse PMI, and soft S_1.*
3. Mitral stenosis/insufficiency. Listen for murmurs.*
4. Pulmonary hypertension. Listen for a loud P2.*
5. Pulmonary stenosis/insufficiency (rare). Listen for murmurs.*
6. Tricuspid stenosis/insufficiency (rare, unless acute). Listen for murmurs and look for AC merger in the JVP pulsations.*
7. Inferior vena cava obstruction (baby; adominal mass, thrombus).
8. Deep vein thrombosis (DVT). Feel for venous cords in the lower extremity. The physical examination of the lower extremity in diagnosing DVT is worthless. Homan's sign is a waste of time; get an ultrasound if it is of concern.
9. Varicose veins; incompetent venous valves.
10. Lymphatic obstruction.

* See Chapter 31.

2. Edema of the face and upper extremities implies a low oncotic pressure or high permeability because gravity (in the upright patient) opposes the venous hydrostatic pressure.

E. Grading edema. There are two parts to grading edema: the extent/location and the pit recovery time.

1. The extent is easily described by noting how far up the edema extends (e.g., edema to the thighs).

TABLE 33-9. Causes of Edema: Low Oncotic Pressure.

1. Kwashiorkor; inadequate protein intake. Look for other signs of malnutrition and vitamin deficiencies.
2. Protein losing enteropathy; abnormal absorption of the protein through the bowel wall. Ask about diarrhea.
3. Cirrhosis. Examine for ascites and other signs of liver failure.
4. Nephrotic syndrome. Examine the urine for protein.
5. Pancreatitis. Protein is lost into the "retroperitoneal burn" that is pancreatitis. Examine for signs of pancreatitis.
6. Burns.
7. Inflammatory bowel disease. Protein is lost from the inflamed bowel wall. Ask about diarrhea.

2. **The pit recovery time (PRT).** Push your finger into the area of edema and hold it for 5 seconds. Release and then measure the amount of time it takes for the pit to return to normal. Each 30 seconds of PRT corresponds to each grade of edema (Figure 33-3). The PRT is useful in distinguishing high hydrostatic pressure from low oncotic pressure/high permeability as a cause of the edema. If the PRT is >60 seconds, the cause is high hydrostatic pressure.

F. Special pearls in diagnosing edema:

1. **Look for sacral edema in bed-bound patients;** the sacrum will be in a more dependent position than the legs, and early edema may collect at the sacrum before it is detected in the legs.
2. **Lipedema**. In the obese patient, excess interstitial fat will retain water. Diuretics will be futile, because the edema is not due to high venous hydrostatic pressure, but rather retention of fluid in the fat in the legs. The clue is that there will be no edema on the dorsum of the feet (because there is no fat there). High hydrostatic venous pressure (i.e., CHF) will cause the feet to swell because they are the most dependent parts of the body.
3. **Nonpitting edema** is due to infiltration of the subdermal tissue with something other than fluid. It appears as a raised, thickened, peau d'orange dimpling over the dorsum of the legs. Causes include:
   a. Graves' disease: antibodies that dock on the TSH receptor to cause hyperthyroidism also attack the subdermal tissue, causing fibrous plaques.

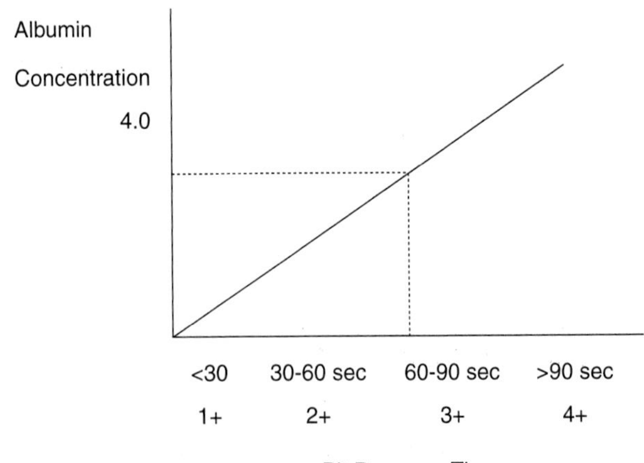

FIGURE 33-3. The correlation of pit recovery time and the serum albumin concentration.

b. Scleroderma is a disease of unknown etiology in which fibrotic tissue is laid down in the interstital space.

VII LYMPH NODES

See Chapter 27.

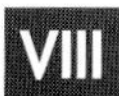

GENERAL RULES OF RHEUMATOLOGY

Rheumatology is the study of liquid that flows from the joints (rheum = to flow). Learn the simple rules of rheumatology, and your attending physicians can teach you the exceptions.

A. Know the roster. There are only a few diseases that affect the joints: osteoarthritis, gout/pseudogout, lupus, rheumatoid arthritis, bacterial infections, and the seronegative arthropathies ("PAIR of diseases:" **p**soriasis, **an**klyosing spondilitis, **in**flammatory bowel disease, **r**eactive arthritis).

B. Joints that bear the greatest weight (knees, hips) and those that are used most frequently (vertebrae, DIPs, and the thumb) wear down the fastest. Osteoarthritis is caused by this wear and tear and it is found in these joints.

C. Systemic disease (rheumatoid arthritis, lupus) affects the whole organism; many joints are likely to be involved. If you see only one joint involved, suspect infection or gout.

D. Joint fluid is filtered fluid. Like other filters in the body, it captures bacteria and antigen-antibody complexes. These impurities cause inflammation and joint pain. Rheumatologic disease results when the body mounts an antibody to a self-antigen. Examples of these autoantibodies include the antinuclear antibody (ANA: lupus) and the rheumatoid factor (an antibody against the F_c portion of the body's normal IgG antibodies). The antigen-antibody complexes get stuck in filters throughout the body such as the glomeruli, small capillaries of the skin, the anterior eye, and the small joints. The symptoms of rheumatologic disease then are: glomerulonephritis, vasculitis, anterior uveititis, and arthritis.

IX PAIN IN THE HANDS

A. Distal interphalangeal joints. The Grand Old Party (GOP) convenes the DIPs:

1. Gout (gutta = a drop of evil humor) is crystallization of uric acid in the joints. Cyrstallization takes place in the coolest joints that are the farthest away from the core body. In order of frequency, gout involves the big toe, the ankle, the knee, and the DIPs (the most distal part of the hand). Think of gout as the "charge of the light brigade." Neutrophils rush into the joint to ingest the crystals and are speared by the spear-shaped crystals. Enzymes are released into the joint, and inflammation results;

thus, pain, redness, and swelling of the joint occur. The joint fluid reveals the presence of these spear-shaped crystals. Repeated bouts of gout will deposit some of these crystals to the side of the joint in a soft, cheesy mass (that glows yellow when you press on it) known as a **tophus.**

2. Osteoarthritis. Every time you pick up something, your DIPs move. Frequently moved joints wear down the cartilage between the bones, resulting in bone on bone friction. When you stimulate bone, it grows. A bony, nontender nodule to the side of a joint (Heberden's or Bruchard's nodules) signify osteoarthritis.
3. Psoriasis is due to an autoimmune attack on the body's skin, resulting in chronic hypertrophic growth of the skin. Skin lesions have multiple layers of skin that flake off prematurely. If you pick one of these scales, you will unroof the dermis, exposing fragile blood vessels, and the skin will bleed (Nikolski's sign). The skin involved is over flexor surfaces (the elbows, knees, behind the ears). These antibodies also involve DIPs. DIP arthritis from psoriasis is almost always accompanied by pitting of the nails (>11 pits per nail) and skin lesions.

B. Proximal interphalangeal joints. This is no-man's territory. It is usually the DIP crew of diseases (GOP) but can also be rheumatoid arthritis/lupus.

C. The metacarpal-interphalangeal joints and wrist are the territory of rheumatoid arthritis and lupus. When involved, the joints are inflamed, red, and tender. These two diseases are protean: to make the diagnosis, you must satisfy 4 of 7 criteria for RA and 4 of 11 for lupus. Table 33-10 has the criteria.

TABLE 33-10. Diagnostic Criteria for Lupus and Rheumatoid Arthritis.

Rheumatoid Arthritis	Lupus
1. Morning stiffness	1. Malar rash
2. Hand joints involved	2. Discoid rash
3. Symmetric joints involved	3. Blood abnormalities
	4. Renal disease
4. Involves three or more joints	5. ANA
	6. Immune phenomenon
5. Radiographic changes	7. Neurologic abnormalities
6. Rheumatoid factor positive	8. Serositis
	9. Oral ulcers
7. Rheumatoid nodules	10. Arthritis
	11. Photosensitivity rash

1. The pearls of RA:
   a. In RA, the RF stimulates a collection of tissue (the panus) just beneath the cartilage lining that erodes into the bone, creating an erosive arthritis. Highly mobile joints pump this RF out of the joint; sedentary joints (such as the MCPs, wrist, elbows, C1-C2) are the most frequently involved.
   b. Rheumatoid nodules are a collection of this RF complexed with other antibodies. They are mobile, nontender round nodules that occur on flexor surfaces of the elbows and wrist.
   c. Eighty percent of the destructive arthritis occurs in the first 2 years. Unlike lupus, RA should be treated early with a disease-modifying drug such as methotrexate, sulfasalazine, infliximab, antimalarials.
   d. Always get neck films on RA patients undergoing surgery to exclude involvement of the C1-C2 spine. The act of flexing the neck during intubation can break the patient's neck.
   e. RA, unlike lupus, rarely involves the kidney or serosal linings (pleuritis, pericarditis).
2. Lupus pearls:
   a. Lupus is caused by ANA antibodies (with the nuclear antigen attached) trapped in the joint space. There is no pannus like in RA, so even though there is inflammation, there is no joint erosion.
   b. When these antibody-antigen complexes deposit in the skin, the cause a photosensitivity rash (see II A 2). The malar rash occurs because the face is the most photosensitive.
   c. Lupus patients will receive many courses of steroids over their lifetime; try to minimize each dose as much as possible. As opposed to RA, treat symptomatically and back off as soon as possible.
   d. Each lupus crisis has a corresponding infection (glomerulonephritis = pyelonephritis; neuritis = meningitis, serositis = pneumonia, pancytopenia = sepsis). Because of her steroid history and the impaired WBCs, always exclude infection before treating a lupus patient with steroids.
   e. Some drugs can induce a similar ANA. Drug-induced lupus only involves the skin and joints; no organs are involved. It goes away with stopping the drug. Another clue is that antihistone antibodies will be positive in drug-induced lupus, but not in de novo lupus.

X Pain of the Wrist

A. Rheumatoid arthritis (see above)
B. Lupus (see above)

C. DeQuervian's tenosynovitis. This is inflammation of the extensor tendons of the thumb. Ask the patient to place his thumb in the palm of the hand, close his fingers tightly over it, and maximally ulnar deviate the wrist (as if casting a fishing line). Finklestein's test stretches these tendons; if they are inflamed, the pain will get worse.

D. Ganglion cyst. Sometimes there is a redundancy in the synovial membrane that contains the joint fluid. When the joint extends, fluid escapes into this out-pocket; when it flexes, it seals off the opening, trapping fluid in this space. This is a ganglion cyst, and it can occur over any joint in the hand or wrist. It is hard, semi-mobile, and painful. It is also known as a Bible cyst, because the only ways to treat it are to (1) surgically remove it, (2) let it go away on its own, or (3) hit it very hard with a Bible so that it pops (not to be done clinically). Because it is filled with synovial fluid, it will transilluminate (glow red) when a halogen light is placed next to it in a dark room.

E. Fractures of the wrist. It is impossible to distinguish a fracture from a strain (stretched ligament) following trauma to the wrist; obtain a radiographic film. One fracture is special, however. Navicular fractures often take 24 to 48 hours before the a positive radiograph is obtained. To make the diagnosis, press on the anatomical snuffbox (the space between the two extensor tendons of the thumb). If tenderness is elicited, a navicular fracture may be present, even if the radiograph is negative.

XI LOSS OF FUNCTION OF THE HAND

This is due to loss of function of one of the three nerves that supply the hand.

A. Median nerve injury. The median nerve passes under the flexor tendon sheath of the wrist. Carpal tunnel syndrome results from prolonged pressure on the wrist (overuse injuries) or trauma that induces compression of this space and thus the median nerve. Use your examination to make the diagnosis.

1. Tinnel's sign: Tap on the flexor tendon sheath at the crease in the wrist. If carpal tunnel syndrome is present, this will irritate the nerve, sending a shock down the first, second and third fingers.
2. Phalen's sign: Ask the patient to maximally flex the wrists for 30 seconds. This will do nothing to a normal median nerve, but the compression will induce numbness of the first, second, and third fingers if the patient has carpal tunnel syndrome.
3. Look for muscle atrophy of the thenar eminence. Loss of nerve stimulation of the muscle causes atrophy.
4. The benediction sign is seen in patients who have had damage to the median nerve higher up in the arm (i.e., not due to carpal tunnel syndrome). Ask the patient to tightly close his fist. Patients with median nerve impairment proximal to where it innervates the flexor muscles of the first, second, and third fingers can flex fingers 4 and 5, but not 1 to 3.

B. Ulnar nerve injury. The ulnar nerve innervates the fourth and fifth fingers and the interosseous muscles that bring the fingers together side by side.

1. Ask the patient to make a fist. Place an index card between two of his fingers. Tell him to squeeze tight. The contraction of the interosseous muscles will prevent removal of the card in a normal hand; it will slide easily out of the hand in an ulnar nerve injury.
2. Over time, the interosseous muscle will atrophy, and the flexor muscles will take over, leading to the "claw hand."
3. Ask the patient to make a tight fist. The fourth and fifth fingers will remain open, as if he is making an "OK" sign.

C. Radial nerve injury. The radial nerve extends the wrist and provides sensation for the dorsal hand and wrist. The patient will be unable to extend his wrist against resistance.

XII Abnormal Skin over the Hand and Wrist

A. Raynaud's disease and Raynaud's phenomenon are due to abnormal vasospasm of the arteries to the hand when exposed to cold. Dunk the patient's hand in a bucket of ice; look for the patriotic pattern: white hands resulting from lack of blood flow, followed by blue hands resulting from cyanosis, then red hands resulting from hyper-reperfusion.

1. Raynaud's disease is not associated with other diseases. The capillary loops on the matrix (see above) are normal.
2. Raynaud's phenomenon is associated with lupus, CREST syndrome, scleroderma, and other diseases. The capillary loops are shaggy or obliterated.

B. Sclerodactaly looks like sausage digits. This is always a sign of a disease that affects the tendons of the fingers. Swelling of the tendons between the joints makes the finger look like a sausage. It is a sign of either scleroderma or CREST syndrome. Scleroderma is an autoimmune disease characterized by diffuse thickening of the skin (sclero = thickining of, derma = skin). Sclerosis also occurs in the esophagus, heart, lungs, and kidneys. The thickening of vessel walls obliterates the capillary loops at the nail matrix (see V B). The normal skin wrinkles over the knuckles are absent because of tightening of the skin. CREST syndrome is a less severe variant of this disease: **C**alcinosis, **R**aynaud's syndrome, **E**sophogeal dysfunction, **S**clerodactyle, **T**elangectasias. Anti-**Scl** antibodies are positive in **scl**eroderma.

C. Polymyositis/dermatositis. This is a vasculitis induced by antibodies that deposit in the skin and muscles. It may be a variant of a paraneoplastic syndrome (a cancer cell makes foreign proteins; the body makes an antibody to these proteins; these Ab-Ag complexes deposit in the skin and muscles). Findings include Gottron's papules (fibrosis over the knuckles) and mechanic's hands.

XIII INFECTED JOINTS

A. The joints, like the lungs and kidneys, are filters of the body; they frequently trap bacteria and are a clue to systemic infection.

B. The involved joint will be warm and tender on examination. Obtaining fluid from the joint (in addition to blood cultures) is the diagnostic test.

C. The most common infections of a joint are *Staphylococcus aureus,* gonorrhea, endocarditis, and Lyme disease.

D. Assume an infected joint is due to *S. aureus* until proven otherwise. Assume also that the organisms arrived there from an embolic source (namely, endocarditis) until proven otherwise.

E. Gonorrhea is rarely cultured from the joint; always obtain a urethral culture (-rrhea = flow, gono = gonads; flow from the gonads). The joint inflammation is largely immune-mediated, and the immune system wanes as the patient ages. Thus, gonorrhea-induced joint disease rarely occurs in patients over the age of 50. Pustules may appear over the affected joints (any joints).

XIV GENERAL PRINCIPLES OF DIAGNOSING ORTHOPEDIC INJURIES

A. Pay particular attention to the mechanism of injury per the history as you examine the bones and joints, because this is often diagnostic.

B. To do the orthopedic examination correctly you have to induce pain. Each maneuver is designed to stretch a particular tendon, ligament, cartilage, or bone. The maneuver that induces the greatest pain or laxity is the one that identifies the damaged tendon, ligament, cartilage, or bone. Do not worry about breaking a ligament or tendon. A ligament or tendon that fragile is going to break soon anyway; it is better to diagnose it in the hospital, where definitive therapy is available.

C. Always begin the examination by assessing the blood supply (warmth of the skin and pulses) and the neurologic function distal to the injury. The skeleton protects the soft tissues. When it is compromised, suspect that the soft tissues may also be compromised.

D. Passive versus active range of motion. All orthopedic injuries are due to either muscles-tendons or joints-ligaments. Muscle and tendon injuries only hurt when the muscle contracts and pulls on the tendon. Because passive movement requires no muscle contraction (the doctor does the moving of the limb), pain with passive movement excludes tendon and muscle etiologies, thereby suggesting a joint-ligament injury. Active motion requires muscle-tendon contraction and bone-ligament movement. Tenderness present with active motion but absent with passive movement implies muscle-tendon injury.

E. Bursitis. Under each tendon is a fluid-filled bursa sac. These keep the tendons from fraying as they move across underlying bones. Overuse of any muscle can inflame the bursa, causing point tenderness over that bursa. It is diagnosed by point tenderness over the bursa. It will hurt with both passive and active motion because both move the tendon across the bursa. Treatments include rest, ice, NSAIDs, and injection of steroids/lidocaine into the bursa.

F. Joints that bear the greatest weight (knees, hips) and those that are used most frequently (vertebrae, DIPs, and the thumb) wear down the fastest. Osteoarthritis is caused by this wear and tear and is found in these joints.

G. Swelling of a joint only occurs with intra-articular injury or inflammation. Damage to a muscle or ligament around (but not in) the joint will be painful and tender, but not swollen.

XV Elbow Pain

A. Lifting and swinging a child by her hands can dislocate the elbow (nursemaid's elbow). In adults, overuse injuries of the tendons that attach near the elbow are the most common cause of elbow pain.

B. Tennis elbow (lateral epicondylitis) is due to overuse of forearm extensor muscles whose tendons cross the lateral epicondyle. Rest the patient's elbow in your hand so that your thumb is on the lateral epicondyle. Ask the patient to extend his wrist while you oppose it with your other hand. Pain at lateral elbow is a positive test.

C. Golfer's elbow (medial epicondylitis) is the same as tennis elbow, except it involves the flexor tendons that cross the medial epicondyle. Shake hands with the patient while resisting the patient's maximum effort to turn the palm down (pronation). Pain at the medial elbow is a positive test.

D. Treatment for both golfer's and tennis elbow is to create a new fulcrum of muscle contraction. Ask the patient to wear an elastic wristband halfway up the arm. This will move the muscles' fulcrum from the elbow to the wristband, thereby relieving the tension at the elbow.

E. Olecranon bursitis. This will appear as a large, painful ball at the tip of the elbow (the olecranon). It usually occurs following repetitive trauma to the area. Although dramatic in appearance, it is clinically benign; it usually resolves with rest.

XVI Shoulder Pain

There are four causes of shoulder pain: dislocation, separation, rotator cuff injuries, and bursitis. The mechanism of injury, the patient's age, and where in the range of motion the pain occurs are diagnostic.

A. Dislocation is rotation of the head of the humerus out of the glenohumural fossa. The mechanism of injury is usually force applied to an outstretched arm (e.g., a football player tackling a running back with his right arm extended). Because the posterior lip of the fossa is larger than the anterior lip, and because the mechanism of force is usually one that pulls the arm backward (the head of the humerus forward), almost all dislocations are anterior. The dislocated shoulder will appear as a ball mass sitting in front of the shoulder; the arm will hang lower and the patient will be holding the arm close to his body to stabilize it. The acute dislocation can be relocated by placing the dislocated arm on the patient's chest (elbow at 90 degrees). Keep the elbow pinned against his side with one of your hands. Grab the wrist with your other hand and very, very slowly begin to abduct the forearm. You must move it so slowly that the patient does not know it is moving. Distract the patient in conversation as you move the arm. If he senses movement, he will anticipate pain, and this will cause the shoulder muscles to spasm, keeping the shoulder dislocated. The lateral rotation will roll the shoulder back into joint. After all relocations, make sure the blood flow and nerve function distal to the injury is intact. Posterior dislocations occur only in the elderly or following seizures or electrocutions. Never attempt a relocation of a posterior shoulder dislocation without surgical assistance; there is a high risk of trapping nerves or vessels during a mechanical relocation.

B. Fractured clavicles and separated shoulders occur from pile-driving injuries, in which the athlete hits an immovable force (e.g., the ground) with the shoulder with great speed. Examples include falling onto the shoulder while skiing.

  1. For all shoulder injuries, begin palpating the clavicle at the sternum, working out. Point tenderness and a cracking sound will become apparent if a clavicular fracture is present. A fragment that displaces inferiorly and posteriorly can potentially rupture the subclavian artery or vein. Make sure you check the distal blood supply on the side of the injury.

  2. The clavicle joins the scapula at the acromioclavicular (AC) joint. This joint is normally not mobile because it is tightly wrapped with ligaments. It can be separated if force is applied directly to it, however, resulting in a separated shoulder. It is manifest by point tenderness and mobility of the joint as you press on it. Surgery is required for complete separations.

C. Rotator cuff injury. The rotator cuff is composed of the tendons of the supraspinatus (the spine refers to the ridge on the back of the scapula), infraspinatus, teres minor, and subscapularis muscles. These tendons keep the humerus head in the socket, especially during rotation of the humoral head. Rotator cuff injuries occur from overuse of rotation (baseball pitchers) or a fall onto a partially rotated shoulder.

  1. First ask the patient to pretend he is holding a soft drink can (elbow flexed to 90 degrees). Ask him to take a drink and then throw the can over his shoulder so that his hand goes above and behind his head. The ability to do both excludes a complete rotator cuff tear.

2. You can also use the drop test. Passively lift the patient's arm 180 degrees above his head. Ask him to lower it slowly. The first 90 degrees is controlled by the deltoids; the rotator cuff takes over at 90 degrees and below. The patient with a rotator cuff injury will suddenly drop his arm to the side at 90 degrees.
3. Use the supraspinatus strength to detect partial tears. With the patient seated, place both arms in a position of 90 degrees of abduction and 30 degrees of forward flexion, with the thumbs pointing down. Push down on both arms as the patient resists. A positive test is lack of resistance.

D. Bursitis. Stabilize the shoulder in your hand. With your thumb, slowly apply point pressure at different parts of the shoulder. Remember that point pressure over the AC joint suggests a separated shoulder. All other point pressure sites are likely to be bursitis.

XVII BACK PAIN

Back pain is the most common orthopedic complaint. The lumbar spine is constantly moving and constantly abused (the back instead of the legs is used for lifting).

A. General rules:

1. Fifty percent of people will have chronic lower back pain. You are unlikely to make it go away, but you can often mitigate the symptoms.
2. Chronic back pain is usually intermittent but persistent. Expect that most people will get better within 4 weeks without treatment.
3. People with back pain want relief. Have nonpharmaceutical solutions to offer, such as buying a good mattress, strengthening back muscles with back exercises, careful lifting techniques, and NSAIDs. Surgery rarely works; try to avoid it if you can.

B. Lumbar spine method:

1. Exclude red flags.
   - **a.** Diskitis is infection of the disk between the vertebrate, osteomyelitis is infection of the veterbrate, and epidural abscess is infection within the spine. Red flags that increase the probability of these diagnoses include **intravenous drug use, fever, and exposure to tuberculosis.**
   - **b.** Metastatic cancer to the spine. Ask about **weight loss, night sweats, and risk factors for cancer.**
   - **c.** Nerve deficits (see Chapter 34)
     - **(1) Sciatica** is pain and paresthesias radiating down the back of the leg. This is due to compression of a dorsal nerve root by either a bulging herniated disk or a bony outgrowth of a vertebra compressing the nerve. **This is not a red flag.** The straight leg test is diagnostic: flex one hip to 90

degrees; pain radiating down the back of the other leg is a positive test. As the right leg flexes, the spine tilts to the left, compressing the left side nerve, with pain radiating down the leg. Herniated disks usually heal on their own (4 to 6 weeks); encourage your patient to maintain activity as tolerated (i.e., not bed rest). No lifting; NSAIDs.

(2) Weakness of the leg with loss of reflexes is a **radiculopathy.** This is due to a nerve compression involving both the dorsal and ventral roots. **This is a red flag, and it warrants an MRI to evaluate the spine.**

(3) Point tenderness elicited by palpating on one spinal vertebra suggests a compression or pathologic (cancer, infection) fracture. Obtain a bone scan to evaluate the vertebrae.

(4) **Cauda equina syndrome.** This is a red flag. Loss of sensation of the buttocks and groin (saddle anesthesia) and urinary/bowel incontinence suggest compression of the cauda equina (peripheral nerves still within the spine). This implies an epidural infection or cancer and requires immediate MRI for evaluation.

(5) Other (non–red flag) patterns of pain radiation. Pain that is localized to the spine is likely degenerative joint disease. Pain sparing the spine but involving the paraspinal muscles is muscle strain. Pain that radiates to the buttocks is a sacral osteoarthritis.

2. Use a graduated approach to avoid wasting time and money.

a. Exclude the red flags listed above. Teach about mattresses, lifting precautions, and back exercises. Give NSAIDs and see the patient again in 4 weeks. Eighty percent of these patients will not return, because the back pain will improve on its own.

b. If the patient returns for a second visit at 4 weeks, order plain films of the spine, more NSAIDs, and acetaminophen with codeine. Return again at 4 weeks. Eighty percent of these patients will not return.

c. If the patient returns for a third visit at 4 weeks, consider ordering a CT scan to further evaluate any abnormalities seen on the spine radiographs. A CT scan can only distinguish soft tissue from non–soft tissue; it cannot distinguish between soft tissues. If you see no bony abnormalities on the CT, order an MRI to look for soft tissue compression. Refer the patient to an orthopedic surgeon or neurosurgeon for evaluation. Make sure she has the study completed before the clinic appointment to avoid wasting one clinic appointment.

d. If the patient does not return for one of these appointments but returns at a later point (say, 1 year later), start the process all over again.

HOT KEY

Infections do not rely on the body's blood supply and can therefore cross into the avascular disk. A mass that involves the vertebra but spares the disk is more likely to be cancer.

Obtain images of the whole spine if you suspect metastatic cancer as a cause of the back pain. You cannot radiate one lesion, only to discover another lesion higher up at a later time and radiate it. The overlap from radiation fields will burn out the spine.

C. Cervical spine osteoarthritis is rare because it is not used as much as the lumbar spine. Use the same red-flag approach with one addition—make sure the patient does not have a history of rheumatoid arthritis. Subluxation of the C1-C2 joint is common. If there has been trauma involving the cervical spine, a cervical fracture or sprain must be radiographically excluded.

D. Sacroiliac joints. The four diseases that involve the sacroiliac joint are the HLA-B27 diseases (a PAIR of diseases): psoriasis, ankylosing spondilitis, inflammatory bowel disease, reactive arthritis. Ask the patient to bend and touch her toes. Decreased mobility in the sacroiliac spine will prevent doing this.

XVIII Hip Pain

A. Trochanteric bursitis (hip pointer). Placc the patient on the unaffected side; press over the trochanter to elicit tenderness in the bursa.

B. Avascular necrosis. Blood supply to the femoral head comes through the trochanter and the femoral neck. Conditions that impair blood flow put the femoral neck at risk for fracture. These include sickle cell anemia (sickled cells plug the vasculature), steroid use, and alcohol use.

C. Hip fracture. The abductor muscles of the leg are much stronger than the adductors. When the hip is fractured, these muscles tighten, shortening the leg and turning the foot laterally.

D. Knee problems. Most hip pain is due to ipsilateral knee damage. The hip suffers damage from compensating for the tender knee, bearing more than 50% of the body weight. Always examine the knee when faced with hip pain.

HOT KEY

Always clear a hip fracture for surgery. The mortality of lying in bed with a broken hip is so high as to warrant immediate surgery.

XIX Knee Pain

There are two types of knee disease: trauma and inflammation.

A. Inflammatory diseases of the joint are marked by erythema, warmth, tenderness, swelling, and an absence of trauma to the joint. Causes include:

1. Infections (see above)
2. Crystal disease (gout, pseudogout) (see above)
3. Degenerative (osteoarthritis)

B. Traumatic knee injuries. There are five traumatic diseases of the knee.

1. Begin with the anterior cruciate ligament. The ligaments in the knee are named for where they insert. The AC ligament (ACL) originates on the posterior femur and inserts on the anterior tibia, preventing the tibia from moving anterior. ACL injuries occur in sports when the lower leg is locked in position (e.g., a cleat that locks in the turf) while the upper body continues to move forward over the knee (e.g., the football player running at full speed gets his cleat stuck in the turf). The player usually hears a "pop," which is the sound of the ruptured tendon. Have the patient lie on the table with the knee flexed and the foot flat on the table. Sit on his foot and grab the back of the proximal tibia with both hands and pull it toward you (Figure 33-4). Pull hard. If the lower leg moves toward you, the ACL is damaged or torn. Lachman's test (on the field) is stabilizing the anterior distal thigh (femur) with your left hand while pulling the posterior tibia toward you (Figure 33-5). Pull hard. If the leg moves, the ACL is torn. Be warned: muscle spasm following an acute injury can stabilize an ACL tear, giving the above tests a false negative result.

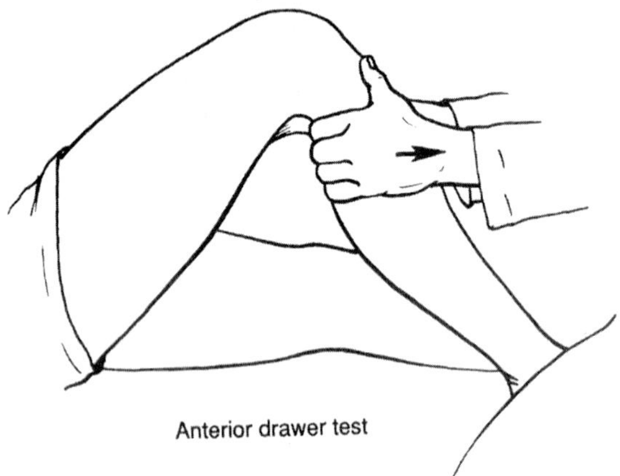

FIGURE 33-4. Testing the anterior cruciate ligament: the anterior drawer test. (From Fu FH, Stone DA, eds. *Sports Injuries: Mechanisms, Prevention, Treatment*, 2nd ed. Philadelphia: Lippincott Williams & Wilkins, 2001.)

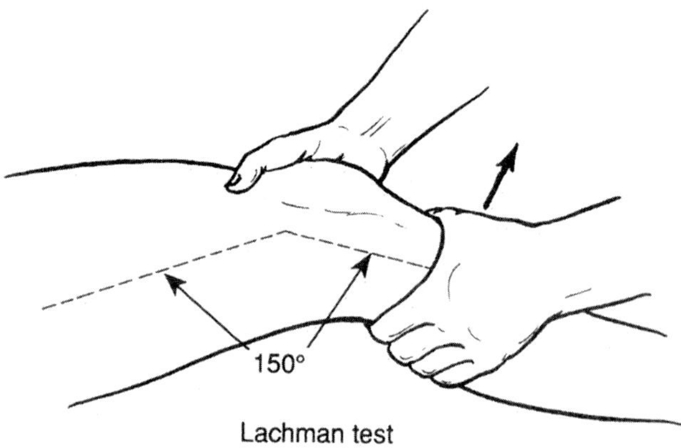

FIGURE 33-5. Testing the anterior cruciate ligament: Lachman's test. (From Fu FH, Stone DA, eds. *Sports Injuries: Mechanisms, Prevention, Treatment,* 2nd ed. Philadelphia: Lippincott Williams & Wilkins, 2001.)

2. Next, test the posterior cruciate ligament (PCL). PCL injuries occur in combination with an ACL injury, as the body moves forward over the locked knee and then slings backward in recoil, tearing the PCL. Isolated PCL tears are rare. Have the patient lie on the table with the knee flexed and the foot flat on the table (Figure 33-6). Sit on his foot and push posteriorly on the proximal

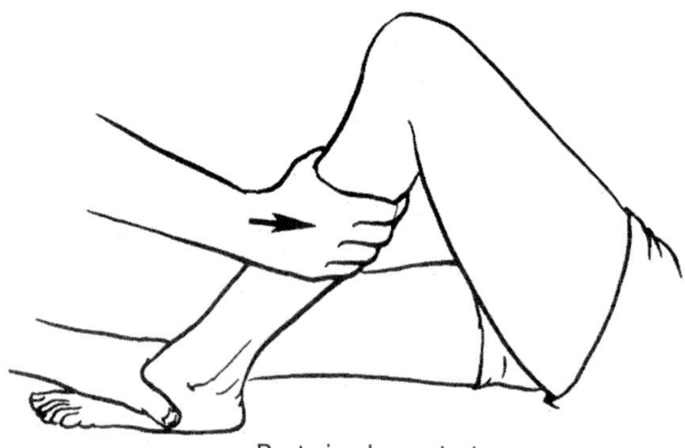

FIGURE 33-6. Testing the posterior cruciate ligament: the posterior drawer. (From Fu FH, Stone DA, eds. *Sports Injuries: Mechanisms, Prevention, Treatment,* 2nd ed. Philadelphia: Lippincott Williams & Wilkins, 2001.)

tibia. If the lower leg moves away from you, the PCL is damaged or torn. PCL injuries are important, because a posterior dislocation can rupture the vessels and nerves behind the knee. Always assess the distal pulse if a PCL injury is suspected.

3. Now test the medial collateral and lateral collateral ligaments. MCL injuries usually occur as a result of a foot that is planted (locking the lower leg) while the upper body twists. Direct trauma to the lateral knee can also induce an MCL tear; direct trauma to the medial knee can cause an LCL (e.g., cut blocks in football).
   a. Have the patient sit on the edge of the table while you sit on a stool. Stabilize his lower leg by grasping it with your knees. Stabilize the distal lateral thigh with your lateral hand; use your other hand to push laterally on the medial proximal tibia. If you feel destabilization or pain, the MCL is injured. MCL injuries also have point tenderness over the ligament.
   b. For LCL injuries, do the same procedure except switch hands: push medially on the proximal tibia.
4. Now evaluate the medial meniscus. The medial meniscus is the cup of cartilage inside the knee that keeps the head of the tibia from moving medially. Injuries are characterized by point tenderness of the medial knee, which is similar to an MCL injury. To distinguish between the two, have the patient lie on his stomach and flex his knee to 90 degrees. Put your knee of the base of his distal femur.
   a. Grasp the ankle and push it down while grinding on it. This will compress the medial meniscus. If it is injured, this will make the pain worse.
   b. Next, grasp the ankle and lift it up. Twist the leg as you lift it. If the medial collateral ligament is damaged, this distraction will cause worsening of the pain.

C. Patellar diseases of the knee.

1. Prepatellar bursitis. People who are regularly on their knees (e.g., plumbers, carpenters, carpet layers, those practicing some religions) can have enough inflammation of this bursa that it becomes irritated and inflamed.
2. Patellofemoral syndrome. The quadriceps muscles of the thigh contribute the tendon that holds the patella in place. The tendon extends inferiorly from the patella to the superior shin. The normal angle of the knee holds the patella in the midline. In young women (before expansion of the hips that occurs between ages 20 to 30 to accommodate childbirth), this angle may be sufficiently off to allow the patella to fall out of place (dislocate) laterally. The out-of-place patella may also "click," especially when walking up stairs and after a period of rest. The risk for dislocation is greatest when the angle is the most shallow and when the quadriceps are fatigued or asleep (e.g., walking up the stairs of a movie theater after the show). Lay the patient supine

and passively flex the knee. Apply medial pressure on the patella as you extend the knee. The patella is unlikely to dislocate, but the sensation of it moving that direction will be all too familiar to the patient. She will stop the test midway in apprehension.

XX Ankle Pain

A. There are two types of traumatic injury to the ankle: sprains (stretching of the medial or lateral collateral ligaments) and fractures. Both occur with a sudden twisting of the ankle with either eversion or inversion.

B. Ankle fractures are a result of the ligament refusing to stretch, pulling the distal part of the tibia or fibular malleolus with it as it moves. Distinguishing between the two requires radiographs, though you can use the following (Ottawa) ankle rules to decide who warrants an x-ray examination. If the patient satisfies one of the following criteria, obtaining a radiograph is warranted.

1. Failure to be able to put any pressure on the ankle at the time of injury or the time of examination. A limp is normal; not being able to limp is not.
2. Point tenderness at the medial or lateral malleolus. Expect tenderness, but not point tenderness.
3. Point tenderness of the anterior foot.

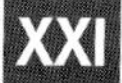

XXI Compartment Syndrome

Compartment syndrome refers to swelling of the soft tissues that occludes blood flow and neurologic function to the distal extremity. It usually occurs with a deep tissue infection or trauma to the calf or forearm. Symptoms include a distal foot or hand that is cool, painless, and pulseless. This requires immediate surgical release, or the extremity will die.

34. The Tier II Neurologic Examination

I THE BIG PICTURE

The Tier II neurologic examination is used to evaluate:

A. Abnormalities discovered during the Tier I examination
   1. Weakness
   2. Gait abnormalities
   3. Sensory loss

B. The six cardinal problems of neurologic function
   1. Stroke
   2. Seizures
   3. Altered mental status
   4. Coma
   5. Movement disorders
   6. Abnormal balance

II WEAKNESS

A. **General considerations.** There are **four major causes** of weakness, as displayed in the iron cross of weakness: neurologic, myositis, electrolytes, inadequate oxygen delivery (Figure 34-1).
   1. **Focal versus diffuse weakness.** Focal weakness suggests a neurologic cause; diffuse weakness suggests one of the other three major causes.
   2. **If the weakness is neurologic in origin, distinguish upper from lower motor neuron disease.**
      a. **Upper motor neurons** originate in the prefrontal cortex, cross at the brainstem, and descend into the spinal cord, where they synapse at the anterior horn in the spinal cord. These fibers also carry fibers that inhibit the reflex arc. Upper motor neuron dysfunction leads to **weakness** (loss of motor input) and a spastic **increase in tone and increased reflexes** (loss of inhibitory neurons).
      b. **Lower motor neurons** originate from the anterior horn and course through the peripheral nerves to the neuromuscular junction. Lower motor neuron dysfunction leads to **weakness** (loss of motor input) **and absent reflexes.**
      c. An important exception occurs in early upper motor neuron weakness (i.e., the first days after a stroke), where reflexes can be decreased and tone normal, mimicking a lower motor neuron lesion.

Cerebral Disease
Stroke
PML

Anterior Horn Disease
Polio or Post-polio
ALS

Spinal Cord Disease
MS
Transverse myelitis
Epidural tumor/abscess
Spinal stenosis
Spinal infarct
HTLV 1

Peripheral nerve
(see below)

NMJ Disease
Myasthenia
Eaton-Lambert

DO_2 = CO x Hgb x Sat%

Muscle

Primary muscle disease
MYOSITIS (see below)

Electrolytes
K+
Mg++
Ca++

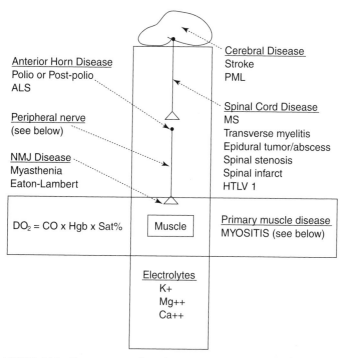

FIGURE 34-1. The iron cross of weakness.

HOT
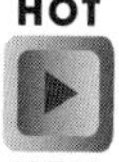
KEY

Spasticity is defined as a velocity-dependent increase in tone during testing. In contrast, rigidity is increased regardless of speed of movement (as seen in Parkinson's).

B. <u>The Top Bar:</u> Nerve input from above. Start at the neuromuscular junction and work backward toward the brain.

1. **Neuromuscular junction.** Weakness in neuromuscular disease results from inhibition of acetylcholine docking at the postsynaptic receptor (Figure 34-2).
    - **a.** Because only the neuromuscular junction is affected, **sensation is preserved.** The **facial and ocular muscles are usually involved.**
    - **b.** There are two diseases that affect the NMJ: myasthenia gravis and Lambert-Eaton.
        - **(1)** Myasthenia is caused by antibodies to the postsynaptic acetylcholine receptor. Even excessive acetylcholine in

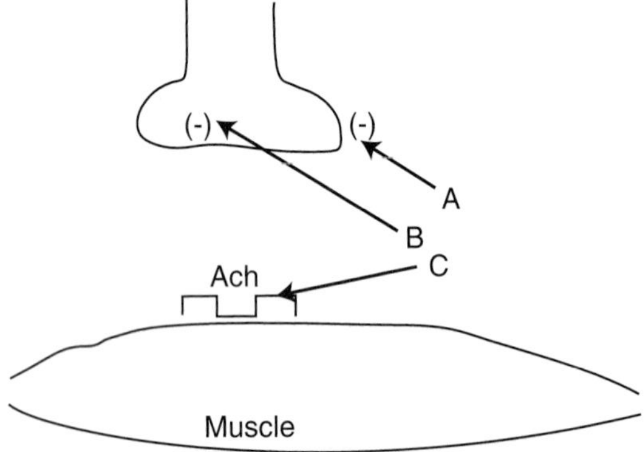

FIGURE 34-2. Neuromuscular junction disease. **A,** Antibody stimulating the presynaptic Ca^{2+} shutoff receptor = **Eaton-Lambert. B,** Toxin inhibits presynaptic release of Ach = **botulism. C,** Antibody to Ach receptor = **myasthenia gravis.**

the NMJ (as occurs with repetitive stimulation) does not increase strength.

(2) Lambert-Eaton is sometimes part of a paraneoplastic syndrome, in which antibodies against the cancer cross-react to a presynaptic calcium channel, preventing calcium dependent release of acetylcholine in the synapse, causing weakness. This can be overridden, however, with repetitive stimulation. The hallmark of Lambert-Eaton is an increase in strength with repetitive motion.

(3) A rare cause of NMJ disease is botulism.

2. **Peripheral nerve.** The peripheral nerve has two components: the axon (axonopathies) and the myelin that insulates the axon, facilitating conduction (demyelinating neuropathies). Peripheral nerve abnormalities can be pure motor, pure sensory, or both (sensorimotor). The DANG THERAPIST mnemonic shows causes of peripheral nerve dysfunction.

Causes of Peripheral Neuropathy **("DANG THERAPIST")**
Diabetes
Alcohol
Nutritional deficiency
Guillain-Barré syndrome
Trauma
Hereditary disorders (e.g., Charcot-Marie-Tooth disease)
Environmental toxins (lead, solvents)
Remote effects of cancer (paraneoplastic syndromes)

Amyloid
Porphyria (acute intermittent porphyria)
Inflammatory conditions (e.g., lupus)
Syphilis
Tuberculosis

3. **Sensory deficits dominate the syndrome.** If the damage to the nerve also involves the motor components, **weakness** and **loss of reflexes** will also be present.
    a. Injury to the peripheral nerve may be localized, affecting a single nerve, or diffuse, affecting multiple nerves.
    b. Localized injury to a single nerve leads to decreased power, sensation, and reflexes in the distribution of that single nerve.
    c. Diffuse injury is caused by lipophilic toxins (such as alcohol or cleaning solvents that infiltrate the lipid-laden Schwann cells) or occlusion of the small vessels that supply the nerves (such as occurs with diabetes and paraneoplastic syndromes). A common pattern is a "stocking and glove" pattern, because the longest and most distal nerves (i.e., the hands and feet) are most affected.

HOT KEY

The **lateral femoral cutaneous nerve** (that serves the lateral thighs) is often impinged by **obese patients** with tight belts. Look for focal lateral thigh numbness.

Carpal tunnel syndrome is an injury to the **median nerve** as it passes through the carpal tunnel at the wrist. The result is weakness in the muscles of the hand innervated by the median nerve and sensory loss in the distribution of the cutaneous branch of the median nerve.

HOT
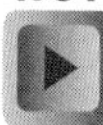
KEY

Cauda Equina Syndrome. The spinal cord ends at L1, but the peripheral nerves from the lower spinal cord stay within the thecal sac until they exit at levels L2-S5. This bundle can be compressed by one lesion within the spine (e.g., a metastatic cancer lesion or an abscess), resulting in a peripheral nerve pattern **(absent reflexes; weakness).** Because these nerves innervate the perineum, bowel, and bladder, patients note **bowel/bladder incontinence and saddle anesthesia.**

4. **Nerve root** (radiculopathy). The nerve root is most commonly injured by a ruptured intervertebral disk.
    a. The key to recognizing a lesion of the nerve root is knowing the motor, reflex, and sensory distributions of the various nerve roots (Figure 34-3).
    b. For example, an injury to the L4 nerve root will cause weakness of the L4 muscles (the dorsiflexor of the ankle and the

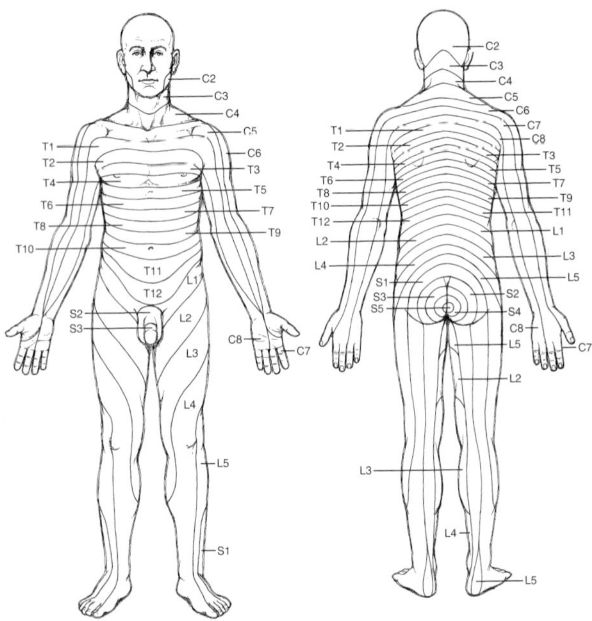

FIGURE 34-3. Distribution of dermatomes on the skin. (From *Stedman's Medical Dictionary*, 27th ed. Baltimore: Lippincott Williams & Wilkins, 2000.)

quadriceps), L4 reflexes (reflex at the knee), and sensation of the L4 dermatome (the medial aspect of the lower leg).

5. **Anterior horn cell.** Lesions of the anterior horn cell are due to polio or amyotrophic lateral sclerosis (ALS: Lou Gehrig's disease).
   a. Because the anterior horn cells are part of the reflex arc, damage results in a **loss of reflexes.** The peripheral nerves are not affected, so **sensory input is preserved.** The loss of neural innervation of the muscles will lead to **decreased bulk in the muscles** innervated by the affected anterior horn cells.
   b. ALS affects both the anterior horn cells and the lateral corticospinal tracts of the spinal cord, leading to a combination of upper and lower motor neuron signs (e.g., loss of reflexes in some areas; increased reflexes in others).
6. **Spinal cord.** The spinal cord brings motor input from the brain to the anterior horn cells and inhibitory fibers from the brain to dampen the reflex arc (peripheral sensation to the anterior horn and back to the muscle via the peripheral nerve). It also delivers sensory input from the extremities to the brain. Spinal cord lesions

are characterized by **weakness** (motor fibers), **hyperreflexia** (inhibitory neurons), and **sensory loss. This pattern distinguishes an upper motor neuron lesion from a lower motor neuron lesion.**

a. A complete transection of the spinal cord will result in loss of all sensory modalities below the spinal cord lesion.

b. Spinal cord lesions will also result in **urinary retention** (hypotonicity of the bladder), and **loss of anal sphincter tone.**

c. Causes of spinal cord disease include multiple sclerosis, trauma or ischemia to the cord, or a mass lesion (cancer or infection) compressing the cord.

> **HOT KEY** Compression of the spinal cord is always a medical emergency. Patients leave the hospital at the nadir of their function: if a patient progresses to being bed-bound, he will leave bed-bound.

7. **Brain and brainstem injuries**, like spinal cord injuries, are upper motor neuron lesions. This will result in **weakness and increased reflexes**, and may include **sensory loss** (if the sensory cortex is also involved in the stroke).
   a. Injury to the motor cortex or pyramidal tracks will result in contralateral weakness of the arm and face more often than the leg. Depending upon location a stroke can also cause aphasia, neglect, and visual field deficits (see V).
   b. Injury to the motor tracks in the brainstem will result in **contralateral weakness of the arm and leg**. Due to crossing of the cranial nerves, the **facial paralysis can be either ipsilateral or contralateral** to the side of the lesion.

C. **Myopathies,** or weakness from muscle disease, occur in a predictable pattern that usually involves the largest, most proximal muscles in a symmetric fashion. **Sensation and reflexes are unaffected**.
   1. Myopathies can be distinguished from weakness due to neuromuscular junction disease by the lack of cranial nerve involvement.
   2. The breakdown of muscle in myopathies may lead to an increase in the creatine kinase level in the blood.
   3. Use the MYOSITIS mnemonic to remember causes of myositis.

The **MYOSITIS** Mnemonic for Causes of Myositis

Muscular disease
V(**Y**)iremia (Influenza, HIV, echovirus, etc.)
Opportunistic pathogens (*Trichinella*)
Steroids
Immune disease (polymyositis)
Tumors/thyroid (paraneoplastic)
Infections (influenza, HIV)
Statins

III Gait Abnormalities (See Chapter 28)

IV Abnormal Sensation

A. **Definition.** Sensation may be decreased or absent, or sensations such as burning or tingling may be present. Sensory examination may yield decreased or increased sensation.

B. **Localization**

1. **Brain lesions.** Lesions of the cortex in the postcentral gyrus of the parietal lobe, as well as lesions deeper in the brain (i.e., thalamus, brainstem) can cause decreased sensation. **All sensory modalities are usually affected.**
2. **Spinal cord.** Spinal cord lesions that affect the entire cord result in a bilateral sensory deficit below that level. A lesion affecting half of the spinal cord (e.g., from a right epidural abscess) will cause contralateral loss of pain and temperature sensation and ipsilateral loss of proprioception (Figure 34-4). Ipsilateral weakness and hyperreflexia will also be present. The most common cause of nontraumatic spinal cord lesions is multiple sclerosis; as the name implies, multiple parts of the spinal cord may be involved, causing multiple deficits on examination.

C. **Sensation of pain and temperature.** Pain and temperature sensation is carried in the small fibers that, on entering the spinal cord, immediately cross and then ascend in the ventral spinothalamic tracts of the spinal cord contralateral to the affected side. These small fibers do not carry motor or reflex information.

D. **Sensation of vibration and joint position** (proprioception). Vibration and proprioception to the extremities are carried in the larger

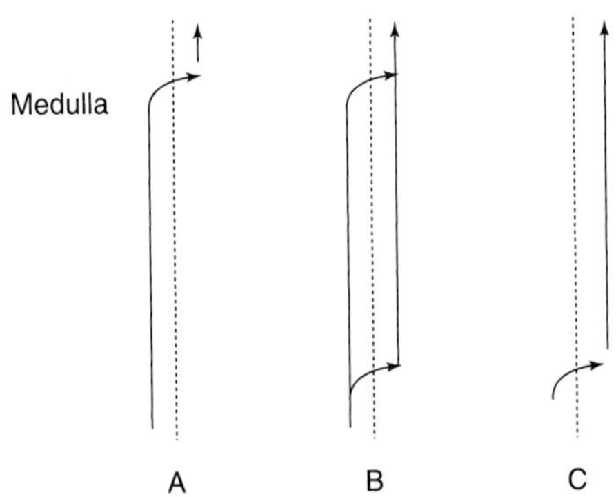

FIGURE 34-4. Crossing patterns of sensory input. **A,** Proprioceptive. **B,** light touch. **C,** Pain and temperature.

fibers that also supply motor function and play a role in stretch reflexes. These fibers run in the dorsal or posterior columns of the spinal cord and do not cross until they reach the brainstem. The most common causes of dorsal column disease are B_{12} deficiency and syphilis.

E. Nerve roots (radiculopathies). As previously discussed (see II B 3), radiculopathies present with sensory loss in the dermatome of that nerve root. The cause is usually compression of the nerve root as it leaves the spinal cord (most commonly from a herniated disc).

F. Peripheral nerves

1. There are numerous causes of peripheral neuropathy (see the "DANG THERAPIST mnemonic"). The two most common causes of a generalized peripheral neuropathy are alcohol abuse and diabetes mellitus.
2. Electromyography and nerve conduction studies can provide objective evidence of nerve dysfunction to supplement the physical examination.

V STROKE

A. Definitions

1. **A stroke is a neurologic deficit resulting from infarction of neural tissue.** Strokes can be divided into ischemic or hemorrhagic infarctions.
2. **A TIA is a neurologic deficit resembling stroke that resolves completely within 24 hours.**

B. Differential diagnosis of stroke. Other entities that mimic stroke must be excluded before making the diagnosis of stroke.

1. **Electrolyte disturbances** such as hypoglycemia may present as a focal deficit that mimics stroke; hence D_{50} (dextrose) is given to patients with a low glucose level and focal deficits.
2. **Todd's paralysis** is focal paralysis following a seizure; its presentation is virtually indistinguishable from stroke.
3. Some forms of **migraine** may also be accompanied by focal deficits resembling stroke.

C. Localizing cerebral lesions. Localization of the lesion is important because it predicts the cause of the stroke and it differentiates stroke from other diseases that may mimic stroke. There are three tools to localize the stroke: (1) motor deficits, (2) sensory deficits, and (3) language.

D. Parietal lobe: The following deficits suggest parietal lobe disease. Parietal lobe lesions are usually due to embolic obstruction of the middle cerebral artery.

1. **Motor deficits**. The central sulcus separates the motor strip (anterior) from the sensory strip. The homunculus is a body-part map that is laid out as if a person stood in the center of the brain and laid over the parietal lobe. Facial weakness suggests a lateral

parietal lesion; upper extremity deficits indicate a superior/medial parietal lesion; lower extremity lesions suggest a medial parietal lesion.

2. Sensory deficits. The same homunculus applies to the sensory strip located posterior to the sulcus.
3. Language. Ninety percent of left-handed patients and 100% of right-handed patients have the language centers on the left side of the brain. A language deficit implies a left-sided stroke; expect any motor deficits to be on the right.

E. Frontal lobe: The frontal lobe controls primitive reflexes, emotion, and personality (hence, a lobotomy renders the patient without personality). Focal damage to the frontal lobe is rare because most emboli lodge in the middle cerebral artery, not the anterior cerebral artery. Cerebral anoxia (e.g., after a cardiac arrest) damages all of the brain and can present with frontal lobe signs. This is especially important in counseling family members who may gain a false sense of hope from a hand grasp in an otherwise brain-dead patient. All of the primitive reflexes are not seen in normal patients because the intact frontal lobe inhibits them. The presence of these reflexes suggests damage to the frontal lobe. Note, that these reflexes are <u>normal</u> in the developing newborn because the brain is still developing.

1. Grasp reflex. Place two fingers in the patient's palm; feel for a grasp.
2. Rooting reflex. Tap the patient's chin with a reflex hammer; look for puckering of the lips.
3. Glabellar reflex. Tap the patient's forehead just above the nose. One eye blink is normal; repetitive eye blinking (hyperreflexia) suggests frontal lobe damage.

F. Occipital lobe: The occipital lobe controls interpretation of visual stimuli. Abnormalities are very rare, though the visual aura of migraine headaches is an example of how a vasospasm of an occipital artery can create a deficit. Occipital strokes can lead to complete absence of vision, because all neurologic pathways connect to the occipital lobe. Do not confuse occipital lobe infarcts with amaurosis fugax ("the lowering of the curtain") that is a nightshade coming down or coming up over the eyes. This is a small stroke of the anterior ophthalmic artery.

VI SEIZURES

A. Definition. A seizure is a neurologic dysfunction resulting from excess excitation of neurons.

B. Classification. This involves distinguishing between seizures that begin in one part of the brain (focal or partial seizures) and seizures that begin in the entire brain simultaneously (primary generalized seizures).

1. **Partial seizures** are further divided into seizures that impair consciousness (complex partial seizures) and seizures in which consciousness is preserved (simple partial seizures).
2. **Generalized seizures**
   a. **Tonic-clonic (grand mal) seizures** are characterized by tonic posturing of all four limbs followed by rhythmic clonic movements of all four extremities. Patients often are incontinent of urine and stool and may injure themselves. Patients may have decreased sensorium for some time after a tonic-clonic seizure (postictal state).
   b. **Absence seizures** (petit mal) are common in children and are often mistaken for staring spells or daydreaming. Patients may pause during speech and stare off into space, usually for less than 30 seconds, before returning to normal without any clue that a spell has occurred.
   e. **Myoclonic seizures** are characterized by very brief, lightening-like jerks of the extremities.
   f. **Atonic seizures** involve the sudden loss of tone in the entire body and can mimic syncope.

C. **Etiology** (See Table 34-1)

VII ALTERED MENTAL STATUS (DELIRIUM)

Delirium is waxing and waning alteration in consciousness. Without the luxury of a good history to guide your diagnosis, you will have to rely upon the 4 P's: Look in the patient's **p**ockets and look for **p**ill bottles. Ask the **p**olice/EMTs who found the patient. Ask the **p**arents/family about the history. Look for medical alert bracelets.

A. Step 1. Make sure you are not dealing with dementia or primary psychiatric disease. Dementia is a global decline in cognitive function that does not wax and wane. The patient is awake and conversant, but cannot complete simple cognitive tasks. Consciousness is rarely impaired in primary psychiatric disease. The patient is awake and conversant, but manifesting disorders of thought and affect (mood).

B. Step 2. Identify the possible causes of AMS. List the causes on the left margin of your admission note, and then sequentially exclude each cause until you have a final diagnosis. See the "SHE STOPS for TIPS on VOWELS" mnemonic for causes of altered mental status.

Mnemonic for causes of altered mental status
("SHE STOPS for TIPS on vowels [AEIOU]")
Sepsis
Hepatic Encephalopathy
Electrolytes (Na^{+}, Ca^{2+})

TABLE 34-1. Causes of Seizures.

Cause	History, Examination, or Radiographic Data
Genetic epilepsy	Family history; birth history.
Drugs and medications	Review the patient's medications thoroughly. In addition, some illicit substances may cause seizures when ingested or as part of a withdrawal syndrome (e.g., alcohol withdrawal).
Infections	Infections of the central nervous system such as encephalitis. Young children may have seizures in the setting of fever.
Electrolyte disturbances	Low sodium, low glucose, low magnesium, and low or high calcium.
Head trauma	Closed head trauma is a risk factor for development of seizures.
Focal brain injury	Any area of damaged brain can serve as a focus for seizure initiation. Strokes, brain surgeries, tumors, and abscesses may predispose to seizures.

Stroke
Trauma
Opiates
Psych
Seizure

Temperature
Infections
Porphyria

Alcohol
Endocrine (thyroid, diabetes, cortisol)
Inflammatory (vasculitis, lupus)
Oxygen
Uremia

Think of the substrates the neurons require to function (oxygen, glucose, thyroid, sodium, calcium). Then consider the etiologies of neuron suppression (alcohol, opiates) and swelling in the head (uremia, hepatic failure, sodium disorders). Finally, consider the causes of neuron death (encephalitis, stroke, seizures, subdural bleeds, temperature extremes, porphyria, trauma, inflammation [lupus, syphilis]).

C. Step 3. Assess the vital signs (ABCDs). Exclude hypoxia, apnea, hypotension, hyperthermia/hypothermia, and hypoglycemia as a cause of AMS.

D. Step 4. Evaluate for head trauma (see below). This is an urgent diagnosis. If there are not obvious signs, complete the following steps and then order a head CT scan to exclude intracerebral bleeds.

E. Step 5. Draw laboratory specimens. Use your differential to guide you.

F. Step 6. While you are waiting for the laboratory results to come back, look for the following physical findings:

1. Asterixis (see Chapter 32). This is a sign of all types of metabolic encephalopathy (hepatic failure, uremia, benzodiazepine overdose).
2. Look for signs of hepatic failure (Chapter 32) and renal failure. Arteriovenous shunts, indwelling catheters, and uremic frost suggest renal failure. Uremic frost is a white powder sheen that is crystallized urea. It is only seen in patients who do not bathe, because bathing will wash it from the body.
3. Look for track marks or other signs of drug use.

VIII DEMENTIA

Dementia is a global decline in cognitive function.

A. Step 1. Exclude disorders that mimic dementia. Make sure that the patient is not suffering from:

1. Delirium (see above)
2. Communication disorders (e.g., aphasia from a stroke)

B. Step 2. Assess the rate of decline in cognitive function. Draw a graph. Ask the patient's family to describe the patient's ability to think and do everyday tasks 1 year ago. Make a mark at the top of the *y* axis as "100%." Divide the *x* axis in 12 segments (one for each month before the current month). Now ask them to describe the percentage of function for each of the previous 12 months. Plot these values. The line should have a constant slope. If there is a sudden drop off in the slope, move to Step 3.

C. Step 3. Exclude reversible causes of dementia. The treatable causes of dementia are in Table 34-2.

IX COMA

A. Coma. Coma is a persistent state of unarousable unawareness. It results from damage to both cerebral hemispheres or damage to the reticular activating system (RAS) in the brainstem. The approach to coma is:

1. Evaluate the cerebral hemispheres.
2. Evaluate the brainstem (RAS).

TABLE 34-2. Reversable Causes of Dementia.

Cause	History, Examination, or Radiographic Data
Depression	Ask the patient: (1) Are you depressed? and (2) What is your mood?
Encephalitis and chronic meningitis	Perform a lumbar puncture.
Mass lesions and external compression	Obtain a head CT scan to exclude chronic subdural hematomas.
Normal pressure hydrocephalus (NPH)	Normal pressure hydrocephalus is obstruction of the arachnoid granulations that reabsorb the CSF. The pressure causes the ventricles to compress the brain, causing dementia. Symptoms begin from top down (in order of onset): (1) dementia, (2) ataxia ("magnetic gait"), (3) incontinence. The diagnosis is confirmed by a CT scan that shows dilated ventricles.
Hypothyroid	Obtain a TSH value.
Iatrogenic drugs	Beta-blockers, sedatives, pain medications, and neuroleptics.
Anemia	Pernicious anemia caused by B_{12} deficiency.
Syphilis (tertiary)	Obtain an RPR value.

3. Assess the severity of the coma. The severity and the etiology of the coma will determine whether you should you continue with supportive care or consider termination of life support.

B. Evaluation of the cerebral hemispheres

1. **Obtain a head CT scan.** A noncontrast CT scan will detect hemorrhage and mass lesions. A contrast CT scan will evaluate mass lesions with surrounding edema (the contrast leaks out around the mass lesion that is causing the edema, thereby identifying the lesion).
2. Infarction of both hemispheres is an unlikely cause of coma because there are two separate blood supplies and the circle of Willis.
3. Cerebral edema due to an intracerebral bleed or mass is a common cause of coma. If the swelling is great enough, the brain will be pushed through the foramen magnum, compressing the brainstem. Because all of the cranial nerves exit from the brainstem, cranial nerve abnormalities in the comatose patient may be warn-

TABLE 34-3. Localization of the Level of Brainstem Compression in Coma.

Level of Impairment	Cranial Nerve Abnormalities
Front brain	I, II
Midbrain	III, IV
Pons	V, VI, VII, VIII
Medulla	IX, X, XI, XII

ing signs that herniation is imminent. While you are waiting on the CT, use your physical examination to assess this risk.

C. **Evaluate the brainstem.** You can localize the deficit to a part of the brainstem using the guide in Table 34-3. Do a level-by-level evaluation of the brainstem. Find the level of greatest function.

D. **Level 1: Front brain/thalamus**

1. Test the **patient's response to pain.** This is part of the **Glasgow Coma Scale** that is used to quantify the depth of coma. See Table 34-4. Look for signs of loss of frontal lobe reflexes.

TABLE 34-4. Glasgow Coma Scale.

Eye Opening (Four Eyes)

1 No eye opening
2 Opens to pain
3 Opens to voice
4 Opens spontaneously

Verbal (V)

1 No voice
2 Incomprehensible
3 Inappropriate
4 Disoriented
5 Normal

Motor (Six Motor)

1 No motor
2 Decerebrate posturing (the patient extends the elbows and wrists) (severe thalamic impairment)
3 Decorticate posturing (the patient makes an "O" by flexing the elbows and wrists) (mild thalamic impairment)
4 Flexion withdrawal
5 Withdrawals to Pain
6 Obeys verbal commands

2. Test CN II.
   a. **Papilledema.** The pressure behind the eye pushes the disc (the end of the optic nerve) toward the cup (cup:disk ratio is small) and blurs the margin of the cup.
   b. **Pupil response.** The light-constriction reflex (see Chapter 8) is a sign of a healthy retina, optic nerve, and brainstem. A unilateral dilated pupil may suggest that the parasympathetic fibers that course along the top part of CN III have been compressed by cerebral herniation (see Chapter 28 for how to assess pupil function).

E. **Level 2. Midbrain. Evaluate CNs III and IV.**
   1. CN III disorders are usually due to a posterior-communicating artery aneurysm or cerebral herniation (swelling of the brain pushes the cerebrum against CN III).
      a. The symptoms of a CN III deficit are loss of all extraocular muscles except the superior oblique (CN IV) and the lateral rectus (CN VI). **The eye is turned down and out.**
      b. Parasympathetic fibers course on top of CN III. The pupil may be dilated in compressive processes (e.g., herniation or aneurysmal compression) resulting from injury to these parasympathetic fibers.
      c. The third nerve also keeps the eyelid open (picture the III pillars of CN III keeping the eye open). When the III nerve is damaged, the **eye droops closed.**
   2. CN IV disorders are rare and are usually due to trauma. The trochlear nerve turns the eye down and out. A deficit results in an eye that cannot look medially and down at the same time.

F. **Level 3. Pons.**
   1. **Evaluate CN V.** Because the sensory nucleus of CN V courses through a large part of the brainstem, it is a sensitive test for brainstem injury. Assessing the motor function of CN V is not helpful because the comatose patient is unable to masticate.
      a. **Corneal reflex test:** brush a wisp of cotton across the cornea. This irritation should cause a reflex stimulation of CN VII to close the eye (thereby protecting the cornea).
   2. **Evaluate CN VI.** The abducens nerve turns the eye out (abducts). A deficit will result in an eye that cannot turn out, but normal primary (forward) gaze is maintained. CN VI is the longest intracerebral nerve in the head and the most prone to trauma or other metabolic abnormalities. This is the reason that it is part of the Wernicke-Korsakoff syndrome.
      a. Wernicke component (reversible): CN VI palsy, ataxia
      b. Korsakoff component (irreversible): dementia
   3. **Evaluate CN VII.** CN VII is part of the corneal reflex examination, which can be tested in coma. It is also one of the most common CN abnormalities in the ambulatory setting (Bell's palsy). Bell's palsy is loss of muscular control of half of the face.

Test this by asking the patient to forcibly close his eyes. Other symptoms include drooling and hyperacusis (CN VII innervates the stapedius muscle that controls the middle ear bones to dampen sound). A stroke of the facial area in the parietal lobe results in paralysis of the lower part of the face (from the eyebrows down). The forehead is spared because it is innervated by both sides of the brain. A peripheral lesion involves all of the facial nerve so that both the upper and lower parts of the face are affected. Causes of peripheral lesions include Lyme disease and herpes zoster (Ramsey-Hunt syndrome), in addition to the more common idiopathic Bell's palsy.

4. CN VIII. Because CN VIII fibers ascend ipsilateral and contralateral to the cerebrum, CN VIII lesions are almost never due to stroke.
5. The most useful tests to assess the midbrain are **doll's eyes** (CNs III, VI, VIII and the MLF) and **cold calorics.** In both tests, findings are observed only if the patient is unconscious (normal input from the cerebrum suppresses these reflexes) and the brainstem is intact.
   a. **The doll's eyes test.** As you turn the patient's head to the right, the right semi-circular canals (SSCs) are stimulated. CN VIII sends a signal through the brainstem to the right CN III and (via the medial longitudinal fasciculus; MLF) to the left CN VI (Figure 34-5). This moves the eyes to the left as the head moves to the right; the eyes stay fixed ahead. If there has been brainstem damage to one of these nerves, the eyes will move with the rotation of the head (Figure 34-6).
   b. **The cold calorics test** (Figure 34-7). Inject 30 ml of cold water into the left ear. This will temporarily paralyze the left SCC. The paralysis of the left SCC is equivalent to the hyperstimulation of the right SCC. The brainstem thinks the head is moving to the right, so it pulls the eyes to the left. A fast nystagmus will bring the eyes back to center in a conscious patient. In a conscious patient, **nystagmus is described by the fast corrective phase** (Cold Opposite, Warm Same [COWS]). However, in an unconscious patient, the calorics test results in a slow drift of gaze toward the ear given cold water. The cold calorics and doll's eyes tests are important because both tests require sensory input to be delivered from CN VIII through the MLF to CN III and CN VI. This evaluates the integrity of the MLF, which is surrounded by the reticular activating system (RAS), which is responsible for consciousness.

D. **Level 4. Medulla.** Observe the patient's breathing pattern (see Chapter 30 VIII).

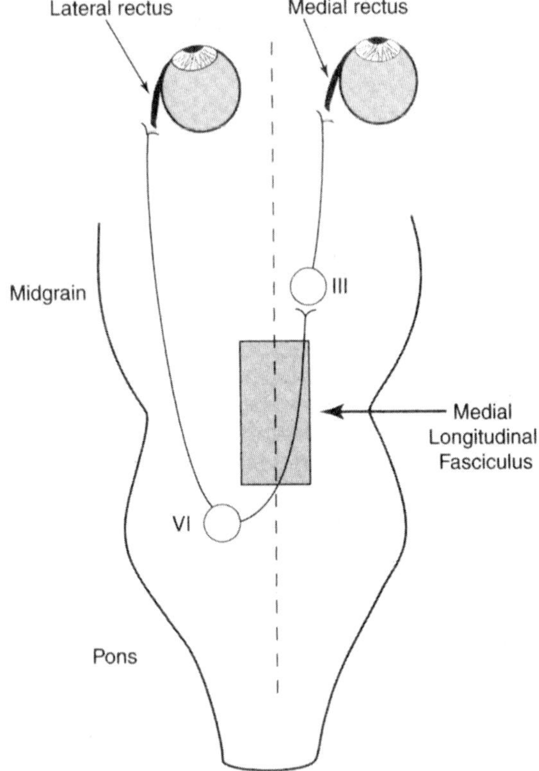

FIGURE 34-5. Horizontal eye movements. (From Weiner HL, Levitt LP, Rae-Grant A: *Neurology*, 6th ed. Philadelphia: Lippincott Williams & Wilkins, 1999.)

E. Using pupil size to assess the level of injury. In addition to the pupil constriction test noted above, the size of the pupils (when symmetric) can also be helpful:

1. Diencephalic (small and reactive)
2. **Mid**brain (fixed, **mid**-positioned midbrain pupils)
3. Tectal (large, fixed pupils)
4. Pons (**pinpoint pons** pupils)

F. Depth of coma. Use the Glasgow Coma Scale to assess the depth of the coma (Table 34-4).

G. Determining real coma from psychiatric etiologies. Use the following tests:

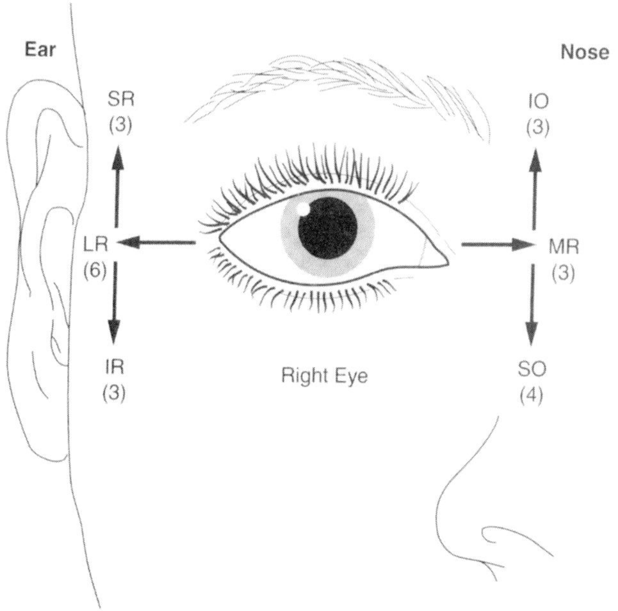

FIGURE 34-6. Primary direction of gaze of extraocular eye muscles. *MR,* Medial rectus; *LR,* lateral rectus; *IO,* inferior oblique; *SO,* superior oblique; *SR,* superior rectus; *IR,* inferior rectus; *3,* 3rd cranial nerve; *4,* 4th cranial nerve; *6,* 6th cranial nerve. (From Cohen ME, Duffner PK: *Weiner & Levitt's Pediatric Neurology,* 4th ed. Philadelphia: Lippincott Williams & Wilkins, 2003.)

1. Open the eyelids and let them go. In coma, the eyelids will slowly return to the closed position. If the coma is nonorganic, the eyelids will immediately shut.
2. Hold the patient's arm above his head and release. The patient without true coma will pull the arm to one side to prevent his arm from hitting him in the face.

X Movement Disorders

A. Definition. Movement disorders are caused by dysfunction of the deep nuclei of the brain. The term *movement disorders* encompasses a broad range of disorders that include diseases in which movement is either impaired or excessive (the latter type is also termed hyperkinetic movement disorders). Some of the most common disorders are parkinsonism, tremor, dystonia, and chorea.

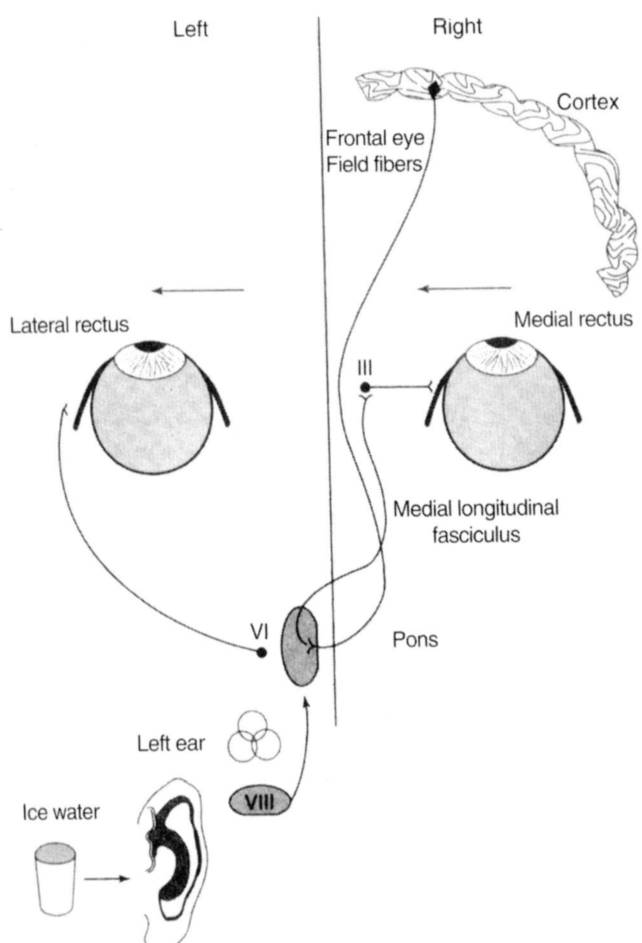

FIGURE 34-7. In the comatose patient with an intact brainstem, ice water in the left ear causes deviation of the eyes to the left. In the awake patient, this deviation is counteracted voluntarily, producing nystagmus to the right. (From Weiner HL, Levitt LP, Rae-Grant A: *Neurology*, 6th ed. Philadelphia: Lippincott Williams & Wilkins, 1999.)

B. Parkinsonism

1. **Cardinal features**
   a. **Resting tremor.** The tremor of parkinsonism is asymmetric and is usually most prominent at rest. Its frequency is usually 3 to 5 Hz.

HOT 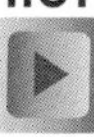 KEY

The tremor of the hands in patients with parkinsonism is described as "pill rolling."

   b. **Bradykinesia.** Movements are slow. Initiation of movement is most commonly impaired disproportionate to continued movement.
   c. **Rigidity.** Tone that is increased uniformly at all velocities. The combination of rigidity and tremor combine to produce a feeling of cogwheeling, that is, a ratcheting, start-stop sensation as you pull on the arm.
   d. **Postural instability.** Patients with parkinsonism are prone to falls as a result of balance problems. The characteristic gait is one of slow, shuffling steps with little arm swing and en bloc turning.
2. **Etiology.** Causes include stroke, metabolic abnormalities, and drugs such as antipsychotics. The most common cause is idiopathic Parkinson's disease, which results in depletion of dopaminergic neurons in the substantia nigra of the midbrain.

C. Tremor

1. **Definition.** A tremor is a rhythmic oscillation of a body part.
2. **Types of tremors**
   a. A **resting tremor** occurs most prominently when the extremity is not in use.
   b. A **postural tremor** of the upper extremities can be demonstrated when a patient is asked to extend the arms and hold this posture.
   c. An **action tremor,** which is classically associated with cerebellar disease, is most pronounced when reaching for a target.
3. **Essential tremor.** This very common type of tremor occurs in persons of all ages, especially the elderly. It is often familial. It is symmetric, has a frequency greater than 7 Hz, is usually postural, and improves with alcohol.

D. Dystonia. Features of dystonia include sustained muscle contractions, causing unusual postures or twisting movements. Dystonias can be isolated to one specific muscle group such as writer's cramp in the hand or torticollis in the neck. Dystonia can also be generalized, affecting all muscle groups, such as in a few rare genetic disorders, or caused by some medications or illicit drugs.

E. **Chorea**

1. **Definition.** The term *chorea* is derived from the Greek word for dance. It is characterized by irregular, brief, jerking movements that occur in multiple body parts in random succession.
2. **Etiology.** Many hereditary, metabolic, toxic, vascular, neoplastic, and even infectious conditions may cause chorea. A classic example of hereditary chorea is Huntington's disease, which is caused by a triplet repeat expansion on chromosome four.

F. **Ballism.** This very rare type of movement disorder is derived from the Greek word "to throw" and consists of flinging arm movements. The most common structure involved in the brain is the subthalamic nucleus, and damage can be secondary to infarction, tumor, or other structural lesions.

XI ABNORMAL BALANCE

Poor balance or coordination results from damage to one of three modalities: visual input, cerebellar input, proprioceptive input.

A. Use the **Romberg test** to distinguishing among the three modalities.

1. **Step 1. Assess visual input.** If the patient can see, visual input is not the cause of his imbalance.
2. **Step 2. Ask the patient to stand with his feet together, his eyes open,** and his arms outstretched. Stand behind him with your arms outstretched (be ready to catch him if he falls). Observe him for 10 seconds to see if he falls. **If he falls with his eyes open** (swaying does not count), **he has a cerebellar lesion.** He will fall toward the side of the damaged cerebellum. Visual and proprioceptive input cannot compensate for a damaged cerebellum because there is nothing there to receive the input.
3. **Step 3. Next, ask him to close his eyes.** This isolates proprioceptive function because it removes visual compensation. By Step 2, you know cerebellar function is intact. Therefore, **if he falls with his eyes closed, his proprioceptive input is damaged.**

B. **Loss of vision** (see Chapter 29)

C. **Loss of proprioception** (see IV D)

D. **Loss of balance resulting from cerebellar dysfunction.** There are three parts to the cerebellum:

1. **The hemispheres receive input from the limbs.** They are responsible for coordinating movement of the limbs. All connections to the cerebellum are ipsilateral; the left arm connects to the left cerebellar hemisphere. The following tests assess the function of the cerebellar hemispheres.
   a. Step 1. **Finger to nose.** Sit two arm-lengths in front of the patient. Hold up one finger and ask her to touch your finger, then her nose, then your finger. It is important that you are two arm-lengths away from the patient so that she is required to completely extend her arm. This prevents the proximal arm

muscles from stabilizing the hand to compensate for the tremor. Now move your finger to a different location and ask her again to touch her nose and then your finger. Repeat this in several quadrants, then with the other hand. Her visual input will enable her to find your finger; the cerebellum is responsible for telling the cerebrum where the finger is in space, so the cerebrum can redirect it to the goal location. An intact cerebellum processes this data quickly, permitting quick adjustments. If it takes more than one or two oscillations to find your finger or her nose, her cerebellum is not keeping up with where her finger is located.

b. Step 2: While the patient is lying in bed, ask her to place her **heel on her shin,** with her foot vertical. Ask her to move her foot up and down her shin, all the while keeping the heel directly on the shin bone. Repeat with the other foot. The cerebellum is responsible for keeping track of where the foot is in space, thereby keeping the moving foot on the shin. Failure to keep the moving foot on the shin implies cerebellar damage.

c. Step 3: **Dysdiadochokinesia.** Ask the patient to hit both thighs with her palms at the same time, then hit the thighs with the back of the palms. Ask her to perform the motion repeatedly; first slow, then progressively faster. If one of the hands cannot keep up with the other, a lesion on that side of the cerebellum is present.

2. **The vermis** sits vertically between the hemispheres of the cerebellum and **is responsible for the axial skeleton** (which keeps the patient vertical). Watch the patient's gait. Ataxic gait may be a function of vermis damage. This is the reason that it is hard to walk a straight line while intoxicated: the vermis is impaired by alcohol.

3. **Vestibular function: nystagmus.** The inner ear has three SCCs. Each canal keeps track of the movement of the head in one of three dimensions: forward/back, left/right, up/down. The movement of fluid within these canals stimulates inner hair fibers that send sensory information to the cerebellum. The key to diagnosing vestibular dysfunction is its intimate connection with the ocular apparatus. When the head moves one direction, a signal is sent to the eyes to move in the opposite direction. Try moving your head side-to-side while reading this text. You are able to do this because the vestibular apparatus senses side-to-side movement and adjusts the eyes so that they can stay focused on the page. Now try moving the page side-to-side while trying to read it. You cannot do this because this relies solely on visual feedback that is too slow to make the necessary adjustments.

a. **When one of the vestibular canals is hyperstimulated** (as occurs with viral infection of the inner ear), the brain is fooled into thinking the head is turning. The eyes are hyperstimulated to turn in the other direction. You have experienced this having come off a merry-go-round. The constant turning of the merry-go-round to the right hyperstimulates the right SCC. When you get off, this canal is still fooled into thinking you are still moving to the right; it tells your eyes to move to the left to maintain straight-on vision. Your visual input, however, tells you that your eyes have moved to the left and readjusts the eyes to midline. But the SSC persists, pulling the eyes to the left; the visual input tries to readjust to the midline. The effect of the eyes moving left to right over and over again creates a sensation that the world is spinning to the left.

b. **Vertigo** is the sensation that the world is spinning and is usually a sign of vestibular dysfunction (and is less commonly a presenting sign of a posterior stroke). Rapid eye movements that may accompany vertigo are termed **nystagmus.** Nystagmus is always a sign of vestibular apparatus abnormalities (or abnormalities of the brainstem that receives this input).

c. **The right and left SSCs are in balance.** Like a set of scales, removing the input from the left SSC is interpreted as more input from the right SSC. Damage to the left SSC (as might occur with gentamicin) has the same nystagmus pattern that would be seen with hyperstimulation of the right SSC.

d. **Method.** Sit in front of the patient and ask her to stare at your finger. Hold her chin with your left hand. Ask her to follow your finger as you slowly move it all the way to the left. She should be able to do this unless the right SSC is being hyperstimulated. A hyperstimulated right SSC (or a damaged left SSC) will pull the eyes to the right, preventing her from maintaining focus on your finger. Repeat this method for the right side. Move your finger slowly as you change positions: two beats of nystagmus is normal when following a rapidly moving target. **A lack of ocular nystagmus excludes the vestibular apparatus as a source of imbalance.**

e. Vestibular dysfunction can occur from abnormalities of the SCCs, abnormalities of CN VIII (peripheral), or abnormalities of the brainstem that receives the input (central). There will also be ringing in the ears (tinnitus) with abnormalities of CN VIII, because auditory input is also affected. Brainstem lesions, on the other hand, usually have vertigo without hearing abnormalities.

f. Causes of peripheral vertigo (Table 34-5).

g. Causes of central nystagmus include multiple sclerosis, acoustic neuroma, and posterior circulation insufficiency (basilary artery stroke or migraine).

TABLE 34-5. Causes of Peripheral Vertigo (Amplitude).

Cause	Historical, Examination, or Radiographic Data
Acoustic neuroma	Acoustic neuromas are a feature of neurofibromatosis. Ask about a family history of drowning. You can imagine how both proprioceptive and visual sensation is lost while underwater. With no vestibular sense, the patient may actually swim downward.
Meniere's disease	Episodic vertigo, sensorineural hearing loss, and tinnitus.
Positional vertigo	Benign positional vertigo (BPV) is due to small stones that form within the SCCs. As the stone rattles around, it stimulates the hair cells, resulting in vertigo. To test for BPV **(Bárnáy maneuver),** sit the patient on the examining table such that when he lies down his head will extend past the edge of the bed. While supporting his head, recline the patient while turning his head to the left so that the head is fully extended off of the edge of the bed. If BPV is present, you will see ocular nystagmus occur after a few seconds. Now sit the patient upright again with the head facing forward. Again look for delayed nystagmus. Repeat the process turning the head to the right.
Labyrinthitis	Usually following an upper respiratory infection or barotrauma (diving).
Inner ear infection	Viral infections.
Trauma	
Psych	
Drugs	Ototoxicity (e.g., furosemide, gentamicin) always begins with vestibular disease before hearing loss. Stumbling in a dark room (i.e., when he does not have visual input to correct for the vestibular loss) precedes hearing loss.
Endocrine	Hypothyroidism.

h. Vertical nystagmus implies either damage to the brainstem from either toxicity (drugs: PCP, phenytoin [Dilantin]) or stroke (supranuclear palsy).

HOT

KEY

Presume that vertigo in an elderly patient is due to a brainstem stroke unless you have definitive evidence of another cause.

HOT
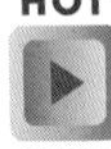
KEY

The vermis is preferentially damaged by alcohol. Alcoholics may have normal cerebellar hemisphere function (finger to nose, heel to shin), but inadequate gait. Always get your patient out of bed to observe her gait.

HOT

KEY

Patients who fall due to cerebellar damage will fall, not collapse. The patient who falls straight down in a collapse (like an imploded building) may be a sign of a nonorganic illness. Patients who have a vestibular disorder will consistently deviate to the side of the lesion. Hysterical gait is deviating to the left, then the right, then the left.

35. Breast Examination

I INTRODUCTION

A. All patients over the age of 40 should be encouraged to self-examine the breast each month and to have physician breast examinations each year. The clinical breast examination provides an opportunity to teach patients how to do the breast self-examination and to emphasize its importance.

B. Mammography should be performed every 1 to 2 years for women 50 and older. Patients with heightened risk should begin mammography at age 40. Risk factors include a history of breast cancer in a mother or sister, a previous breast biopsy revealing atypical hyperplasia, and first childbirth after age 30.

C. The breast is composed of glandular tissue that can mimic breast lumps. Familiarity with normal breast tissue is the key to distinguishing between a new lump and fibrocystic disease, and this is accomplished by encouraging patients to become familiar with their own breast tissue. Patients should perform self-examinations 3 to 4 days after the first day of the menstrual cycle (when cystic enlargement is the least) or the first day of the month for women who are postmenopausal.

D. When clinical breast examinations are conducted by male physicians, and perhaps even female physicians, female chaperones should be present.

II OBSERVATION OF THE BREAST TISSUE

A. Adequate lighting is essential. With the patient seated, ask her to remove her gown to the waist. Inspect the breasts for any skin abnormalities. As a breast cancer grows, it retracts surrounding tissue and may cause the skin overlying the mass to change. Skin changes include:

1. Dimpling or puckering
2. Erythema or color variations
3. Ulceration, changes in moles or scars
4. Unilateral vascularity or edema
5. Peau d'orange (orange peel appearance)
6. Ridging of breast tissue (blocked lymphatic)
7. Lumps

B. Any irregularity should be investigated with a mammogram. Even if not confirmed by mammogram, note the irregularity in the physician's notes for future comparison.

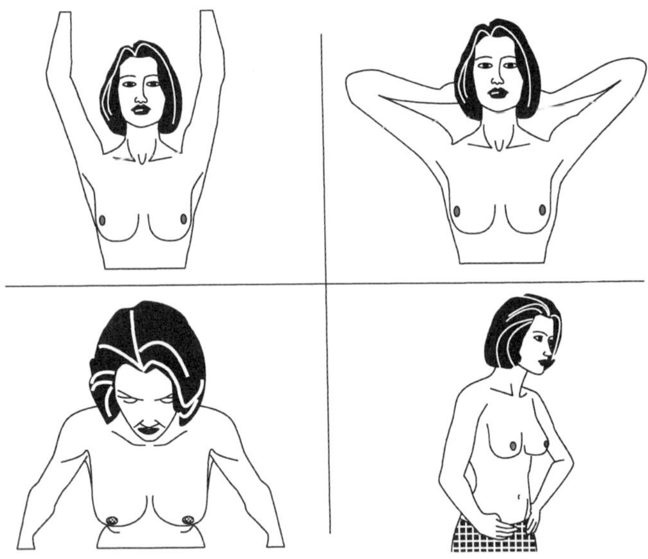

FIGURE 35-1. Observation of breast tissue.

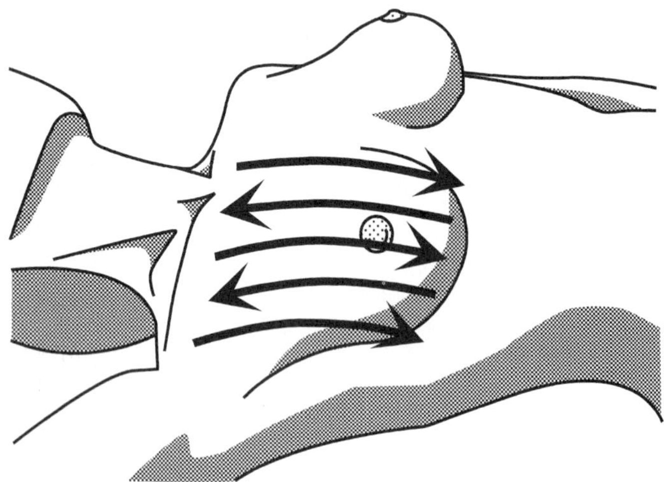

FIGURE 35-2. Z-technique for palpating the breast.

C. **Inspect both breasts from four positions** (Figure 35-1). Each of these four maneuvers changes the contour of the breast tissue and may augment any retractions or skin dimpling not previously apparent.
   1. Ask the patient to raise her arms over her head.
   2. With the patient's hands on her hips, ask her to push in at the waist to contract the pectoral muscles.
   3. Ask the patient to lock her fingers behind her neck and try to pull them apart.
   4. Ask the patient to lean forward from the waist so you may observe symmetry of the breasts from above.

D. **Inspect for nipple for areolar changes.**
   1. **Discharge** (especially unilateral, spontaneous, or in older women)
   2. **Crusting or scaling**
   3. **Retraction or deviation**
   4. **Thickening**

III PALPATE THE BREAST TISSUE

A. Ask the patient to lie on her back with her hand behind her head. Place a small pillow or towel under the scapula. If she has very large breasts, have her roll her hips in the direction opposite the breast you are examining. These maneuvers will expose the lateral part of the breast and better distribute the breast tissue on the chest wall.

B. Rest the right breast flat in the palm of your left hand (reverse for left breast).

C. Begin at the superior lateral aspect of the breast. Palpate by making small circles using the pads of three fingers. Use light, moderate, and then deep palpation. Move left to right a "Z" pattern: from the top of the breast to the sternal boarder, then back to the lateral breast (Figure 35-2).

D. Alternatively, you may use a spiral, grid, or spokes pattern (Figure 35-3). Whatever pattern you use, be consistent.

E. Depress the nipple with pads of two fingers to ensure that there is no discharge, mass, or pain.

F. Repeat the same procedure with the other breast.

IV PALPATE THE LYMPH NODES

Breast cancer, like other adenocarcinomas (cancers from gland-forming organs), travels lymphatically when it spreads. The axillary lymph nodes are the first to be involved in breast cancer. Although the tissue type of the breast cancer is important, the number of lymph nodes involved is most important; as a general rule, the 5-year survival of breast cancer can be estimated by the number of lymph nodes involved (subtract 10% from 100% for each node positive). For this reason, palpation of the lymph nodes is very important.

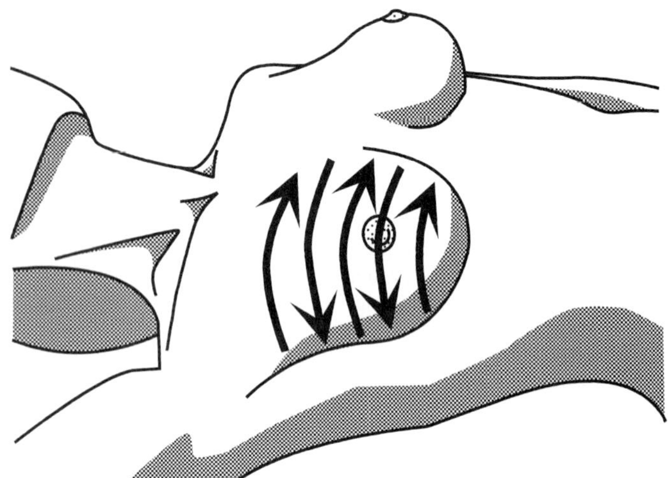

FIGURE 35-3. Linear technique for palpating the breast.

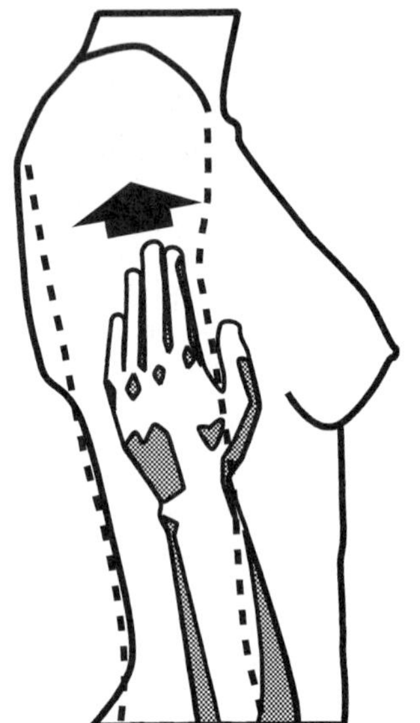

FIGURE 35-4. Palpating axillary lymph nodes.

A. Ask the patient to sit up again and place her arms at her sides.
B. Support the patient's relaxed arm on your forearm and insert your fingers deep into the axilla (Figure 35-4).
C. Start in the central region each time and palpate down to the bra line, to the elbow, behind the pectoralis, and subscapular at the back wall of the axilla. Palpate for masses in the tail of the breast.

36. Genitourinary and Gynecologic Examinations (Tier II Only)

I OVERVIEW OF THE MALE GENITOURINARY EXAMINATION

A. **The Tier I genitourinary examination is simply inspection for ulcers or masses.** For men between the ages of 16 and 30, palpation of the testicles (for testicular cancer) is a Tier I examination. Even if nothing is found, this emphasizes to the patient the importance of doing self-examinations (i.e., if it matters to you, it should matter to him).

B. **Genitourinary diseases vary according to age.** The "-celes" (i.e., varicocele, spermatocele, hydrocele) are due to congenital predispositions and most often occur at young ages (10 to 30 years). Sexually transmitted diseases can occur at any age but are most common during sexual peaks (20 to 40 years). Prostate disease is rare until after age 50.

II THE MALE GENITOURINARY EXAMINATION

Palpate the testicle by placing it between your thumb and fingers and gently rolling it between your fingers: a mass will become immediately apparent. If you find a mass, transilluminate (see below). Now rotate your fingers to the top of the testicle. The small fleshy mass where the vas deferens and arteries/veins enter the testicle is the epididymis (Figure 36-1A). The slightest pressure will cause great tenderness if the epididymis is infected (epididymitis, see below).

A. **Testicular pain**

1. **Testicular torsion.** Torsion occurs when the testis is not attached to the tunica vaginalis that normally lines the inside of the scrotum, attaching it to the scrotal wall (Figure 36-1A). When unattached, the testicle can twist about the spermatic cord, allowing arterial blood into the trapped testicle, but preventing venous blood from leaving (Figure 36-1B). **The torsed testicle will be swollen and painful.** The testicles always torse from lateral to medial; therefore, correction (which is usually performed surgically) involves rotation of the affected testicle from medial to

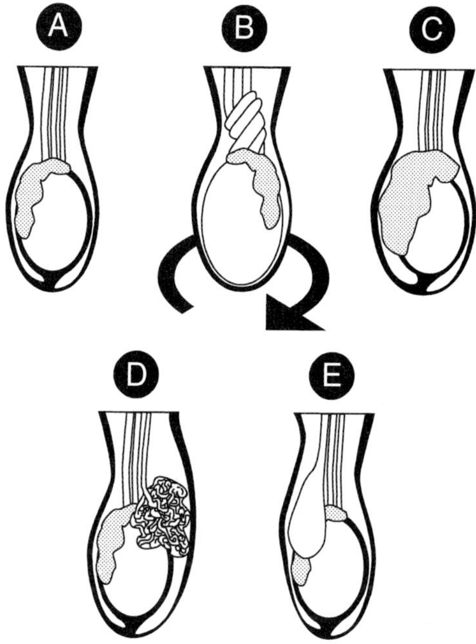

FIGURE 36-1. Testis in the scrotum.

lateral (as if you were opening a book). This is a congenital abnormality, and thus it usually only affects younger men (15 to 25 years).

HOT 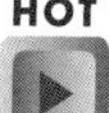 KEY

Testicular torsion is a surgical emergency, because impaired blood flow can lead to ischemia and loss of the testicle. Surgical repair includes correction of the torsion and anchoring of both testicles (because the congenital defect affects both sides).

2. **Orchitis** is infection of the testicles (e.g., due to mumps). The epididymis is unaffected, and the infection is usually preceded by viral symptoms. Both testicles will be tender, but usually not swollen.
3. **Epididymitis** results from retrograde transmission of gonorrhea, chlamydia, or enteric bacteria through the urethra to the epididymis. The epididymis is very tender and may be enlarged, and the remaining testicle is normal (Figure 36-1C).
4. **Varicoceles** are masses of venous engorgement resulting from obstruction of the left testicular vein. Blood makes its way into

the testicle, but venous outflow is prevented. This venous dilation feels like a bag of worms in the scrotum (Figure 36-1D).

a. Varicoceles almost always occur on the **left testicle,** where venous drainage is to the left renal artery (in contrast to the right testicle, where venous drainage is to the iliac vein).

b. **Venous dilation develops over the course of days, not hours.** Varicoceles do not transilluminate. The testicles are not affected and are minimally tender, if at all.

B. **Scrotal or testicular masses.** If you find a mass, **determine whether it transilluminates.** Place a light directly on the mass. A mass that is full of clear serous fluid glows bright red. A mass that is full of anything else (e.g., semen, blood, pus) or is solid absorbs the light and does not transilluminate. A halogen light works better than a pen light, but use caution because halogen lights are very hot.

1. **Testicular cancer** presents as a hard, nontender nodule and generally does not transilluminate. Any suspicion of testicular cancer should prompt referral to a urologist.
2. **Spermatoceles** are engorged masses of semen just superior to the epididymis. They are soft (unlike testicular cancer), nontender (unlike epididymitis), and they do not transilluminate (Figure 36-1E). Spermatoceles, which are due to an obstruction of the vas deferens, usually resolve spontaneously.
3. **Hydroceles** are cystic masses within the scrotum. They are benign, painless masses of serous clear fluid that transilluminate. No therapy is required.
4. **Varicoceles** (see above)
5. **Scrotal edema.** The inguinal canal connects the abdominal cavity and the scrotum. Any ascites in the abdomen also collects in the scrotum. An athletic supporter can be used to compress the scrotum and push this fluid back into the abdomen.

C. **Prostate.** There are three abnormalities of the prostate: prostate nodules, prostatic hypertrophy, and prostatitis.

1. **Prostate examination.** To examine the prostate, place your gloved, *lubricated* first finger at the entrance of the anus, with the flexor side of the finger facing anteriorly. Apply slight pressure and hold it there; the anal sphincter will initially oppose your pressure. Wait for the sphincter muscle to tire. When you feel the sphincter relax (but not before), insert your finger until you feel the superior margin of the prostate.

   a. Practice on your own hand to learn how the prostate should feel. Close your left hand in a tight fist with the thumb folded into the palm. Squeeze hard. With your right index finger, palpate the thenar eminence (the muscle at the base of thumb). This is the consistency and size of a normal prostate.

   b. Now relax your fist but keep your thumb folded into the palm. Again palpate the thenar eminence; this is the consistency of a boggy prostate of prostatitis.

c. Tighten your fist again. Palpate the thenar eminence and walk your finger up over the knuckle of your thumb. This hard bony mass is the consistency of a prostate nodule.

2. **Benign prostatic hypertrophy.** The most common cause of post-renal obstruction is prostatic enlargement. Benign prostatic hypertrophy occurs in all men if they live long enough. Unless it obstructs urinary flow, it is of little consequence. Obstruction causes symptoms such as urinary frequency, hesitancy, and dribbling.
3. **Prostate cancer.** A hard prostate nodule on palpation suggests cancer. However, only one third of the prostate can be palpated.
4. **Prostatitis.** The swelling of an acutely infected prostate will create a boggy sensation on palpation. The prostate will also be very tender. Acute prostatitis is usually due to an ascending urinary tract infection. Chronic prostatitis is less painful; symptoms include a dull perineal pressure during urination or defecation.

D. **Hernia.** A hernia is the expression of abdominal contents through a rift in the abdominal wall. Any surgical scar is a potential rift. Three naturally occurring weak spots in the abdominal wall are the inguinal canal, the femoral canal, and the umbilicus.

1. **Inguinal canal.** The normal inguinal canal is so small that it allows only the spermatic cord to enter the abdomen. Repeated abdominal pressure (as in weight lifters or the chronically constipated) may cause this opening to enlarge, allowing a segment of bowel to move into the canal. Complications arise only when the bowel becomes trapped in the canal, or incarcerated, causing a bowel obstruction.
   a. To palpate for an inguinal hernia, ask the patient to stand while you sit on a stool facing him. Begin with the right inguinal canal. Use the index finger of your left hand.
   b. Insert your first finger into the scrotum, where it joins the lower abdominal wall until you feel the spermatic cord. Follow the cord with your finger into the inguinal canal until you feel a small ridge; this is the inguinal ring. Ask the patient to bear down or cough. Pay attention to the tip and middle part of your finger. An indirect hernia pushes the bowel into the inguinal canal through the inguinal ring; you will feel a pressure on your fingertip. A direct hernia pushes the small bowel directly through the side of the inguinal canal wall; you will feel a pressure against the middle part of your finger.
2. **Femoral canal.** Another potential space in the abdomen is the opening of the femoral vessels as they enter the thigh space. This weak spot causes the less common femoral hernia.
3. **Umbilicus** (see Chapter 32)

E. **Penile pain**

1. **Priapism.** This is a constant erection caused by arterial blood in the penis. Venous blood cannot escape. A urology consult is warranted.

2. **Peyronie's disease.** Fibrosis of one side of the corpus cavernosum causes the penis to bend to one side. It is of cosmetic importance only.
3. **Ulcers** (see below)
4. **Phimosis** or **paraphimosis.** Phimosis is infection under the foreskin. Paraphimosis is foreskin trapped behind the head of the penis during erection, inducing a localized priapism of the penile head.

III THE FEMALE GENITOURINARY EXAMINATION

The pelvic examination is a Tier II examination for most women, but is also a regular part of screening. Women should have yearly pelvic examinations after the onset of intercourse, because the risk of cervical cancer escalates proportionally to the risk of exposure to human papilloma virus (a sexually transmitted disease). When pelvic examinations are conducted by male physicians, and perhaps even female physicians, female chaperones should be present.

A. **Position the patient** at a 45-degree angle to allow eye contact with the patient throughout the examination. This will also relax the abdominal muscles for easier palpation.
   1. The buttocks should be at the edge of the examining table. Ask the patient to place her heels in the stirrups, which should be positioned so you have full vision of the vulva.
   2. To maintain privacy, place a drape from the lower part of the abdomen to the knees. Push down on the middle portion of the drape so that you can maintain eye contact with the patient; this alleviates anxiety and allows you to see any facial grimacing due to pain. Position yourself on a rolling stool with a light over your shoulder.

B. Tell the patient you are going to touch her inner thigh at the knee. Move your hand along the inner thigh to the vulva. This allows the patient to anticipate the location of your hand. **Spread the labia majora** with your first two fingers so you can see the labia minora, the clitoris, and the urethra. Look for ulcers, lice, warts, swelling, and erythema. Vulvar cancer is rare, but look carefully when examining older women because it is more common in this population.

C. Tell the patient you are going to **insert your index finger into the vaginal vault.** Insert the finger and pull back. Use the thumb of the same hand (which is external to the vaginal vault) to lightly palpate at 5 and 7 o'clock. Bartholin's glands are located at 5 and 7 o'clock at the introitus; these are responsible for vaginal lubrication. Obstruction of these glands leads to pain, enlargement, and discharge.

D. Perform a **speculum examination.**
   1. **Lubricate the speculum** using warm water, not the K-Y gel. The gel may taint any cultures obtained during the examination.

2. Spread the vulva with the first two fingers of your left hand. Make sure the speculum is closed (the two pieces are together). Turn the speculum 90 degrees counterclockwise so that its wide dimension is now vertical (Figure 36-2). Pain with insertion of the speculum comes with touching the urethra. **Insert the speculum** with your right hand, putting pressure on the posterior introitus with the speculum (i.e., away from the urethra) as you enter. Angle the speculum slightly inferior and posterior, following the course of the vagina as it descends into pelvis.
3. Once inserted, slowly rotate the speculum 90 degrees clockwise so the wide dimension is horizontal. **Open the speculum,** being careful not to pinch the skin. Use your left index finger to stabilize the speculum so that it does not touch the urethra. The cervix should be visible between the bills of the speculum. If it is not, close the speculum, and reinsert it at a more posterior angle. Note the color, shape, and position of the cervix. Look for ulcers, masses, lacerations, or discharge.
   a. Pap smear
      (1) Brush. Insert the brush into the cervical os and gently twist it. Remove the brush and swab onto a glass slide.

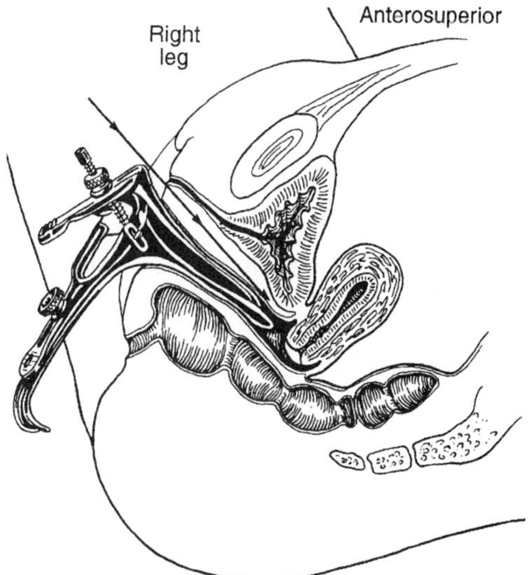

FIGURE 36-2. The pelvic examination: speculum examination. (From Beckmann CRB, Ling FW, Laube DW, et al: *Obstetrics and Gynecology*, 4th ed. Baltimore: Lippincott Williams & Wilkins, 2002.)

(2) **Pap stick,** which has a notched end that resembles a mitten. Insert the thumb of the mitten into the os and turn it 360 degrees. Remove the stick and swab onto a glass slide. Send these to the laboratory.

b. **Cultures.** If you see discharge in the vaginal vault or from the os, use a cotton swab to collect a sample and place this onto the chocolate agar plate (or culture tube). Repeat the process with a *Chlamydia* swab, placing the swab in a special culture tube.

4. **Close the speculum,** and rotate it 90 degrees counterclockwise back to vertical. Remove it slowly, applying pressure on the posterior introitus as it is withdrawn (again, to avoid contact with the urethra).
5. At this point, ask the patient if she needs to urinate before proceeding to the bimanual examination. The bladder must be empty to adequately perform the bimanual examination.

E. **Perform a bimanual examination,** which allows you to feel the adnexal structures along the vagina and to palpate the cervix.

1. **Lubricate** the first two fingers of your right hand. Approach the introitus as described previously (i.e., descend along the thigh with the back of your hand). Insert the two fingers into the vagina, placing pressure on the posterior introitus, away from the urethra as you enter. Supinate your hand so the palm faces up. With the two fingers slightly spread, find the cervix between your fingers. There may be slight tenderness; exquisite tenderness suggests pelvic inflammatory disease.
2. Place your left hand on the patient's lower abdomen. The base of your hand should be on the pubis, and the palm should be on the abdomen so that your fingers extend to the area of the abdomen halfway from the umbilicus to the symphysis pubis. Position the first two fingers of your right hand under the cervix and lift up slightly. **Bring your two hands together to palpate the uterus** (Figure 36-3). Feel for uterine size (pregnancy), masses (fibroids, cancer), and tenderness. The nonpregnant uterus is 4 to 6 cm from the pubis. If the base of your left hand is on the pelvic brim, the edge of the uterus should not extend past your fingers.
3. **Palpate the right ovary** by moving the first two fingers of your right hand to the right vaginal wall. Place your left hand on the abdomen and depress slightly until your right and left hands meet. Gently roll your hands back and forth; this should trap the ovary between the hands. Be gentle; the ovaries are very sensitive. The left hand should do the moving, and the right (vaginal) hand should be the sensor. Keep the fingers of the vaginal hand straight. The normal ovary is 1 to 3 cm. Larger ovaries suggest ovarian cysts or carcinoma. To palpate the left ovary, repeat the process.
4. **Palpate the lateral vaginal wall** using the same technique. Because the fallopian tubes open into the abdominal cavity, infec-

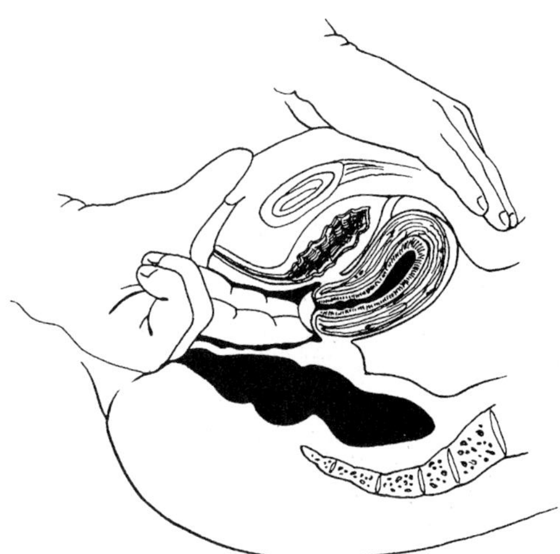

FIGURE 36-3. The pelvic examination: bimanual examination. (From Beckmann CRB, Ling FW, Laube DW, et al: *Obstetrics and Gynecology*, 4th ed. Baltimore: Lippincott Williams & Wilkins, 2002.)

tions may take the form of tubo-ovarian abscesses along the vaginal wall. If they are present, you may feel an enlarged, tender mass.

5. **Remove your gloved hand slowly,** applying pressure posteriorly.

F. **Consider performing a rectovaginal examination.** This examination should be performed if colon cancer, incontinence, rectocele, or cul-de-sac tumors or infections are suspected. Change your gloves, and lubricate the first two fingers of your right hand. Insert the index finger into the vagina (using the approach above) and the middle finger into the rectum. Use the technique described in the male genitourinary examination for entering the rectum (see II C 1 a). Apply steady pressure; insert your finger only when you feel the sphincter fatigue. Ask the patient to bear down as if having a bowel movement. You are feeling for tumors or masses between your two fingers. Remove your fingers slowly.

G. Redrape the patient after completing the examination, and ask her to move her buttocks onto the examination table before taking her feet out of the stirrups. Always remove your gloves outside of the view of the patient. Offer a tissue, tampon, or sanitary napkin after the examination. Allow the patient to get dressed before discussing the findings. If the findings are normal, tell her immediately.

IV Abnormalities Observed in Both the Male and Female Examinations

A. **Genital ulcers and sexually transmitted diseases.** Any of the first four infections listed below can cause reactive inguinal lymphadenopathy.

1. **Herpes.** The herpes virus lies dormant in the dorsal root ganglion after its initial infection of a sensory nerve. Intermittently, the virus descends the sensory nerve to destroy the tissue, causing an ulcer. Because the sensory nerves are involved, **the ulcer is painful.** There can be many of them or only a few; the anus may be involved, as well as the labia or penis. Fever and malaise can accompany infections. The diagnosis is confirmed by scraping the ulcer to look for giant multinuclear cells or on clinical grounds alone.
2. **Syphilis.** A spirochete burrows into vessel walls, destroys the vessel, and causes ischemia to the tissue and thus an ulcer. Because the nerves to this area of the skin are also destroyed, **the ulcer is painless.** Syphilis may also present as flat plaques (condylomata lata). The diagnosis is confirmed by obtaining a serum RPR or MHATP test.
3. **Bubo.** *Haemophilus ducreyi* is quickly absorbed by the lymphatic system and taken to the inguinal lymph nodes. The inflammation in the nodes creates an ulcerative mass overlying the inguinal nodes (bubo). The diagnosis is confirmed by culture of the urethra.
4. **Gonorrhea.** Purulent discharge and urinary pain are consistent with the diagnosis. The disease, caused by *Neisseria gonorrhoeae,* is frequently cotransmitted with *Chlamydia* organisms. This disease is also known as the "clap" (from the red-light Le Clapier district of Paris). The diagnosis is confirmed by urethral culture.
5. **Condylomata acuminata (warts)** are caused by infection with the human papilloma virus. Acuminata warts are pedunculated, as opposed to condylomata lata (syphilis), which are flat plaques. Diagnosing warts is important, because cervical cancer is largely due to infection with this virus.
6. **Pubic lice.** These organisms feed on the skin four times a day. The pruritus associated with the infection is due to a reaction to lice saliva and is maximal during these feeding periods.
   a. Lice are difficult to see unless you look closely. They live close to the skin and may look like freckles. The pubis is not exposed to the sun; therefore, it should not have freckles. Lice resembling freckles flake off with a comb or fingernail.
   b. Many therapeutic creams and shampoos exist, although shaving the pubic hair is the only foolproof method of eradication.

Most treatments are neurotoxins; if the patient does not rinse the treatment after application, the neurotoxin can induce pruritus similar to that from the infection.

HOT 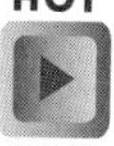 KEY

RPR is an antibody that forms in response to a normally occurring protein buried within the vessel wall. As the syphilis spirochete burrows into the vessel wall, it exposes the protein to the immune system. A positive RPR is synonymous with syphilis, although any vasculitis (e.g., lupus) or damage to a vessel wall (e.g., intravenous drug use) can cause a positive RPR.

B. Perineal skin infections

1. **Tinea cruris** ("jock itch") is due to a fungal infection. It is characterized by erythema, pruritus, and pain. Satellite lesions (small, circular lesions on the periphery of the main erythema) are common, and the scrotum is frequently spared.
2. **Erythrasma.** This is due to a *Corynebacterium* infection. The rash will glow blue under a Wood's lamp (black lamp). The scrotum is frequently involved, and there are no satellite lesions.
3. **Fournier's gangrene.** This deep skin infection is due to folliculitis. If the staphylococcal or streptococcal infection extends into the deep fascia, necrotizing fasciitis can result.

PART V

Approaching the Core Clerkships

37. Internal Medicine

I INTRODUCTION Internal medicine encompasses every adult disease that does not require surgery or involve pregnancy. **Compulsive attention to detail marks the great internist and determines in large part how well you do in this rotation.** After an internal medicine intervention is instituted (e.g., an intravenous beta-blocker), it usually cannot be taken back. Therefore, whenever you begin a new therapy, always ask, "What am I looking for to see if this works? What side effects am I looking for?"

II THE TEAM Each patient on the internal medicine service is assigned to either an intern or an intern and a medical student. Students are assigned to patients with an intern but are expected to act as each patient's primary physician, making decisions and then checking these decisions with the resident or intern before acting on them. Although direct involvement by the attending physician varies, **the attending physician is officially responsible for the entire service** and all medical decisions.

III WHAT TO EXPECT

A. Typical schedule. The schedule of the typical medicine day is shown in Table 37-1.

B. Tasks. There are two parts of the day best suited for accomplishing the following tasks: the early morning and the afternoon. Prioritization is vital; orders placed before the flood of orders from other services are placed (i.e., before 9 AM and just after 1:00 PM) will be executed immediately; orders after 10:00 AM in the morning and 2:00 PM in the afternoon may not be executed until much later. **By maximizing efficiency, you will have more time for your patients,** which is the key for doing well in this rotation. Prioritize as follows:

1. Talk with social workers. Most of their contacts (nursing homes, shelters, government agencies) close at 4:00 PM.

TABLE 37-1. Schedule for a Typical Day During Your Internal Medicine Rotation.

Time	Activity
7:00 AM	Pre-rounds (when you see patient by yourself)
8:00 AM	Work rounds
9:00 AM	Morning report
10:00 AM	Attending rounds
12:00 PM	Noon conference
1:00 PM	Work time
5:00 PM	Sign-out to cross-cover

2. Order consults and tests. If consults were requested yesterday or in the morning, call the consult for the recommendations. If tests have been suggested, order them now.
3. Check laboratory results, especially cultures. Act on the findings.
4. See your patients again in the afternoon. This is the time to provide reassurance and listen to their concerns. If they become accustomed to your afternoon visits, they will require less attention during the busy morning pre-round time. Ideally, you should see your patients at least twice a day.
5. Get your patient out of bed. Get help if necessary. Patients' natural inclination is to remain in bed. Even very ill patients benefit from sitting in a chair for a time. Walk your patient if you can.
6. Every day, ask yourself, "What is keeping this patient from going home?" If you have no valid reason to keep the patient, ask your resident to discuss possible discharge.
7. Write your progress notes (see Chapter 15).

IV General Features of the Internal Medicine Rotation

A. **Primary skills.** While the skills discussed in Chapters 10 to 21 are important for all services, they are absolutely vital for internal medicine. Nowhere else will your clinical reasoning ability and your documentation of your clinical reasoning (in oral and written form) be put to test like on your internal medicine rotation. Read these chapters carefully before beginning your internal medicine clerkship.

B. **Multiple rounds.** The nature of internal medicine is to assess, act, reassess, and then act again. Medication takes time to work, so the consequences will be delayed (unlike surgery, in which the consequences are usually immediate). Early detection of side effects makes all the difference in correcting the mistake. For this reason, expect to round several times a day on your patient; sometimes with your team, sometimes alone.

C. **Vastness.** Internal medicine encompasses all diseases, and even rare diseases may play a role. To be successful in internal medicine, focus on the most common diseases (Table 37-2).

HOT KEY An atypical presentation of a common disease is more common than a typical presentation of an uncommon disease. Older patients and those with other comorbid diseases (e.g., HIV or steroid-dependent patients) often present with atypical variations of common diseases.

D. **Comorbidity**

1. **Patients on the internal medicine service frequently have more than one disease**, although it is usually only one disease or event that has prompted the admission. Common comorbid diseases include hypertension, COPD, HIV, diabetes, renal insufficiency, liver disease, congestive heart failure, and coronary artery disease. Identify the primary reason for admission (e.g., pneumonia) and focus your efforts on this diagnosis. Devote remaining time to diseases to make sure comorbid diseases do not interfere with or become affected by the treatment of the primary disease.
2. **Treating one disease can exacerbate another.** After diagnosing the disease, your task is twofold: treat the diagnosed disease, and then think about the implications of this treatment on other comorbid diseases. For example, gentamicin may be indicated for a gram-negative infection, but how will this affect the patient's chronic renal failure? Always anticipate before you act.

E. **Chronic disease management.** Patients in internal medicine are likely to take their disease home with them (i.e., diabetic patients will remain diabetic after discharge). Spend time with patients who have chronic diseases, making sure they understand their disease and how to manage it when they leave the hospital. This is the key to preventing early readmissions for the same disease.

F. **Recognizing truly "sick" patients.** Over time, you will be able to distinguish patients who are ill but likely to get better on their own from those patients who are truly sick. **Distinguishing the patient who is merely ill from the one who is about to die is one of the most important lessons you will learn in medical school.** The internal medicine rotation is a valuable time to learn this skill, because patients are much more ill on the internal medicine service

TABLE 37-2. Recommended Topics That a Third-Year Medical Student Should Know (from the Clerkship Directors in Internal Medicine).

Topic	Inpatient	Ambulatory
General Skills		
Diagnostic decision making	X	X
Case presentation skills	X	X
History taking and physical examination	X	X
Communication and relationships with patients and colleagues	X	X
Test interpretation	X	X
Therapeutic decision making	X	
Bioethics of care		X
Self-directed learning	X	X
Prevention		X
Coordination of care	X	X
Basic procedures	X	
Geriatric care		X
Nutrition		X
Advanced procedures	X	
Specific Problems or Diseases		
Abdominal pain	X	
Acute myocardial infarction	X	
Acute renal failure	X	
Altered mental status	X	
Anemia	X	
Back pain		X
Chest pain	X	
Common cancers		X
Congestive heart failure	X	
Cough		X
Chronic obstructive pulmonary disease/obstructive airway disease	X	
Depression		X
Diabetes mellitus	X	X
Dyslipidemias		X
Deep venous thrombosis and pulmonary embolism	X	
Dyspnea	X	
Dysuria		X
Gastrointestinal bleeding	X	
HIV infection	X	X
Hypertension		X
Joint pain		X
Liver disease	X	
Nosocomial infection	X	
Pneumonia	X	
Smoking cessation		X
Substance abuse	X	X

than on other services. In the course of the rotation, ask your resident, "Is this patient truly sick?"

G. **Heuristics.** Because the differential diagnosis for internal medicine complaints is so vast, clinical reasoning is vital in discarding the extraneous diagnoses to get to the "smart list" of diagnoses that will guide your subsequent testing (see Chapter 10). Small errors in your clinical reasoning can be disastrous in internal medicine practice. Beware of heuristics (also known as "cognitive shortcuts"), which are influences that may corrupt your clinical reasoning because of past experiences.
   1. **Recent memory.** Example: If you have recently seen a case of tuberculosis, all new cases seem more like tuberculosis.
   2. **Knowledge.** Example: A hematologist knows hematology, and that physician's vision of the world is selectively more oriented to hematology diagnoses.
   3. **Tragedy.** A bad outcome artificially inflates your suspicion of the same diagnosis in subsequent patients. Example: If you saw a patient who died of aortic dissection last week, now every patient with chest pain appears to have an aortic dissection.

V USING MEDICATIONS

A. There are no formal surgical procedures in internal medicine practice; thus, the interventions you will encounter during this clerkship will often center upon the administration of medications.

B. Having a strategy for the use of medications is important, because after you give a medication, it can rarely be taken back.

C. One such strategy is to visualize medications as tools. Start with a small toolbox of medications and become intimately familiar with them; know their indications, doses, expected benefits, and side effects and be familiar with other medications with which they are not compatible. Make your tools cheap and easy to use; choose those that have multiple indications. This will simplify your life. **Remember that one of the most common reasons for noncompliance is cost.**

VI TOPICS AND SKILLS YOU WILL NEED TO KNOW: RECOMMENDATIONS FROM THE CLERKSHIP DIRECTORS IN INTERNAL MEDICINE

The knowledge and skills covered in an internal medicine rotation are beyond the scope of this book. Because of the vastness of the field of internal medicine, however, knowing where to spend your time is the key to doing well in this rotation. Table 37-2 has the most important learning objectives, as identified by the Clerkship Directors in Internal Medicine. Use the reading strategies in Chapter 44, along with the sources provided in Chapter 45, to address each topic.

38. Surgery

I INTRODUCTION

A. As a general rule, the goal of the surgical rotation is to be in the operating room (OR). Your job is to maximize the efficiency of taking care of patients on the wards (i.e., preoperative or postoperative patients) to enable you to spend as much time as possible in the OR. You cannot learn surgery without being in the OR.

B. The surgical rotation often involves long periods of assistance with basic tasks in the OR. You may find yourself holding retractors or performing simple incisions or ties. Do not be disappointed. Your role is to learn the basic surgical skills. These skills are the foundation for complex surgical techniques should you choose a career in surgery and for procedural skills if you choose another specialty.

II THE TEAM

Surgical services require a well-defined and strong hierarchy. The time frame for decisions is very short in surgery, and decisiveness is important. The instructions of the attending physician must be followed promptly. This does not mean that you cannot ask questions, but wait until the appropriate time. For example, asking questions in the middle of an operation that has just gone awry is not ideal; hold your questions until after rounds and then ask.

III WHAT TO EXPECT

A. Typical day. The schedule of the typical surgery day is shown in Table 38-1.

B. Surgical "limbo." You may have unscheduled time after work rounds and before the first OR case or days when you have not been invited to the operating room. Use this time wisely; there is much to be done.

1. Prioritize jobs so that orders with a long lag time (e.g., consults or radiographic tests) or those for tests that may affect treatment (e.g., a CBC for a transfusion) are completed first.
2. If you have extra time, read about the cases for the day. Focus as much on the anatomy of the procedure (i.e., dust off your anatomy atlas) as the indications for and the possible complications of the procedure. If you are asked questions in the OR, they are likely to concern the anatomy involved.
3. Surgical days are long and begin early. There will be less "at home reading time" than on other rotations. To prevent falling

TABLE 38-1. Schedule for Typical Day in Surgery Rotation.

Time	Activity
5:30 AM	Pre-rounds
6:00 AM	Work rounds
7:00 AM	Operating room
12:00 PM	Noon conference/ lunch
1:00 PM	Operating room
5:00 PM	Afternoon work rounds
6:00 PM	Afternoon rounds

behind, it is important that you have something to read while at the hospital during surgical downtime (Chapter 45).

C. **End of the day.** Before you go home, make sure that preoperative tasks are set for the next day so important morning time is not wasted on unexpected events.

1. Review all consults and act on the physicians' recommendations. Review late laboratory results, especially cultures. Start therapy where indicated.
2. See all postoperative patients one more time. Check drains and pain control.
3. See the preoperative patients and make sure they are ready for the next day.
4. Make sure laboratory tests are ordered for the next day.
5. Check the OR schedule for the next day. Look for cases that interest you. If you are assigned a case, go home and review the anatomy.

IV Surgical Rounds

A. **Pre-rounds** (see Chapter 3). As you see each patient in the morning, ask yourself, "What would my senior resident want to know about this patient to advance his or her care?" Focus on the surgical wound, the organ system related to the wound, drains, and bowel function. Almost all patients who have had general anesthesia, especially those who have had abdominal surgery, have a postoperative ileus (e.g., the bowel is anesthetized as well). Until bowel motility resumes, ingested food may back up and lead to vomiting. Part of pre-rounds is determining if the ileus has resolved.

1. Each day, ask the patient, "Have you passed gas or had a bowel movement today?" If the answer is "yes," you can advance the patient's diet. Most patients begin with clear sips (clear liquids, ice chips), advance to a liquid diet, and then resume a regular

diet. If the patient's progress is slower than expected, assess for other causes (e.g., infection, obstruction, pain).

2. Do not remove a wound dressing unless your senior resident has given you permission to do so.
3. Other vital data for surgical patients include I&O and any tube drainage. Be prepared to answer the question, "Why is this patient still in the hospital?"

B. Surgical rounds presentation

1. Identify the patient (e.g., "This is Mr. Hernandez, a 45-year-old man who is 2 days status-post cholecystectomy.").
2. Describe what was notable about the patient's course overnight.
3. Note vital signs.
4. Note I&O, including drain output.
5. Report findings of a focused physical examination. Say "normal" if it is normal.
6. Name only the antibiotics and those medications you think the senior resident might change.
7. Be prepared to present a plan for the day. Time is precious, so be very focused and brief.
   - **a.** Focus on the wound and complications. Note any plans to remove or place drains or catheters. Note the antibiotic regimen and plans for ambulation or physical therapy.
   - **b.** Briefly discuss the fluids, electrolytes (laboratory findings), and nutrition.
   - **c.** Note comorbid diseases and their management only if the comorbid disease is active (e.g., the patient is short of breath because of his heart failure). If this is extensive, suggest a medicine consult.
   - **d.** If repeat surgery seems possible, note the criteria that warrant returning to the OR.
   - **e.** Discuss anticipated discharge and any necessary arrangements.

C. Surgical work rounds

1. Look for ways to maximize efficiency. Consider assembling the service's charts on a mobile chart rack or wheelchair to take around on rounds (as long as this is not disruptive to the nursing station). Orders should be written immediately or, at the very latest, before the team breaks to go to the OR.
2. Make a scut list for the entire service as rounds proceed (see Chapter 20 IV).

D. Surgical notes. Notes should be completed before rounds, although on busy services they may be completed during rounds. Either way, there is no time for extensive notes. Surgical patients who are not in the ICU are usually reasonably healthy; otherwise, they would not be surgical candidates. In your notes, focus on the components of your oral presentation.

V Informed Consent for Surgical Procedures

A. Basic components

1. Provision of warning of the risks of the procedure
2. Information on the planned procedure and the alternatives
3. Patient permission to perform the procedure

B. Additional component of surgical consent. The consent must encompass all planned as well as potential procedures. An unconscious patient is unable to consent to an additional procedure if a complication or an unexpected finding is encountered.

C. Obtaining informed consent

1. Make sure you understand all components of the procedure before you try to explain it. Always include the generic risks of any procedure, including anesthesia-related problems, bleeding, infection, and transfusion.
2. When describing a procedure, use language the patient can understand (eighth-grade level). Avoid jargon and complicated descriptions. Ask the patient to repeat the plans back to you.

D. Role of the witness. The consent must be signed by a witness, who should hear the explanation of the procedure and see the patient signing the consent. Ask someone who is not involved in the procedure or with the patient (i.e., not a team or family member) to serve as a witness. Document in the preoperative note that risks and benefits and alternatives have been explained and that consent has been obtained.

VI Admission to the Surgical Service

Admission to the surgical service is the same as for other services with the following exceptions:

A. Many admissions are for planned or elective procedures. Depending on the procedure and the hospital, these patients are admitted either the morning of their surgery or the day before their surgery. Your resident tells you which admissions are planned for the day. These patients are admitted through the admissions office and assigned a bed. When patients have arrived at their beds, your resident is notified.

1. To expedite the process, you or your resident will go to the admissions office in the morning and write admission orders for all elective patients scheduled to be admitted that day.
2. These orders are the same as those listed in Chapter 20, with special emphasis on admission laboratory tests (CBC, electrolytes, PT/PTT, urinalysis, type and screen), ECG, chest radiograph, and old medical records.

B. Same-day surgery patients are admitted on the day of their surgery. If there are no complications, they are discharged later the same day. These patients usually have simple procedures with low complication rates. Two important factors must be considered with same-day surgery patients.

1. If you see the patient the morning of the procedure, begin the history (before you say anything else) by asking if he has had anything to eat or drink since midnight. If the answer is "yes," immediately notify your senior resident so that OR space can be opened up; the surgery will likely be canceled.
2. Make sure the patient has someone to pick him up at the end of the day. Regardless of how well the procedure goes, no same-day surgery patient can drive himself home.

C. Emergent surgeries come from two sources:

1. Patients from other hospital services (e.g., medicine or obstetrics) will have a medical chart documenting their history and physical examination, as well as the events that have lead up to the emergent surgery. Because the procedure is emergent, you may not have the luxury of obtaining your own full history and physical examination. Begin by talking with the physician in charge of the patient on that service. Then collect as much data as possible from the chart. If time allows, see the patient and take your own history.
2. Patients admitted to the operating room directly from the ER. Speak directly with the ER physician to obtain as much information as possible. The key components of the history include the time course of the disease, including the mechanism of injury (if applicable), and a detailed medication and drug allergy history. The patient's family may be a valuable source of information.

VII Scrubbing and Gowning Techniques

A. Scrubbing

1. Be sure to remove all jewelry before entering the operating room. This includes necklaces, earrings, watches, and rings. Clip your fingernails; long fingernails will puncture the gloves.
2. Before scrubbing, find a gown that is your size, as well as two sets of gloves that are your size. Give these to the circulating nurse to hand off to the scrub technician.
3. Put on your mask before you enter the operating room and before you begin scrubbing; after you are scrubbed you cannot touch anything that is not sterile (e.g., the mask). Make sure the nose-piece is molded around your nose and the top border is snug across your face. If it is not, your breath will fog your glasses. You should be able to breathe easily. The knots in the back should be well tied. Tie the top one first.
4. If you wear glasses, wash them and your face before you begin scrubbing. This helps prevent fogging and removes the oil that causes the glasses to slip on your nose. If the procedure is likely

to result in a splatter of bodily fluids, ask for a face shield. Your resident can guide you as to which procedures (if not all) require a face shield.

5. The general rule of scrubbing is that everything from the fingernail to the elbow should be scrubbed. Spend extra time on the fingernails.
6. Scrub the forearms and elbows first. If you do the hands first, the contaminated water from the elbows will run down onto your previously scrubbed hands.
7. The general rule is to continue scrubbing until the attending and resident have completed their scrubbing (even if your started before they did). This will allow them to enter the operating room before you and begin preparations for surgery, without you getting in their way.
8. After you are scrubbed, you must remain sterile. This means that your hands must not touch anything that is not sterile.

To stay sterile after scrubbing, always keep your hands where you can see them. This prevents you from touching your face, touching below your waist, or leaning on things.

B. Gowning technique. After scrubbing, you enter the OR. You must touch nothing from the moment you enter. To keep your eyes on your hands, never let your hands drop below your waist.

1. Hold your hands in front of you, and open the door by backing into it. The scrub nurse will have your gown. If you enter at the same time as the attending or resident, you will be the last to be gowned. Wait patiently. Do not touch anything.
2. The nurse will hold the gown so that the arm holes face you. Insert one arm at a time. At this point, it is not necessary that your hands come out the sleeves.
3. In front of you on the gown is a waist-tie. The two pieces of the tie are attached to the gown, with the left much shorter than the right. The two are connected by a piece of paper. Grab the paper with your right hand and hand it to the scrub nurse (if your hand is outside the arm of the gown, touch only the paper; do not touch the tie. If your hand is still within the arm of the gown, grab wherever you like). Slowly turn yourself around 360 degrees so that you are again facing the scrub nurse, who will tie the two waist ties together. You are now ready to glove.

C. Gloving technique. The scrub nurse will ask you what size glove you wear. If you have small hands, try size 6. If you have large hands, try size 8. See how the gloves fit, and adjust your size next time. There are many types of gloves. Use the standard variety unless you know you have a latex allergy or unless you develop a rash.

1. If the scrub nurse gloves for you, she will hold the glove by the edges in front of you. This is your signal. With the left hand, insert your hand straight down into the glove with your thumb pointed forward and downward. Insert rapidly, and the glove will snap nicely around your wrist.
2. If you miss a finger (e.g., four of your five fingers find their way into the fingers of the glove), do not panic. Glove the other hand, and then use the sterile glove of one hand to adjust the glove of the other. Grasp the glove finger that missed and pull on it until your finger can extend into the hold.
3. If the scrub nurse lays out your gloves instead of gloving you, follow this technique. Both gloves will have a cuff at the wrist. With your dominant hand pick up the opposite glove by the cuff. This part of the glove will eventually be against your skin or gown, so it is OK to touch here. Do not touch any part of the glove that could potentially touch the patient. Hold the glove so that you can insert your nondominant hand directly into the glove (the fingers should be pointing downward). For your dominant hand, use your now gloved hand to pick up the remaining glove from the outside, under the folded lip of the glove.

VIII Working in the Operating Room

A. **Approaching the wound.** Introduce yourself to the scrub nurse immediately. Tell him that you are a medical student scrubbing in on the case and ask where you should stand. This is also a good time to volunteer to do any of the preoperative tasks (e.g., placing a Foley catheter, "prepping" the abdomen).

B. **Surgical tasks**
  1. **Holding retractors.** You may be asked to hold one of the retractors to improve the surgeon's visual field. There is nothing glamorous about this task, but there are two important rules.
     a. Keep your eyes on the retractor. You cannot let it slip out of the wound or let it drift into the surgical field. Indeed, this is one of the reasons you may be asked to hold the retractor: to occupy your hands to prevent them from becoming nonsterile and to keep your mind on the operation at hand.
     b. Do not rock back on your heels with arms outstretched to allow your legs to relieve your tired arms. This locks your knees, compressing the veins from the lower leg. This decreases your preload, which decreases your cardiac output, thus decreasing your cerebral perfusion: you may pass out.
  2. **Suctioning.** You may be asked to hold a Yankauer (a rigid plastic suction tube) to suction smoke (from the cautery), blood, or secretions. There are three important rules.
     a. Never let the suction get in the way of the surgeon's visual field.

b. Never enter the wound while the surgeon is working there unless you are told to do so. The exception may be during simple ties. When you do enter, enter from the side, just over the surface of the wound.
c. Suction as much as you need to but not more than you have to.

3. **Cutting sutures.** The surgeons will frequently tie knots as they close incisions or tie off bleeding vessels. You may be asked to cut the excess suture material distal to the knot. When cutting, always make sure the large screw on your suture scissors is pointing up; this ensures proper cutting (and not fraying) of the suture. In general, braided sutures (e.g., Vicryl, silk, etc.) should be cut close to the knot, whereas monofilaments (e.g., PDS, Prolene, Nylon) are cut with a 1- to 2-cm "tail," avoiding the possibility of their unraveling. If in doubt, too long is better than too short. Avoid cutting the knot, which would slow the progress of the operation.
4. **Stapling.** Larger incisions are often closed using staples. You may be asked to staple the skin closed. The resident will approximate the two flaps of skin with pick-ups and then present them to you. Keep the notch at the end of the stapler in line with the incision and then fire the stapler to staple the edges together.

C. Scrubbing out

1. If you know you have to scrub out at a certain time (e.g., you have a mandatory lecture at 1:00 PM), tell the surgeon at the beginning of the case. This allows the surgical team to make provisions for your absence, and it allows you to focus on the case instead of worrying about finding an opportune time to tell the team you have to leave.
2. If you have to scrub out unexpectedly (e.g., you have to urinate), wait for a timeout in the procedure. This will be signaled by the surgeon's hands coming out of the wound, or reaching for a tie. Simply announce, "Dr. Cameron, I have to scrub out for 5 minutes." It is better to scrub out than to pass out.
3. A few medical students pass out in the OR. This does not mean that they cannot be surgeons.
   a. If you begin to feel lightheaded, let the attending physician know immediately so that you can be helped to a chair (rather than falling into the surgical field).
   b. If you do pass out, do not be distressed. Fainting is usually a one-time vasovagal response to seeing something to which you are not accustomed. It does not suggest that it will occur again. Prolonged standing can cause pooling of blood in the inactive muscles of the lower extremities, increasing the chance of fainting. Consider intermittently contracting your leg muscles while standing to promote venous return and to reduce the chances of feeling faint.

D. Needle sticks. The OR involves a host of body fluids and sharp objects. Many precautions are taken to prevent exposure to body fluids, and needle sticks are very rare. However, they do occasionally occur.

1. The best way to prevent a needle stick is to keep your eyes focused on the wound at all times and to keep your hands in front of you (i.e., within vision) at all times. Most needle sticks occur when a hand inadvertently enters the surgical area out of sight of its owner.
2. If a needle stick does occur, announce it immediately. It may be embarrassing to announce a needle stick during the surgery, but your health is of great importance. The breech in the glove will only allow more blood to enter your wound if you do not scrub out and cleanse the wound immediately. Your resident will tell you how to get appropriate care.

IX Operative Notes and Orders

Writing these notes and orders can save a lot of time for the team. The more time you save, the more time you will have in the OR.

A. Preoperative note (see Chapter 15).
B. Postoperative dictation and note (see Chapter 15). The surgeon or senior resident will do the dictation, but you can do the note.
C. Preoperative orders (see Chapter 19).
D. Postoperative orders (see Chapter 19).

X Dressings and Wound Care

A. Operative wounds. Never remove an operative dressing until your resident tells you to do so. The operative dressing usually remains in place for 2 to 3 days, unless there is postoperative fever or excessive wound pain requiring inspection to exclude infection or wound dehiscence.

B. Lacerations

1. **Wound healing**
   a. **Primary closure** is used only for clean wounds and refers to immediate closure of the wound (within 8 hours of the laceration) with sutures, staples, or glue. The wound must be completely irrigated and explored to ensure that no bacteria or foreign material are trapped inside the closed wound. If you cannot completely see the bottom crevice of the laceration, obtain a radiograph to exclude foreign bodies (especially if glass is involved in the injury).
   b. **Delayed primary closure** is used for contaminated wounds in which closure might create an infection. The wound is left open and packed with gauze, with closure at 48 to 72 hours.

c. **Secondary intention** is used for dirty wounds, for wounds in which the time since injury is prolonged, and for drained abscesses. The wound is left to close on its own. Packing with gauze occupies the dead space in the wound. This is important, because dead space, where it is difficult for antibiotics and WBCs to reach the wound, is advantageous for bacteria. Packing prevents the wound from closing, and allows it to heal from the bottom to the top.
   (1) Infected or necrotic wounds are dressed with wet-to-dry dressings (*damp*-to-dry dressings). Moisten the gauze with sterile saline and pack it into the wound. Then apply a dry dressing and then tape. The damp dressing adheres to the necrotic tissue, and with daily removal of these dressings, the necrotic tissue adherent to the moist dressing is removed.
   (2) These dressings are changed each day, and the patient must be taught how to do this or must return to the wound care clinic each day.

2. Wound healing tips
   a. Do not use iodine in wounds; it slows wound healing.
   b. Antibiotics are not routinely indicated; use your judgment. If the wound is contaminated, or if a there is surrounding erythema, combine wound care with an antibiotic that covers staphylococcal and streptococcal infections (e.g., cephalosporin, dicloxacillin).
   c. Give a tetanus-diphtheria (Td) booster to any patient who has not received one within the past 10 years.
   d. Never close animal bites that are puncture wounds, because of a high risk of infection.

C. **Abscess.** An abscess is a loculated pocket of pus that insulates the infection from antibiotics and WBCs that would ordinarily eliminate the infection. The pocket may be in an anatomically enclosed space (e.g., joints, pleural space), in a walled-off pseudocyst (e.g., pancreatitis, appendicitis), or in a fascial plane (e.g., arm). Wherever it is, it must be surgically drained. The key to distinguishing an abscess from cellulitis or other tissue infection is fluctuance.
   1. The tissue must feel boggy to touch to be worth draining. If it is not, begin antibiotics and observe.
   2. Larger abscesses, those that will require significant pain medication, or those that are adjacent to critical structures (nerves, blood vessels) may require draining in the operating room.
   3. When opening an abscess, make sure the incision is wide enough to establish a portal for exploration, drainage, and adequate packing. Never explore a blind skin wound with your fingers; needle fragments are not uncommon.

D. **Joint infections.** An infected joint behaves like an abscess (enclosed space). A drain must be placed or the joint must be flushed each day.

E. Necrotizing fasciitis. This condition is an extension of an infection (cellulitis, folliculitis) into the fascial plane between the dermis and muscular tissue. Because this represents a potential space (although small), bacteria can extend longitudinally in short time (especially *Streptococcus,* with its hyaluronidase enzymes). As the bacteria extend, they damage the nerves and vessels that are in this space. The result is physical findings such as anesthesia, ecchymosis, and vesicles (swelling on the surface lifts the overlying skin). Any of these findings with a cellulitis should prompt an immediate ultrasound or surgical exploration.

XII SUTURING

A. General rules

1. Absorbable sutures are typically used, although these can induce more of a reaction than nonabsorbable sutures. Table 38-2 gives the absorption time for various absorbable suture materials. Reasons to use nonabsorbable sutures include the following:
   a. Strength is required (e.g., fascia, anastomosis). Table 38-3 lists various nonabsorbable sutures and their decreasing tensile strength.
   b. Scarring is an issue. The reaction to absorbable sutures causes increased scarring.
   c. Infection is present. Nonabsorbable sutures are foreign bodies to which bacteria cling.
2. Braided sutures are easier to tie (the braid keeps them from slipping through the knots).

B. Learning to tie sutures. Remember the following key points:

1. Do not crush tissue with instruments. An instrument can be used to pick up a piece of tissue, but it should not be used to grasp a piece of tissue forcibly.
2. Obtain good light and visualization of the entire wound before you begin.
3. During the procedure, always keep your eye on the needle. Bring the needle close to the wound so that both the needle and the

TABLE 38-2. Absorbable Sutures.

Absorbable	Absorption Time
Chromic	3 months
Monofilament	6 months
Plain	2 months
Silk	2 years
Vicryl	2 months

TABLE 38-3. Nonabsorbable Sutures.

Nonabsorbable	Decline in Tensile Strength
Cotton	50% decrease per 6 months
Ethilon; nylon	20% decrease per year
Nurolon	20% decrease per year
Ethibond/Mersilene	Infinite
Prolene	Infinite
Steel	Infinite

wound are in your field of vision at the same time. If you must divert your sight from the wound (e.g., to reach for something on the procedure tray), take the needle out of the needle driver and leave it on the sterile drape next to the wound. Remember that poor vision, fatigue, and lack of concentration are what cause most needle sticks.

4. Hold the needle in the needle driver at a 45-degree angle. Enter the tissue with the tip of the needle perpendicular to the skin surface. Then supinate your hand so that the needle enters and turns toward the wound. Enter the skin 2 mm from the laceration line. This will keep the skin from bending into the laceration after you tie the suture, thereby preventing scarring (Figure 38-1).
5. Enter one side of the laceration at a time (except for very small lacerations, when it may be suitable to go through both sides with one needle stroke). When you see the needle poke through the wall inside of the laceration, release the needle from the needle driver. Grasp the tip of the needle inside of the laceration and pull your suture almost completely through; leave enough suture outside of the laceration to enable you to easily tie the knot when you are finished (8 cm).
6. Enter the opposite wall of the laceration at a 90-degree angle. Supinating your hand should result in the needle tip poking through the skin surface at the same distance from the laceration from the initial needle insertion (2 mm) (Figure 38-1).
7. When the needle is through the opposite side of the laceration, grasp the suture remaining on the other side of the laceration and pull the suture completely through until the wound edges approximate each other. The edges of the laceration should bow outward as you pull the two suture ends tight. With your scissors, clip the suture 8 cm from the wound. Tie the knot as described below.

C. Tying sutures

1. Practice tying sutures. Do not take unopened sutures from the OR or the wards; these cost money. Ask the scrub nurse for extra

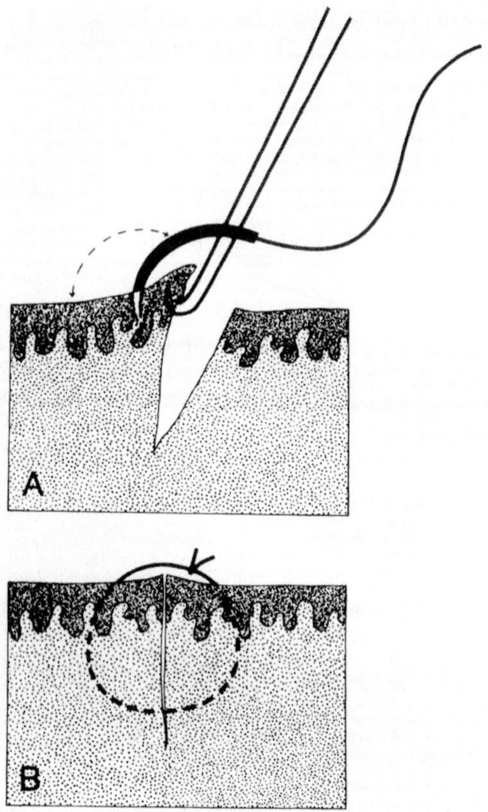

FIGURE 38-1. A, Reflection of the wound edge permits passage of the needle so that it incorporates more tissue at the base of the suture loop than at the top and aids in eversion of the wound edge. This is especially useful in thin skin over wrinkle lines or creases, which tend to invert. In this figure, the skin hook is shown reflecting the wound edge. **B,** This technique incorporates more tissue in the lower half of the suture loop than in the top and permits eversion of the wound edges when the suture loop is tied. (From Simon RR, Brenner BE: *Emergency Procedures and Techniques,* 3rd ed. Baltimore: Williams & Wilkins, 1994.)

sutures that you may have for practice. Make sure you try at least the following: a braided silk suture, a regular silk suture, and a synthetic suture (Ethilon). Learn and be comfortable with the tensile strength of each so you know how much tension you can put on each suture type before it snaps. Be familiar with the slippage of a synthetic suture.

2. Practice needle insertion on an orange or thick loaf of bread. Make a small incision, and then proceed. Make sure that your insertion and exit sites are equidistant from the laceration and that both are far enough from the wound (3 mm) so that when you make the knot taut, the wound edges evert (point up). This prevents dead airspace (and thus bacteria) from being trapped in the laceration.
3. Learn to tie a surgeons' knot, or a square knot.
   a. Using the two ends of the suture, form a half-knot by passing the right strand over the left. As you do this, make sure the knot has not twisted 180 degrees. Make sure you can clearly see the right-over-left twist when you look at your half-knot. Now pass the strand that is *currently* in your left hand (not the original left strand) over the right. Alternate back and forth.
   b. If you deviate from this method and tie two successive right-over-left, right-over-left half-knots, you have tied a slip knot that will loosen over time, exposing the laceration.
   c. The key throw is the first throw, especially with nylon sutures. You must make the first half-knot tight enough that it does not slip (thereby allowing the laceration to open) as you tie the second half-knot to lock it down. This is why practicing with the different suture types is important. You must be familiar with your own strength and how much tension you can apply to a silk (or nylon) suture before it breaks.

D. Suture removal. Most other sutures are removed after 7 days. Exceptions include the following:
1. Cosmetic sutures (face, which are removed after 5 days)
2. Sutures at pressure points (e.g., skinfolds), which are removed after 10 days

XIV POSTOPERATIVE DRAIN CARE

A. Never pull a drain or catheter until specifically told to do so. Boluses of fluid are occasionally used to open clogged drains. Never apply a bolus to a drain that is inserted into a fresh anastomosis, because this increases the risk of rupturing the anastomosis.

B. There are five types of drains.
1. **Straight drains.** These drains are designed to drain the wound around the procedure. They are left to drain via gravity, without suction.

a. **Penrose drains.** This is a straight drain into the wound to allow serosanguineous drainage to escape. Usually this tube has a large safety pin inserted into it or a large adhesive bandage to keep it from being drawn into and subsequently lost in the wound.

b. **Oral feeding or nasogastric tubes.** These tubes frequently clog, especially when food is delivered through them. If they clog, irrigate the tube to dislodge the clot. If this does not work, replace the tube. Do not reinsert the guidewire. Cola and pineapple juice are both highly acidic and can sometimes unclog a feeding tube.

2. **Self-suction drains.** These drains are attached to a self-suction device (e.g., Jackson-Pratt drain). These low-suction drains are used when drainage around the procedure is required but when the risks associated with a high-suction tube are to be avoided. The low suction causes these drains to clot frequently.
3. **Sump drains.** These drains have two lumina, the aspiration port that goes to the space of interest (e.g., stomach), and the continuous air circuit open to the air that prevents the aspiration port from sucking closed.
4. **T tubes.** These drains are inserted into a lumen within the body. For example, the T part of the tube is inserted into the bile duct with the straight piece draining out of the abdomen). Never pull a T tube, lest you pull out the entire bile duct.
5. **Chest tubes,** which are used to drain the pleural space. They are attached to a box with three chambers. The tube connects directly to the drainage chamber that collects the blood, pus, or air from the chest. The drainage chamber is connected to an empty-space chamber, which prevents the wound drainage from being sucked into the water seal chamber and the wall suction. This in turn is connected to the water seal chamber, which regulates how much suction is delivered to the pleural space based on how much water is put in the container. It prevents air from leaking back into the chest cavity should the wall suction become unhooked.

XV Other Postoperative Issues

A. Fever in postoperative patients is predictable, and the etiology is predictable based on the number of postoperative days. Possible causes can be remembered using a mnemonic known as the "five Ws."

1. **Day 1. W**ind (atelectasis). Order incentive spirometry. Nothing else needs be done unless the patient appears ill or is hypotensive.
2. **Days 2 to 3: W**ater (urinary tract infection). Order a urinalysis and culture. Treat appropriately.

3. **Days 4 to 6: W**ound infections. Carefully inspect the wound. Look for fluctuance.
4. **Day 7+: W**alking. Consider a pulmonary embolism. Order a V/Q scan or spiral CT.
5. **Day 7+: W**onder drug. Consider a drug reaction.
   a. If the patient does not respond to antibiotics, consider retained pus or a new pulmonary embolism as a cause of the fever (remember that a thrombus can cause fever).
   b. Draw new cultures, including those through central lines. Consider obtaining additional cultures from effusions, ascites, and urine.

B. Get the patient out of bed as soon as possible. Atelectasis and pulmonary embolism result from being bed-bound, and pneumonia results from atelectasis. Normal bowel motility resumes sooner if the patient begins to move, thus decreasing aspiration risk from parenteral feeding.

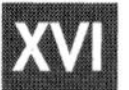

Laparoscopic Surgery: How to Drive a Camer-A

In laparoscopic cases, you may be responsible for holding the laparoscope and repositioning it to follow the surgeon's movements of the instruments.

A. The equipment. The equipment for the laparoscope consists of two components.

1. The patient component consists of the laparoscope camera that collects images from inside the patient. The laparoscope is made up of a long metal rod that contains the lens.
2. The second component is the cart, which holds the light source, monitor, and camera control box. On the camera there are two buttons and two dials. The buttons are used to set the contrast or "white balance" in the camera. The dials are used to focus and zoom the lens.

B. Using the laparoscope

1. Usually the scrub nurse will set up the laparoscope for you, but you should take the opportunity either before or after a laparoscopic case to learn how to focus, zoom, and white balance the camera.
2. After everything is set up, the camera is placed into a small incision in the abdomen. Typically, the surgeon will look around with the camera to inspect the abdomen.
3. The next step is the establishment of the other incisions (ports) to insert the instruments used for the surgical procedure. These incisions are made with the assistance of the laparoscope. The visual image from within the body allows the surgeon to avoid major vessels and organs while making additional incisions on the abdomen surface.

C. Operating the 0-degree laparoscope. The 0-degree laparoscope is so named because its end is flat, which means that you point it straight at what you want to image.

1. **Acquire and center** the area you want to image by moving the entire laparoscope. All you need to do is point the laparoscope straight at what you want to see on the monitor. Note that the port through which the laparoscope is inserted through acts as a fulcrum. Moving your hands in one direction moves the laparoscope's end (and thus, the image on the monitor) in the opposite direction.
2. **Zoom in and out.** The zoom control on the camera is infrequently used. Zoom in and out by adjusting the distance between the end of the laparoscope and the area you are imaging by pulling back or pushing in on the laparoscope.
3. **Maintain the horizon** by rotating the camera around the end of the laparoscope. Generally, you'll want to keep the buttons on the top of the camera pointed up.

D. Operating the 30-degree laparoscope

1. The 30-degree laparoscope's end is angled at 30 degrees, which means that you **do not** point it straight at what you want to image. When you point this laparoscope straight ahead, you'll be looking slightly up at an angle of 30 degrees.
2. The 30-degree laparoscope is much harder to use, but it is becoming more popular because it allows the surgeon to look straight up, straight down, and around corners, none of which you can do with the 0-degree laparoscope. Operations that require moving the 0-degree laparoscope in and out of different ports several times can be performed while leaving the 30-degree laparoscope in a single port for the entire operation.
3. **Acquire and center** the area you want to image by moving the entire laparoscope *and by rotating the entire laparoscope.* The light cord runs down the center of the laparoscope; use this as your reference point. The end of the laparoscope will point away from the light cord at a 30-degree angle.
   a. When the laparoscope is rotated so that the light cord points down, the end of the laparoscope will be angled up at 30 degrees.
   b. When the laparoscope is rotated so that the light cord points to the left, the end of the laparoscope will be angled to the right at 30 degrees and vice versa.
4. **Zoom in and out** the same way as with the 0-degree laparoscope (i.e., push in or pull back on the scope).
5. **Maintain the horizon** the same way as with the 0-degree laparoscope. The laparoscope and the camera must be rotated separately because they control two different things.

E. Getting the best image during the procedure

1. **Listen to the operator.** This rule always supersedes rules 2 to 5. Most surgeons will tell you what they want you to do (e.g., "Push in on the laparoscope.").

2. **Center the surgical activity on the monitor.** *Keep the instruments that the surgeon is actually using centered on the monitor.* There may be many more instruments within the patient that are not moving and thus do not need to be viewed.
3. **Limit shaking and jerking.** When the scope is not moving, steady the camera port with one hand while holding the laparoscope with the other hand. When you move the scope, try to move in one fluid motion instead of a series of rapid, jerking motions.
4. **Keep an appropriate distance.** The surgeon will usually let you know when to "move in a little" and "move out a little." When in doubt, try to keep the camera distance so that the area of focus (where the surgical action is occurring) is half the area of the entire monitor screen.
5. **Maintain the horizon.** The surgeon will want things that are actually "up" in the abdomen to be "up" on the monitor. The horizon can be maintained at all times by **keeping the buttons on the camera pointed toward the ceiling.** You can also obtain visual cues from things inside the body that are affected by gravity. For example, the surfaces lines of fluid pools should appear perfectly horizontal on the monitor. On the other hand, suture strings and leaking fluids should hang or drip perfectly vertical on the monitor.

F. **Cleaning the lens.** Sometimes the lens gets fogged up. The fog can be cleared by:
1. The laparoscope can be withdrawn so that the end of the lens can be wiped with a commercial antifog solution.
2. The end of the laparoscope can be wiped clear on liver or bowel. **Ask or wait to be told before doing either.**

G. **Adding ports and changing instruments.** During the course of most procedures, new incisions will be made to add additional ports and instruments will be exchanged through existing ports.
1. When new ports are placed, focus the camera on the insertion point from the inside of the body so that the surgeon can see that he is not penetrating significant arteries or other structures.
2. When instruments are exchanged through existing ports, keep the camera focused on the instrument being taken in or out of the abdomen. This will allow the surgeon to follow the removed instruments in or out of the field to protect organs as the instruments pass.

H. **Final tip: Do not forget your role.** You are positioning the camera to acquire images for the surgeon's benefit. Do not make the mistake of moving the laparoscope to see something about which you are curious or want to "check out." You must stay focused on the area where the surgeon is working.

39. Obstetrics and Gynecology

I Introduction

A. Obstetrics and gynecology, or OB/GYN, has **both inpatient and outpatient components.** The inpatient service is divided into obstetrics, benign gynecology, and gynecologic oncology. The outpatient service is mainly spent between routine obstetrics and gynecologic evaluations.

B. This chapter will give you an overview of the important skills on the rotation to make you comfortable. A complete description of OB/GYN is beyond the scope of this book; use an OB/GYN textbook (Chapter 45) and your residents to fill you in on the details.

II The Team

The inpatient OB/GYN service is usually dominated by a **strong hierarchy.** The attending physician has the last word, especially when it comes to patients in active labor or surgical patients. The chief resident is generally in charge of everyone else.

III What to Expect

A. The schedule of the typical OB/GYN day is shown in Table 39-1.

B. The inpatient service operates much like a **surgical service.** Notes should be written before work rounds and are routinely repeated (but shorter) in the afternoon. OB patients are young, and for this reason tend to be in reasonably good health, presenting with one problem. **Focus your notes.**

C. The goal is always to get the floor work done to get to the OR or to the L&D suite. If you do not insist in being in the L&D/OR and if you are not aggressive in getting there, you will be easily shut out. You cannot learn OB/GYN unless you get there, however, so you must be efficient on the wards.

IV Inpatient Obstetrics

There is usually a ward consisting of antepartum and postpartum patients.

A. Antepartum patients. These patients are hospitalized before delivery because of high-risk conditions such as preeclampsia, preterm labor and premature rupture of the membranes, placenta previa, acute surgical and medical conditions during pregnancy, and multiple gestations.

TABLE 39-1. Schedule of the Typical OB/GYN Day.

Time	Activity
6:00 AM	Pre-rounds
7:00 AM	Work rounds
8:00 AM	OR/L&D
12:00 PM	Noon conference/lunch
1:00 PM	OR/L&D or OB/GYN clinic
5:00 PM	Afternoon notes/work rounds

1. **Know everything about these patients,** including all vital signs, daily laboratories, ultrasounds, and studies. These women are the most complicated and sickest patients on the obstetrics service.
2. Know patients' gestational age, and comment in every progress note on fetal status. **Remember, in obstetrics, you always have two patients to consider**.
3. Develop an overall short-term plan and long-term plan for each patient. If you are on call or on L&D and are asked to see one of the antepartum patients, always **evaluate her promptly.** The status of both the woman and the fetus can deteriorate rapidly, and this is why they are hospitalized.
4. You will usually see the antepartum patients on pre-rounds, discuss your notes with the intern or resident during work rounds, and then go on attending rounds with a perinatologist or attending obstetrician. During rounds, concisely present your daily evaluation of the patient and plan. Read before rounds so that you know the pathophysiology and management of your patients.
5. Never perform a pelvic examination or other procedures on these patients without first speaking with your resident.

B. Postpartum patients. After seeing the antepartum patients, you will then round on the patients who have delivered. Most patients who have had vaginal deliveries stay in the hospital 24 to 48 hours, and those who have had cesarean sections stay 48 to 72 hours.

1. Before going into the patient's room, make sure you know the information in Table 39-2. Spend extra pre-round time if necessary to know this information; it can usually be found in the delivery summary/parturition records.
2. Include the following in your evaluation.
   a. **Breasts.** Normally, breasts are nontender and nonengorged.
   b. **Fundus.** A normal, nongravid fundus is firm, nontender, and below the umbilicus.
   c. **Perineum and lochia.** It is helpful to inspect the perineum for swelling and to look on the pad for lochia, especially if the woman has had a laceration. (Check with your resident at

TABLE 39-2. Checklist of Information to Know Before Seeing Postpartum Patients.

Date and time of delivery
Sex of infant
Type of delivery
Term versus preterm delivery
Type of incision/episiotomy (if any)
Labor anesthesia
Prenatal laboratory findings and history. Note any complications or high-risk conditions such as diabetes or preeclampsia.
Medications that the patient is taking (e.g., magnesium, antibiotics, insulin)

the beginning of the rotation to see whether you should do this part of the examination.)

3. Your progress note should contain all of the information in Table 39-2, as well as your findings on the breast, fundus, and perineum/lochia examination. In addition, be sure to note:
   - **a.** Whether the patient is breastfeeding
   - **b.** Any pain or new symptoms
   - **c.** Whether the patient wishes to be released from the hospital or not
   - **d.** Always write the prenatal laboratory findings in the side margin and alert the resident if the patient needs orders for any intervention (e.g., administration of RhoGAM or rubella vaccine).
   - **e.** On day of discharge, discuss contraception with the patient. Document this discussion.
4. **Cesarean sections.** All patients who have had cesarean sections require a full cardiovascular, pulmonary, and abdominal examination in addition to the postpartum examination.
   - **a.** You should also **inspect the incision daily.** Make sure it is clean, dry, and intact and comment on whether staples or sutures are present.
   - **b.** All vital signs, I&O, and O_2 saturation should be recorded, as in any surgical patient.
   - **c.** For a Pfannenstiel incision, typically the staples come out and Steri-Strips are placed on postoperative day 2 or 3. (Often, this occurs immediately before discharge.)

V Labor and Delivery

A. After making all rounds, the day will begin with the off-going residents signing out patients to the oncoming teams.

1. This process is rapid but important, because this is the only sign-out you will receive before caring for these patients.
2. **Key points to giving a board sign-out** include:
   a. Patient's last name, gravity, parity, gestational age, and reason for being on L&D (e.g., post-dates induction)
   b. Briefly mention any relevant medical problems (e.g., diabetes)
   c. Concise summary of the labor course thus far, finishing with a plan (e.g., next check, will place internal monitors)
3. Concisely state only the important facts. However, know everything about the patient in case you are asked questions.
4. Do not act apologetic or unclear of the plan during board sign-out.
5. Find out any information you do not know before sign-out to avoid embarrassing yourself in front of a large group.

VI PRENATAL CARE

A. Initial history and examination. Determine the patient's gravity and parity. Use the "**G**eorgia **P**ower **A**nd **L**ight" mnemonic:

Gravidity: number of pregnancies (twins count as one pregnancy)
Parity: number of term and preterm deliveries
Abortions: number of elective and spontaneous abortions
Living children: number

B. Time of conception. It is important to know when conception occurred, because all decisions and prenatal care depend on the estimated date of confinement, or due date.

1. If the menstrual cycle was normal and the woman was not using oral contraceptive pills or breastfeeding in the 6 months before the LMP, you can estimate the date of conception based on the first date of the LMP (use a pregnancy wheel).
2. **Quickening,** or the date of first fetal movement, occurs 18 to 20 weeks after conception for first pregnancies and 16 weeks after conception for subsequent pregnancies.
3. **Fetal heart tones** are first heard at 16 weeks.
4. **Fundal height.** Measure the distance in centimeters from the symphysis pubis. To estimate the weeks of the pregnancy, add 12 to this distance.
5. **Ultrasound is the best method for estimating dates.** See an obstetrics textbook for the specific parameters (Chapter 45).

C. High-risk pregnancies. The following conditions warrant referral to a high-risk pregnancy clinic.

1. History of pregnancy loss between 14 and 20 weeks
2. History of preterm deliveries (<36 weeks) or intrauterine fetal demise
3. Multiple gestations

4. Third-trimester bleeding or placenta previa
5. Isoimmunization. Mothers with Rh-negative blood may give birth to Rh-positive infants (the Rh-positive protein comes from the father's DNA). The mother may develop an antibody to the infant's antigen (if maternal-fetal blood sharing occurs). The first pregnancy merely produces the mother's immune response. However, the second pregnancy can elicit the mother's immune system to attack the fetus.
   b. Perform Rh testing according to Table 39-3. If the mother is Rh-positive, do nothing. If she is Rh-negative, you must determine the infant's blood type.
   c. If the infant's blood is Rh-positive, you must block the mother's development of antibodies with RhoGAM. A micro-dose is used antepartum for events that may risk maternal-fetal blood sharing (e.g., abortion, miscarriage, vaginal hemorrhage, ectopic pregnancy, or abdominal trauma during the first 12 weeks of gestation). All unimmunized Rh-negative women receive standard-dose RhoGAM at 28 weeks and another standard dose within 72 hours of delivery of Rh-positive infants.
6. Significant medical comorbidities. These diseases include hypertension, diabetes, and renal, pulmonary, and cardiac disease.

D. **Prenatal assessment.** Prenatal visits are scheduled every month until 28 weeks, every 2 weeks until 36 weeks, and every week thereafter until delivery. At each visit, assess the following:
   1. **Weight.** Patients should gain $^1/_2$ lb for the each of the first 28 weeks and then 1 lb per week thereafter. Give dietary advice to all patients (limit processed carbohydrates, snacks, and fats) to mothers who gain more weight. Artificial sweeteners are acceptable. Gaining more than 5 lb per week implies water weight gain and suggests preeclampsia. Weight loss from one visit to the next is of concern.
   2. **Blood pressure.** The blood pressure should be **less than 140/90 mm Hg** on all visits. Expect the blood pressure to increase in the third trimester, but it should still remain below 140/90 mm Hg. See below for management of pregnancy-induced hypertension (XII B).
   3. **Fetal height, heart rate, and movement.** These fetal characteristics are assessed by ultrasound. Your obstetrics textbook has the parameters to follow.
   4. **Urine protein testing.** Values of 1+ or less are acceptable. If protein is present, exclude urinary tract infection via a urine culture. **If the value is 2+ or more, or if there is associated hypertension, suspect preeclampsia.** Diabetes screening is not performed until 28 weeks. However, if the urine dipstick is more than 2+, it should be done earlier.

E. **Timing of prenatal testing** (see Table 39-3)

TABLE 39-3. Schedule for Prenatal Testing.

Weeks	Test	Notes
12 weeks	Ultrasound for dating and Pap smear	
16 weeks	Genetic testing (if indicated)	
20 weeks	Triple screen: estradiol, human chorionic gonadotropin, and α-fetoprotein.	All values will elevate as the gestational age increases and if twins are present. If any value is >2.5 normal for the estimated date, an ultrasound should be performed to confirm dates. Amniocentesis should be offered if levels are still greater than expected after confirming correct gestational age to exclude a neural tube defect. Amniocentesis should also be offered if any value is <0.5 to exclude a chromosomal abnormality.
28 weeks	Screen for gestational diabetes	Give 50 g of glucose, then test the serum after 1 hour. If the glucose is >140 mg/dl, perform a 3-hour glucose tolerance test (100 g/day × 3 hours). Abnormal values are >95 mg/dl (fasting), 190 mg/dl (1 hour), 165 mg/dl (2 hours), and 145 mg/dl (3 hours). If two or more of these values are exceeded, refer the woman to a high-risk clinic.
	Check Rh status	See VI C 5 in the text. If the screen is positive, immediately refer to a high-risk clinic.
	Check a hemoglobin. If the patient is anemic, order a ferritin level.	If anemic and the ferritin is <100, begin iron supplementation. If anemic and the ferritin is >100, order a hemoglobin electrophoresis to exclude sickle cell anemia or β-thalassemia.

(Continued)

TABLE 39-3. Continued

Weeks	Test	Notes
	Check for HIV, hepatitis, and rubella	All require intervention at labor, so test now so preparation can be made. AZT at birth reduces transmission by 80%. If the mother is positive for hepatitis B e antigen (HBeAg), the neonate should be given immune globulin at birth and hepatitis vaccination. Women not immune to rubella should be vaccinated upon discharge postpartum.

F. Edema. This condition is of little concern unless it is associated with proteinuria or hypertension, or unless weight gain is more than 5 lb per week.

G. Urinary tract infection. This condition can be treated as in nonpregnant women with the following caveats:

1. Avoid tetracycline and fluoroquinolones (teratogenicity) in all trimesters.
2. Avoid metronidazole during the first trimester, and avoid sulfa drugs (kernicterus) and nitrofurantoin (fetal hemolytic anemia) during the third trimester.
3. Vaginal infections are treated only if symptomatic.

H. Responding to contractions. After 24 weeks, patients should call their obstetrician if they experience more than four contractions per hour for more than 2 consecutive hours. Less frequent contractions are likely **false labor (Braxton Hicks contractions) due to uterine stretch.** Round ligament pain, so named because it occurs along the lateral uterus, is also due to uterine stretching and is benign.

VII FETAL HEART RATE MONITORING

Methods include placing an electrode directly on the fetal head if the membranes are ruptured or using ultrasound if the membranes are intact. The **normal heart rate is 110** to **160 bpm.**

A. Tachycardia suggests either prematurity, fetal hypoxia, or maternal distress (drugs, hyperthyroidism, arrhythmias, fever). Persistent tachycardia may be an indication for cesarean section.

TABLE 39-4. Fetal Heart Rate Monitoring Decelerations.

	Duration of Deceleration		
Beats per minute	<30 seconds	30 to 60 seconds	>60 seconds
>80	Mild	Mild	Moderate
70 to 80	Mild	Moderate	Severe
<70	Moderate	Severe	Severe

B. Variability. The fetal heart rate should vary in two dimensions.

1. **Short-term variability** is beat-to-beat changes in the heart rate. On the tracing, it looks like noise. Loss of short-term variability causes concern for diminishing fetal reserve and, thus, fetal demise.
2. **Long-term variability** is a change of 2 to 6 cycles per minute. Sedation and fetal rest are the most common causes of absence of long-term variability. Other causes include drugs, hypoxia, and prematurity.
3. Variable decelerations in the heart rate suggest umbilical cord compression.

C. Late decelerations are repetitive decelerations in the fetal heart rate that occur during uterine contractions. These suggest ureteroplacental ischemia due to uterine contraction. Table 39-4 classifies the severity of late decelerations. For severe prolonged variable decelerations or late decelerations, change the maternal position, elevate the presenting part, administer oxygen, and decrease uterine activity (decrease oxytocin if infused). If these are ineffective, prepare for cesarean section.

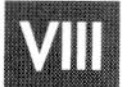

VIII Induction of Labor

Labor is induced in three circumstances: electively, after premature rupture of membranes, or postterm. Most patients are induced at 24 hours postrupture or at 7 to 14 days postterm. Ten percent of women rupture the membranes before the onset of labor, although labor begins in 90% of these women within 24 hours. The **risk of chorioamnionitis increases as the time from rupture to delivery increases.**

A. Oxytocin or manual rupture of the membranes is used to **induce labor.** Use the fetal heart tracings to monitor oxytocin dosing, because of the risk of excessive uterine contractions and uteroplacental ischemia. Ask your resident how to escalate the oxytocin dose to induce labor.

B. The **Bishop scale** is used to determine the **probability that induction will be successful** (Table 39-5). A score of 9 or above is predictive of success, and a score of less than 4 usually warrants insertion of a prostaglandin gel to ripen (dilate) the cervix. Prostaglandin

TABLE 39-5. The Bishop Score.

Dilation	Effacement (%)	Consistency	Cervix Position	Station	Score
<1 cm	<40	Firm	Posterior	<−2	0
1 to 2 cm	40 to 50	Medium	Midposition 1	−2 to −1	1
3 to 4	60 to 70	Soft	Anterior	Engaged	2
>5 cm	>80	?	?	>+1	3

gel should not be used when the uterus is already contracting or simultaneously with oxytocin.

IX LABOR AND THE OBSTETRIC ADMISSION NOTE

Take advantage of the records of prenatal visits; these contain most of the past medical history required. Tailor your history to the circumstances. For example, if the woman is in active labor, it makes little sense to determine the exact date of conception or past Pap smears; focus on the labor.

A. **History.** The first line of the note and presentation should list the patient's age, reproductive history (GPAL), estimated date of conception and how determined (LMP, ultrasound), and chief complaint. The chief complaint is usually premature rupture of membranes or contractions. Ask about dysuria, vaginal discharge or bleeding, and symptoms of preeclampsia. In addition, note the extent of previous prenatal care and whether the ultrasound is consistent with dates.

B. **Past medical history** is similar to that described in Chapter 3, with a special emphasis on medical diseases that may complicate the delivery, such as hypertension, diabetes, coronary disease, asthma, seizures, and sickle cell anemia. Note if oral contraceptive pills were used within 6 months of the LMP, because this may alter the dates. Past obstetric history should include details of each past pregnancy, including maternal age, method of delivery, complications, and outcome.

C. **Examination.** The examination should focus on the vital signs, fundal height, fetal heart tones, estimated fetal weight, and contractions. Perform a pelvic examination to assess the extent of labor.

1. **Cervical dilatation** refers to the size of the cervical os and ranges from closed to 10 cm (complete cervical dilatation).
2. **Station** is the distance from the lowest bony fetal part to the ischial spines. A value of −5 cm is 5 cm above the spines, and +5 is 5 cm below the spines.
3. **Effacement** (%) is the thickness of the cervix (normally 2 to 3 cm = 0%). As the fetus descends, the cervix thins. A completely thinned cervix represents 100% effacement.
4. **Presenting part.** At 5+ cm dilatation, the cranial sutures of the fetal head can be palpated through the cervix. If you see anything other than vertex (head presenting), call your attending physician.
5. **Status of membranes** (ruptured or unruptured). If there is fluid gushing from the vagina (ruptured membranes), note whether it is clear or meconium-stained.
   a. To distinguish urine from amniotic fluid, test its pH with a Nitrazine dipstick. Amniotic fluid has a pH of 7.2 to 7.4; urine is much more acidic. Amniotic fluid also crystallizes on a glass slide, forming a fernlike pattern (ferning).

b. Meconium is fetal stool, and, if aspirated, it can result in pneumonia. The pediatric team should be prepared to deal with this fetal condition following delivery.

D. **Laboratory tests.** Ensure that all prenatal laboratory tests have been obtained. If not, obtain them now. CBC, coagulation studies, and electrolytes should be ordered.

E. **Assessment.** The assessment should document:

1. Whether labor is true or false
   a. **True labor** is contractions that **occur at regular and gradually shortening intervals; the contractions gradually increase in frequency.** Pain is in the back and abdomen. It is associated with cervical dilation, and the contractions are not stopped by sedation.
   b. **False labor (Braxton Hicks contractions) occurs at irregularly regular intervals that have the same intensity.** Discomfort is in the lower abdomen. There is no cervical dilatation, and the contractions are relieved by sedation.
2. The stage of labor and the time elapsed thus far (Table 39-6).

F. **Plan.** Most patients are admitted for monitoring for spontaneous vaginal birth.

1. **Prolonged latent phase.** Oxytocin infusion induces uterine contractions, and the latent phase becomes the active phase.
2. **Prolonged active phase** resulting from the **three Ps: Power, Passenger, and Pelvis**
   a. Inadequate contractions **(power).** Active labor contractions should occur every 2 minutes. Contractions that occur too infrequently can be accelerated with oxytocin. Contractions that occur too frequently ($>$10 per 5 minutes) can compromise uterine blood flow, reducing uterine contractile strength. Placing the patient in a lateral decubitus position (on her left side) and hydration or oxygen will help. The most common problem is inadequate contractile strength.
   b. Cervical–pelvic disproportion (**p**assenger and **p**elvis) is confirmed when the cervix has reached at least 4 cm dilatation, and there has been no descent or further dilatation for 2 hours. The treatment is cesarean section.

G. **Labor notes.** Use SOAP note format.

1. **Subjective.** Include pain.
2. **Objective.** Always list vital signs. After the initial complete physical examination and estimated fetal weight, always include:
   a. Fetal heart tones (FHTs), including baseline, variability, reactivity, and presence of decelerations.
   b. Tocometer. List frequency of contractions and Montevideo units if an internal monitor is present.
   c. Findings on sterile vaginal examination. Usually the resident performs this, but you can include it in your notes. Mention dilatation, effacement, and station (e.g., 6/complete/–1).

TABLE 39-6. Stages of Labor.

Stage	Criteria	Time in Stage
First stage	Begins with effacement and dilatation	
Latent	Cervical change with regular contractions	20 hours in nulliparas; 14 hours in multiparas
Active	Rapid cervical dilatation	12 hours in nulliparas; 5 hours in multiparas
Second stage	Begins with complete dilatation and ends with the birth of the infant	3 hours in nulliparas, 1 hour in multiparas
Third stage	Ends with delivery of the placenta	

d. In the margin of each progress note, always write all medications the patient is taking, including oxytocin, and whether an epidural is present, and which internal monitors are in place.

4. **Assessment.** In each assessment, always comment on the following:
   a. Labor progress
   b. Fetal status
   c. Pain
   d. Risk status. If the woman has any high-risk conditions, these should be addressed.
5. **Plan** as determined by your findings with the above information.

X DELIVERY

Learning to deliver infants is best learned by doing it. Do not be afraid of the experience; most non–high-risk deliveries require very little assistance.

A. It is important to determine the **orientation** of the fetus. If the presentation is anything other than vertex, notify your attending physician.

B. **Do not be intimidated by a cesarean section.** Use the methods described in Chapter 38 for preparation for this operative procedure. Your resident will demonstrate the technique.

C. Be familiar with the stages of labor. Table 39-7 has the **seven cardinal movements of labor.**

D. **Your primary task is coaching the woman regarding breathing and pushing.** Your resident will show you how. After delivery, place the newborn on the mother's stomach. Double clamp the umbilical cord and cut it between the clamps. If cord blood is to be drawn, do this now.

E. The placenta should deliver within 20 minutes.

F. Uterine atony is failure of the uterus to contract after delivery to occlude the bleeding from the placental insertion site. After delivery of the placenta, gently massage the uterus to stimulate contraction.

TABLE 39-7. The Seven Cardinal Movements of Labor.

1. Engagement. The head abuts the cervix.
2. Descent
3. Flexion of the fetal head
4. Internal rotation
5. Extension
6. External rotation
7. Expulsion
   a. Delivery of the anterior shoulder
   b. Delivery of the posterior shoulder

TABLE 39-8. Components of the Delivery Note.

1. Exact time and date of the delivery and the type of birth (spontaneous, induced, cesarean section)
2. Physicians present: the obstetrician, the anesthesiologists, the residents, and yourself
3. Anesthesia used
4. Amount of blood lost
5. Method of placental delivery (spontaneous or manual)
6. Episiotomy, lacerations, and method of repair. Note that the rectum was examined and was intact or made so via repair.
7. Note the mother's blood type, and if Rh-negative, if RhoGAM was administered.
8. Sex and condition of newborn. Use the Apgar scale (see Table 39–9). A score >7 requires no assistance, 3 to 6 requires vigorous stimulation; and <3 requires immediate intervention.

If bleeding continues for more than 2 minutes, oxytocin can be infused to induce spasm. If bleeding still persists, notify the attending: this may represent retained placenta.

G. **Episiotomy** is an incision in the posterior vaginal wall to enlarge the birth canal. Ask your resident to show you the methods and indications. The degree of the episiotomy is important, because different surgical techniques are required to correct it after the birth.
   1. First-degree: break in the skin or vaginal mucosa
   2. Second-degree: tear to deeper tissues
   3. Third-degree: tear of the anal sphincter
   4. Fourth-degree: tear of the rectal mucosa

H. **Delivery note** (Table 39-8)

XI POSTDELIVERY

A. **Postdelivery orders**
   1. Order oxytocin IM or IV to induce uterine spasms to reduce bleeding if bleeding does not stop with uterine massage.

TABLE 39-9. Apgar Scale.

	0	1	2
Respiratory effort	None	Weak	Good
Pulse (bpm)	None	<100	>100
Muscle tone	Flaccid	Some flexion	Good flexion
Color	All blue	Blue in extremities	All pink
Reflex irritability	None	Grimacing	Crying

2. Order pain relief. Acetaminophen with codeine (Tylenol #3) is usually sufficient. Avoid NSAIDs, because they can increase bleeding. Cold sitz baths are used for the first 24 hours.
3. Check vital signs every 4 hours for the first day, then every 8 hours.
4. Give IV fluids with normal saline.
5. Advance the diet as the patient tolerates.
6. Be sure that RhoGAM is given to Rh-negative women with Rh-positive infants within the first 24 hours. Immunize rubella-negative women before discharge.
7. Order a CBC for the first postoperative day in patients who have had cesarean sections.
8. For the patient who has had cesarean sections, follow the method of writing postoperative orders in Chapter 19.

B. Postdelivery day No. 1. Follow the standard SOAP note format, with a focus on the following:

1. Breast engorgement, cracking, or erythema
2. The uterus should be at or below the level of the umbilicus. An enlarged uterus suggests intrauterine wall hemorrhage.
3. Lochia (vaginal discharge) should be less than 2 pads per hour. An amount in excess of this suggests uterine atony.
4. Examine the episiotomy only if the woman is complaining of fever or pain.
5. Ensure that the woman has received RhoGAM if she is Rh-negative.
6. Discuss breastfeeding versus bottle feeding. If breastfeeding is chosen, obtain an educational consult. Encourage breastfeeding because it increases the immunity of the neonate (fewer ear and throat infections, even in early childhood) and provides some natural contraception for a few months.
7. Discuss contraception. Offer medroxyprogesterone immediately or norethindrone at 4 weeks postdelivery. These progesterone-only contraceptives do not impede breast milk production.

XII Complications of Pregnancy

A. Preterm labor is uterine contractions with cervical dilatation after 20 weeks and before 37 weeks.

1. **All causes of abdominal pain can mimic preterm labor,** and many patients attribute true preterm labor to other causes of abdominal pain (e.g., diarrhea, urinary tract infection, back pain).
2. **The most effective therapy is bed rest.** Terbutaline, a β_2-agonist, decreases uterine smooth muscle tone, thereby relieving the contraction. Magnesium sulfate increases the membrane potential of the cell, thereby decreasing uterine muscle contraction. When active labor is progressing, neither drug is effective.

B. **Pregnancy-induced hypertension (preeclampsia)** applies to patients who are not hypertensive before pregnancy but **develop blood pressure greater than 140/90 mm Hg during pregnancy and have more than 2+ proteinuria.**
   1. **Eclampsia** is associated with the development of **seizures or neurologic symptoms.** Laboratory findings may include renal failure and HELLP (a form of disseminated intravascular coagulation with **h**emolytic anemia, **e**levated **l**iver enzymes, **l**ow **p**latelets).
   2. **Treatment for severe eclampsia is delivery of the fetus at any age,** because the condition worsens as pregnancy proceeds. Seizure prophylaxis with magnesium sulfate should be provided with severe disease as the patient approaches delivery.

C. **Magnesium sulfate** is the **treatment for both preeclampsia and preterm labor.** A loading dose of 4 to 6 g is given at the rate of 2 g/hr. The magnesium level and the patient's response guide therapy (Table 39-10). Look carefully for signs of toxicity (diminished reflexes), especially if concomitant renal insufficiency is present. Treat toxicity with calcium.

XIII GYNECOLOGY CLINIC

The basic skills necessary for succeeding in the gynecology clinic are presented in Chapter 42. There are eight topics you must know: amenorrhea, dysmenorrhea, uterine bleeding, sexually transmitted disease/pelvic inflammatory disease (see Chapter 36), menopause, Pap smears (see Chapter 36), endometriosis, and contraception. Your OB/GYN book discusses each topic.

XIV GYNECOLOGIC ONCOLOGY

The principles of surgery described in Chapter 38 apply here as well.

A. The key to gynecologic oncology is knowing **every** detail about your patients. **Gynecologic oncology incorporates both medicine**

TABLE 39-10. Serum Magnesium Levels in Magnesium Sulfate Therapy.

Serum Magnesium Level	Significance
4.5 to 8.5	Therapeutic
>8	Central nervous system depression/lethargy
10	Diminished reflexes
15	Respiratory paralysis
17	Coma
>20	Cardiac arrest

and surgery. Carrying around a good medicine reference book is key. This is a good rotation to observe surgery with good visualization of anatomy.

B. Topics that are important to know about each patient include the following:

1. All recent laboratory values, current medications, and type of treatment (e.g., specific chemotherapeutic agent). Look up and know all of the side effects.
2. The type of surgery she had or planned
3. The cancer staging for her type of cancer
4. The anatomy: review the blood supply, lymph node locations, and nerve supply to the pelvis. In addition, review the anatomy of the gastrointestinal system.

40. Pediatrics

I Introduction

A. Pediatrics encompasses the care of healthy and ill patients from birth through young adulthood (18 to 23 years of age). Pediatrics is unique in that the approach to the patient as well as to the disease and its treatment frequently varies depending on the developmental and chronologic age of the patient. In addition, perhaps more than other medical field, pediatrics requires healthcare providers to involve the patient's caregivers and to interact with them and their social support system.

B. The pediatric clerkship generally includes experiences in the inpatient ward, nursery, and outpatient clinic. Pediatricians often do not wear white coats, because these garments may inadvertently frighten their patients. You may want to bring your white coat on the first day of the rotation, but be prepared to remove it if the rest of your team is not wearing them. Instead, use a waist pack for hands-free storage. Consider including stickers, small plastic toys that can be cleaned, and a calculator.

C. This chapter addresses the general approach to the pediatric patient; aspects of the history and physical examination; the inpatient ward service; the nursery service; the outpatient clinic; and the adolescent patient.

II General Approach to the Pediatric Patient

A successful encounter with a pediatric patient requires that you address both the patient and the caregiver.

A. Regardless of the patient's age, acknowledge or comment on the patient first (e.g., coo at a baby, comment on a school-aged child's clothes).

B. Try to lower yourself to the patient's eye level; sit, squat, or kneel. Tell the patient and caregiver who you are and what to expect (e.g., "I am a student doctor, we will speak for a few minutes, and I will return with my supervisor later."). A caregiver with a sick child or a hungry child may be impatient, and you will generally gain her confidence by being forthright.

C. Address school-aged children directly; you will likely engage both patients and caregivers better. For younger patients, much of the history inevitably comes from the caregiver. Regardless of the patient's age, it is helpful to explicitly ask the caregiver about her concerns because they may differ from those of the patient.

D. Observe pediatric patients when they are calm. This should be the first thing you do when you walk in the room, because it may be your last chance! Is the child alert and looking around or struggling to stay awake? Is he breathing fast, is he or limping, is he consolable? Your evaluation may change dramatically after you start your examination if the child becomes frightened or starts crying.

E. Be flexible with the order of your physical examination, and allow it to proceed following the opportunities that arise.

1. If a child is sleeping, complete the cardiac, pulmonary, and abdominal examination.
2. If the child is crying, look in the oropharynx.

F. Do not let a crying child inhibit you from gathering information. If you need to restrain a child to complete the examination, have your supervisor present so you can both examine the child at once.

G. Complete parts of the examination with the patient in the caregiver's lap if the child is more comfortable there.

HOT
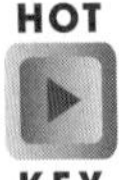
KEY

If a patient appears ill or you suspect child abuse, find a supervisor immediately. Several diseases (e.g., meningitis, sepsis) have a rapid course, and the symptoms and signs may be subtle.

H. Include the caregiver in formulating the treatment plan. The caregiver often has information that may not be readily apparent. For example, the child may not be able or willing to take pills or the home has several flights of stairs, making a wheelchair impractical.

III ASPECTS OF THE PEDIATRIC HISTORY AND PHYSICAL EXAMINATION

A. History. Several topics are unique to the pediatric history. Depending on the child's complaint, you may not include all these topics in your actual presentation. However, you should ask the child or family about all topics.

1. **Birth history.** Depending on the child's complaint, maternal and childbirth history can be important. This history should be obtained for any child younger than 3 years of age or for any child in whom the current condition may relate to the birth history (e.g., developmental delay). Ask about any complications during childbirth (e.g., prematurity, cesarean section, number of days in the nursery, use of oxygen).
2. **Developmental history.** Failure to develop can be subtle, so milestones by age have been designed to assess normal child development. It is useful to have a sense of the major milestones, which are categorized by gross motor, fine motor, speech and

language, and social and adaptive skills (Table 40-1). The Denver Developmental Scale is a widely used developmental assessment screening tool with which you should be familiar. Remember that you can gain much information regarding development by observing a child. However, pediatricians generally rely heavily on caregivers' reports, because children may not accurately depict their development during the visit, especially if they are ill or frightened.

3. **Dietary history.** Ask about the volume and type of nutrition. Breast-fed infants (0 to 6 months) should feed 10 to 12 times in 24 hours (approximately every 2 to 3 hours). Bottle-fed infants should feed an average of 2 to 3 oz every 2 to 3 hours. Make sure the formula is iron fortified. Infants should have a minimum of six wet diapers in 24 hours, and stools are yellow, seedy, and soft. Solid foods should not be introduced until 4 to 6 months of age, and animal milk should not be consumed until after 12 months of age. From 1 to 2 years of age, children should drink whole milk to provide the additional fat needed for proper brain development. After 2 years of age, they should switch to low-fat milk. Animal milk consumption should be limited to a maximum of 24 ounces a day to prevent iron deficiency anemia.
4. **Immunizations.** At present, most schools require vaccinations against the following 10 diseases: diphtheria, tetanus, pertussis, measles, mumps, rubella, varicella, polio, *Haemophilus influenzae,* and hepatitis B. In addition, vaccines against pneumococcus, influenza, and hepatitis A are available to children. In febrile infants and young children, the *H. influenzae* and pneumococcal vaccines have greatly decreased the risk of serious bacterial infections; thus, it is critical to know if such children have received the complete series of these vaccines. The most recent guidelines endorsed by the Centers for Disease Control and Prevention and the American Academy of Pediatrics are shown in Figure 40-1.
5. **Family history.** Genetics plays an important role in pediatric medicine. Atopy (e.g., asthma, eczema, allergies) is a very common condition that runs in families. A variety of diseases such as sickle cell disease, cystic fibrosis, congenital heart disease, rheumatologic conditions, and metabolic disorders are also inherited.
6. **Social history.** Find out the identity of everyone in the examination room. Do not make assumptions. Ask about who lives in the home, whether there are siblings, and who cares for the child. Ask about smoking in the home and whether the child attends day care. In general, children older than 12 years of age should be spoken with alone at some point during the interview (see VII).

B. Physical examination

1. **General considerations**

   a. In general, the basic physical examination of a child is similar to that of an adult. However, examining a child can be a

TABLE 40-1. Developmental Milestones (Harriet Lane).

Age	Gross Motor	Visual-Motor/ Problem Solving	Language	Social/Adaptive
1 month	Raises head from prone position	Birth: Visually fixes 1 month: Has tight grasp, follows to midline	Alerts to sound	Regards face
2 months	Holds head in midline, lifts chest off table	No longer clenches fists tightly, follows object past midline	Smiles socially (after being stroked or talked to)	Recognizes parent
3 months	Supports on forearms in prone position, holds head up steadily	Holds hands open at rest, follows in circular fashion, responds to visual threat	Coos (produces long vowel sounds in musical fashion)	Reaches for familiar people or objects, anticipates feeding
4 months	Rolls over, supports on wrists, and shifts weight	Reaches with arms in unison, brings hands to midline	Laughs, orients to voice	Enjoys looking around
6 months	Sits unsupported, puts feet in mouth in supine position	Unilateral reach, uses raking grasp, transfers objects	Babbles, ah-goo, razz, lateral orientation to bell	Recognizes that someone is a stranger
9 months	Pivots when sitting, crawls well, pulls to stand, cruises	Uses immature pincer grasp, probes with forefinger, holds bottle, throws objects	Says "mama, dada" indiscriminately, gestures, waves bye-bye, understands "no"	Starts exploring environment, plays gesture games (e.g., pat-a-cake)
12 months	Walks alone	Uses mature pincer grasp, can make a crayon mark, releases voluntarily	Uses two words other than mama/dada or proper nouns, jargoning (runs several unintelligible words	Imitates actions, comes when called, cooperates with dressing

			together with tone or inflection), one-step command with gesture	
15 months	Creeps up stairs, walks backward independently	Scribbles in imitation, builds tower of two blocks in imitation	Uses 4 to 6 words, follows one-step command without gesture	*15 to 18 months:* Uses spoon and cup
18 months	Runs, throws objects from standing without falling	Scribbles spontaneously, builds tower of three blocks, turns two three pages at a time	Mature jargoning (includes intelligible words), 7- to 10-word vocabulary, knows 5 body parts	Copies parent in tasks (sweeping, dusting), plays in company of other children
24 months	Walks up and down steps without help	Imitates stroke with pencil, builds tower of seven blocks, turns pages one at a time, removes shoes, pants, etc.	Uses pronouns (I, you, me) inappropriately, follows two-step commands, has a 50-word vocabulary, uses two-word sentences	Parallel play
3 years	Can alternate feet when going up steps, pedals tricycle	Copies a circle, undresses completely, dresses partially, dries hands if reminded, unbuttons	Uses minimum of 250 words, 3-word sentences, uses plurals, knows all pronouns, repeats two digits	Group play, shares toys, takes turns, plays well with others, knows full name, age, gender
4 years	Hops, skips, alternates feet going down steps	Copies a square, buttons clothing, dresses self completely, catches ball	Knows colors, says song or poem from memory, asks questions	Tells "all tales," plays cooperatively with a group of children
5 years	Skips, alternating feet; jumps over low obstacles	Copies triangle, ties shoes, spreads with knife	Prints first name, asks what a word means	Plays competitive games, abides by rules, likes to help in household tasks

From Capute AJ, Biehl RF: *Pediatr Clin North Am* 20:3, 1973 (with permission from Elsevier); Capute AJ, Accardo PJ: *Clin Pediatr* 17:847, 1978; and Capute AJ, et al: *Am J Dis Child* 140:694, 1986. Rounded norms from Capute AJ, et al. *Dev Med Child Neurol* 28:762, 1986. Used with permission.

Recommended Childhood and Adolescent Immunization Schedule UNITED STATES • 2005

Vaccine ▼ / Age ▶	Birth	1 month	2 months	4 months	6 months	12 months	15 months	18 months	24 months	4–6 years	11–12 years	13–18 years
Hepatitis B[1]	HepB #1		HepB #2			HepB #3				HepB Series		
Diphtheria, Tetanus, Pertussis[2]			DTaP	DTaP	DTaP		DTaP			DTaP	Td	Td
Haemophilus influenzae type b[3]			Hib	Hib	Hib	Hib						
Inactivated Poliovirus			IPV	IPV		IPV				IPV		
Measles, Mumps, Rubella[4]						MMR #1				MMR #2	MMR #2	
Varicella[5]							Varicella			Varicella		
Pneumococcal[6]			PCV	PCV	PCV	PCV			PCV	PPV		
Influenza[7]						Influenza (Yearly)					Influenza (Yearly)	
Vaccines below red line are for selected populations												
Hepatitis A[8]											Hepatitis A Series	

FIGURE 40-1. Recommended childhood and adolescent immunization schedule (United States, 2005). *(Figure continued)*

This schedule indicates the recommended ages for routine administration of currently licensed childhood vaccines, as of December 1, 2004, for children through age 18 years. Any dose not administered at the recommended age should be administered at any subsequent visit when indicated and feasible.

■ Indicates age groups that warrant special effort to administer those vaccines not previously administered. Additional vaccines may be licensed and recommended during the year. Licensed combination vaccines may be used whenever any components of the combination are indicated and other components of the vaccine are not contraindicated. Providers should consult the manufacturers' package inserts for detailed recommendations. Clinically significant adverse events that follow immunization should be reported to the Vaccine Adverse Event Reporting System (VAERS). Guidance about how to obtain and complete a VAERS form are available at **www.vaers.org** or by telephone, **800-822-7967**.

Range of recommended ages | **Only if mother HBsAg(−)**

Preadolescent assessment | **Catch-up immunization**

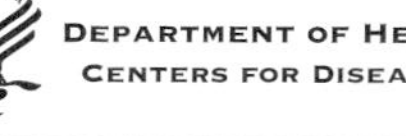

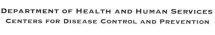

DEPARTMENT OF HEALTH AND HUMAN SERVICES
CENTERS FOR DISEASE CONTROL AND PREVENTION

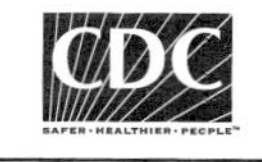

The Childhood and Adolescent Immunization Schedule is approved by:
Advisory Committee on Immunization Practices www.cdc.gov/nip/acip
American Academy of Pediatrics www.aap.org
American Academy of Family Physicians www.aafp.org

Footnotes
Recommended Childhood and Adolescent Immunization Schedule
UNITED STATES • 2005

1. **Hepatitis B (HepB) vaccine.** All infants should receive the first dose of HepB vaccine soon after birth and before hospital discharge; the first dose may also be administered by age 2 months if the mother is hepatitis B surface antigen (HBsAg) negative. Only monovalent HepB may be used for the birth dose. Monovalent or combination vaccine containing HepB may be used to complete the series. Four doses of vaccine may be administered when a birth dose is given. The second dose should be administered at least 4 weeks after the first dose, except for combination vaccines which cannot be administered before age 6 weeks. The third dose should be given at least 16 weeks after the first dose and at least 8 weeks after the second dose. The last dose in the vaccination series (third or fourth dose) should not be administered before age 24 weeks.

   Infants born to HBsAg-positive mothers should receive HepB and 0.5 mL of hepatitis B immune globulin (HBIG) at separate sites within 12 hours of birth. The second dose is recommended at age 1–2 months. The final dose in the immunization series should not be administered before age 24 weeks. These infants should be tested for HBsAg and antibody to HBsAg (anti-HBs) at age 9–15 months. (*Figure continued*)

Infants born to mothers whose HBsAg status is unknown should receive the first dose of the HepB series within 12 hours of birth. Maternal blood should be drawn as soon as possible to determine the mother's HBsAg status; if the HBsAg test is positive, the infant should receive HBIG as soon as possible (no later than age 1 week). The second dose is recommended at age 1–2 months. The last dose in the immunization series should not be administered before age 24 weeks.

2. **Diphtheria and tetanus toxoids and acellular pertussis (DTaP) vaccine.** The fourth dose of DTaP may be administered as early as age 12 months, provided 6 months have elapsed since the third dose and the child is unlikely to return at age 15–18 months. The final dose in the series should be given at age ≥4 years. **Tetanus and diphtheria toxoids (Td)** is recommended at age 11–12 years if at least 5 years have elapsed since the last dose of tetanus and diphtheria toxoid-containing vaccine. Subsequent routine Td boosters are recommended every 10 years.

3. ***Haemophilus influenzae type b (Hib) conjugate vaccine.*** Three Hib conjugate vaccines are licensed for infant use. If PRP-OMP (PedvaxHIB® or ComVax® [Merck]) is administered at ages 2 and 4 months, a dose at age 6 months is not required. DTaP/Hib combination products should not be used for primary immunization in infants at ages 2, 4 or 6 months but can be used as boosters after any Hib vaccine. The final dose in the series should be administered at age ≥12 months.

4. **Measles, mumps, and rubella vaccine (MMR).** The second dose of MMR is recommended routinely at age 4–6 years but may be administered during any visit, provided at least 4 weeks have elapsed since the first dose and both doses are administered beginning at or after age 12 months. Those who have not previously received the second dose should complete the schedule by age 11–12 years.

5. **Varicella vaccine.** Varicella vaccine is recommended at any visit at or after age 12 months for susceptible children (i.e., those who lack a reliable history of chickenpox). Susceptible persons aged ≥13 years should receive 2 doses administered at least 4 weeks apart. (*Figure continued*)

6. **Pneumococcal vaccine.** The heptavalent **pneumococcal conjugate vaccine (PCV)** is recommended for all children aged 2–23 months and for certain children aged 24–59 months. The final dose in the series should be given at age ≥12 months. **Pneumococcal polysaccharide vaccine (PPV)** is recommended in addition to PCV for certain high-risk groups. See *MMWR* 2000;49(RR-9):1-35.
7. **Influenza vaccine.** Influenza vaccine is recommended annually for children aged ≥6 months with certain risk factors (including, but not limited to, asthma, cardiac disease, sickle cell disease, human immunodeficiency virus [HIV], and diabetes), healthcare workers, and other persons (including household members) in close contact with persons in groups at high risk (see *MMWR* 2004;53[RR-6]:1-40). In addition, healthy children aged 6–23 months and close contacts of healthy children aged 0–23 months are recommended to receive influenza vaccine because children in this age group are at substantially increased risk for influenza-related hospitalizations. For healthy persons aged 5–49 years, the intranasally administered, live, attenuated influenza vaccine (LAIV) is an acceptable alternative to the intramuscular trivalent inactivated influenza vaccine (TIV). See *MMWR* 2004;53(RR-6):1-40. Children receiving TIV should be administered a dosage appropriate for their age (0.25 mL if aged 6–35 months or 0.5 mL if aged ≥3 years). Children aged ≤8 years who are receiving influenza vaccine for the first time should receive 2 doses (separated by at least 4 weeks for TIV and at least 6 weeks for LAIV).
8. **Hepatitis A vaccine.** Hepatitis A vaccine is recommended for children and adolescents in selected states and regions and for certain high-risk groups; consult your local public health authority. Children and adolescents in these states, regions, and high-risk groups who have not been immunized against hepatitis A can begin the hepatitis A immunization series during any visit. The 2 doses in the series should be administered at least 6 months apart. See *MMWR* 1999; 48(RR-12):1-37.

challenge. Take advantage of opportunities as they present themselves (see II). In most cases, have the caregiver remove **all** of the child's clothing.

b. Hygiene should be considered. Infectious diseases are prevalent in the pediatric patient, and nosocomial spread is a risk. As with all patients, make sure you wash you hands properly before and after the examination. Also, clean your stethoscope with alcohol or other antiseptic solution before and after each examination. If you are ill but still working (e.g., you have an upper respiratory tract infection), make sure you wear a mask.

2. Vital signs. Do not forget to report the vital signs, including temperature and how it was measured. (In infants, temperature should be measured rectally.) Most strictly, fever is defined as a central (rectal or oral) temperature >38.0°C. That said, in some clinical contexts (e.g., older children), temperatures as high as 39° or 39.5°C degrees may not be fully evaluated as fevers. The age-specific parameters for pulse, blood pressure, and respiratory rate are shown in Table 40-2.

3. Growth

a. Weight, height, and head circumference (birth to 3 years) are used to assess growth. Growth charts to plot these parameters are part of each admission and clinic visit. These charts include lines that represent percentiles for age (e.g., 5%, 10%, 25%, 50%).

(1) Ideally, you should plot a patient's growth parameters at every visit, enabling comparison with norms and gaining a sense of trends (e.g., weight loss over the past few months). These trends are as important as the absolute numbers. In general, any growth curve that crosses two of the marked percentile lines in either direction is a red flag.

(2) At the very least, report a patient's body weight.

b. Newborns are allowed to lose up to 10% of their birth weight, but they should be at least at birth weight by 2 weeks of age. When newborns begin to gain weight, they should gain 20 to 30 g/day from birth to 6 months and 10 to 15 g/day from 6 to 12 months. Toddlers gain only a few pounds (1 kg) a year (30 g = 1 oz; 2.2 lb = 1 kg).

4. Genital examination. When performing a genital examination in pediatric patients, have the parent in the room unless the patient is an adolescent (see VII). A supervisor should always be present during the genital examination of noninfants. Explain to preschool-aged children, as well as older ones, that you are examining their private areas because you are a doctor, and remind them that their caregiver is in the room.

TABLE 40-2. Pediatric Vital Signs.

Normal Values for Respiratory Rates in Children (breaths/min)

Age	Respiratory rate (breaths/min)
Birth to 6 weeks	45 to 60
6 weeks to 2 years	40
2 to 6 years	30
6 to 10 years	25
>10 years	20

From Adams FH, Emmanoulides GC (editors): *Moss' heart disease in infants, children, and adolescents*, ed. 3, Baltimore: Williams & Wilkins, 1983.

Acceptable Heart Rates in Children (beats/min)

Age	Awake	Asleep	Exercise/fever
Newborn	100 to 180	80 to 160	<220
1 week to 3 months	100 to 220	80 to 200	<220
3 months to 2 years	80 to 150	70 to 120	<200
2 to 10 years	70 to 110	60 to 90	<200
> 10 years	55 to 90	50 to 90	<200

From Adams FH, Emmanoulides GC (editors): *Moss' heart disease in infants, children, and adolescents*, ed. 3, Baltimore: Williams & Wilkins, 1983.

Normal Vital Signs by Age

Age	Weight (kg)	SBP (mm Hg)	DBP (mm Hg)
Newborn	1	40 to 60	20 to 36
Newborn	2 to 3	50 to 70	30 to 45
1 month	4	64 to 96	30 to 62
6 month	7	60 to 118	50 to 70
1 year	10	66 to 126	41 to 91
2 to 3 years	12 to 14	74 to 124	39 to 89
4 to 5 years	16 to 18	79 to 119	45 to 85
6 to 8 years	20 to 26	80 to 124	45 to 85
10 to 12 years	32 to 42	85 to 135	55 to 88
> 14 years	>50	90 to 140	60 to 90
Adult	70	90 to 140	60 to 90

From *PALS Pocket Survival Guide*. International Medical Publishing, 1995. Used with permission.
http://www.vh.org/adult/provider/anesthesia/ProceduralSedation/pedvitalsigns.html Pediatric Vital Signs: Age-Adjusted Normal Values Tara Hata, MD, Ellen J. Nickel, PharmD, BCPS, Brad Hindman, MD, Doug Morgan, MS, RPh. Peer Review Status: Internally Peer Reviewed by The University of Iowa Hospitals Procedural Sedation Committee.
SBP, Systolic blood pressure; DBP, diastolic blood pressure.

IV Inpatient Ward Service

A. General considerations

1. The inpatient pediatric service is similar to that for general adult internal medicine, with the same process of admission, rounds, and discharges. However, there are several important differences between the way children and adults are evaluated, monitored, and treated.
2. At the beginning of your rotation, ask your attending physician and senior resident what they expect of students. Do they want presentations on topics? What is the average patient load? What kind of presentations should you make on rounds? Should you report to the interns or senior resident directly? You will gain more from the rotation and receive better evaluations if the expectations are clarified at the outset.

B. Admission and orders.

Use the same format shown for adults, as described in Chapter 13. Note the following differences:

1. **Vital signs.** The "normal" ranges for vital signs vary significantly for children and must be specific to the child's age. A respiratory rate of 40 breaths per minute is normal in a newborn but an indicator of respiratory distress in a 12-year-old child. A table of normal ranges is presented in Table 40-2.
2. **Diet.** Children are picky eaters. Ask the caregiver what the child eats at home (e.g., breast milk, particular brand of formula) and try to provide it. It is also good to use daily weight to monitor adequate intake in infants.
   a. IV fluids must be adjusted according to weight. Most clinicians use the rule of 100 ml/kg/day for the first 10 kg, 50 ml/kg/day for the next 10 kg, and 25 ml/kg/day thereafter. This roughly translates into the "4-2-1" rule for calculating the IV fluid rate. For each of the first 10 kg, a child is given 4 ml/hr; for each of the next 10 kg, 2 ml/hr; and for each kg thereafter, 1 ml/hr. For example, a 12-kg child would get a total of 44 ml/hr; 40 ml per hour for the first 10 kg (4 ml/hr $\times$ 10 kg), and then 4 more for the next 2 kg (2 ml/hr $\times$ 2 kg).
   b. Children require less salt than adults. Newborns generally receive $D_{10}W$ as their fluid for the first days; infants beyond the first few days of life, $D_{5}{}^{1}/_{4}NS$; and all other children, generally $D_{5}{}^{1}/_{2}NS$. Always use NS as a bolus for hypovolemia in children, regardless of age.
3. **I&Os.** With rare exception, strict records of the I&Os of all pediatric inpatients should be kept.
   a. In any child in whom feeding or growth is an issue, you should report the infant's intake in terms of ml/kg/day, or, ideally, calories/kg/day and describe the route (e.g., NG tube for formula, breast-feeding). Normal values for infants vary by their

weight and age, but the intake of a healthy newborn should be 120 ml/kg/day to ensure growth by the first week. Obviously, if the child is breast-feeding, it is not possible to report intake in ml/kg/day, so report frequency and duration of feeds.

b. Similarly, it is a good habit in all but very well children to report urine output in terms of ml/kg/hr, with a minimum of 2 ml/kg/hr being adequate.

4. Medications. With very rare exceptions, medication dosages are calculated using weight. Some chemotherapeutic agents are dosed based on total body surface area. It is a good habit to write the order in a standard format, with the actual dose in weight, route, and frequency (20 mg IV q6h), but follow it with the dose per weight desired along with the patient's weight to allow the pharmacy to double-check your work.

5. Laboratory tests. Pediatricians generally try to minimize routine laboratory tests in children, and ordering routine morning laboratory tests is avoided, if possible. Laboratory tests are generally more difficult to perform in children and are usually much more psychologically traumatic. In neonates with small blood volumes, routine tests can even lead to need for transfusion. Before you write any laboratory order, ask yourself if you think the result is likely to change the management. If not, reconsider the order.

C. Rounds. Ask your senior resident how she likes to run rounds and what she likes in presentations from students (e.g., full examination or just pertinent negatives and positives; see Chapter 10).

1. Examine your patient every morning before rounds. In general, do not wake a sleeping infant; careful observation of respiratory effort with gentle auscultation can be enough.

2. Presentations will depend on the style of your senior resident. Consider using the SOAP format presented in Chapter 16.

a. Focused report of events of the night.

b. Report strict I&Os, weight, and vital signs.

c. The greatest pitfall of the A&P section is to turn it into a passive summary.

(1) Force yourself to make a one-sentence assessment that includes the diagnosis (or the most likely diagnosis). If this is the patient's admission presentation, include a few of the most probable diagnoses and what makes one more likely than the other.

(2) Always ask yourself if the patient is doing better or worse and convey that idea.

(3) Devise and present a concrete plan of action and decision making. Tell what tests you plan to order or check, what therapeutic interventions you will continue or stop, and your estimate date of discharge.

(4) As in all inpatient services, be the expert on your patients. Take the most detailed history on admission. Know what happened overnight by talking to the postcall intern. Talk to the nurses, read through the nursing notes and flow sheet carefully, and check all the laboratory results. More often than you might think, it is the careful work of medical students that is the clue to tricky diagnoses.

(5) Keep children's parents informed of all daily activities and include them in decision making if possible.

(6) Think ahead to discharge and what support or training will be needed. For example, for a new patient with asthma, you should make sure that education about how to use an inhaler with a spacer is provided as soon as possible, not on the day of discharge.

V NURSERY

The nursery is usually a very busy and exciting place, unique in the hospital in that is filled primarily with healthy patients. To many students, newborns seem a bit foreign and fragile. However, you stand to gain a lot if you are open to working with them.

A. History. Presentation of the history of a newborn is fairly standardized, although there are some institutional variations.

1. Begin with an introductory sentence that tells how premature, or term, the infant is, and also notes the mode of birth (vaginal or cesarean section), birth weight, maternal age, and the mother's past obstetric history (gravida, para).
2. Provide a list of pertinent prenatal laboratory findings, beginning with maternal blood type and Rh status, followed by a number of studies, including antibody status to determine the child's risk for hemolytic disease, rapid plasma reagin to exclude maternal syphilis infection, and hepatitis B antigen status. Many hospitals screen for gonorrhea, chlamydia, and most recently, group B streptococcal status.
3. Comment on events during the delivery and whatever you did to resuscitate the infant. Apgar scores (see Table 39-9) are by custom calculated at 1 and 5 minutes. For example, you might say: "Baby X is a 5200-g boy born at 41 weeks to a G_3P_2-1, 42-year-old mother who is O-positive, antibody-negative, RPR-negative, hepatitis B surface antigen (HbsAg)–negative, PPD-positive, chest radiograph–negative, gonorrhea-negative, and chlamydia-negative. Pregnancy was complicated by first-trimester radiation exposure and occasional marijuana use. Pediatric personnel were at the delivery because of late decelerations, but the child was vigorous on delivery and given only warmth, drying, and tactile stimulation before being handed to the mother. Apgar scores were 8 and 9."

B. Newborn examination. Although the newborn examination is fundamentally similar to that of an older child or adult, there are some differences worth noting. Find a warm place to examine the child (ideally a radiant warmer table, but a sunny spot in the room can suffice). Be sure to undress the infant, leaving only the diaper until the genital examination. Always wash your hands and clean your stethoscope before and after examining every infant. The following text includes highlights, some tips, and important things to look for in the newborn examination. Supplement these tips by reading the chapter on the newborn examination in a standard pediatric text.

1. **Heart.** It is best to begin with the heart examination while the child is most likely to be calm. Some murmurs are present at birth, whereas others declare themselves over the first 24 to 48 hours; you want to make a good examination each time. Palpate the inguinal canal to ascertain a strong femoral pulse to exclude a coarctation of the aorta, which leads to diminished distal pulses (you may also feel the pedal pulses).
2. **Lungs.** Likewise, have a good "listen" before crying starts. At birth, an infant's lungs may sound congested before fetal fluid has been resorbed, but if you listen over the next few minutes it should become entirely clear. Palpate the clavicles to feel for crepitus that might indicate a fracture from a difficult delivery.
3. **Head.** Feel the head for the suture lines, fontanelles, and any swellings. Cephalohematomas are collections of blood in the periosteum that feel like fluid-filled balloons and honor suture lines. They are important to note as a risk factor for jaundice as the blood is gradually resorbed. Another common sign of mild trauma is caput succedaneum, which is edema of the scalp that crosses sutures lines. Palpate the fontanelle and feel for sutures that override.
4. **Eyes.** You must check both eyes for a red reflex with the ophthalmoscope. It is nearly impossible to open a crying infant's eyes forcefully, so try keeping the child calm, moving into a dark room from a light one or gently eliciting a Moro reflex. Examine the nares to see if they are patent and the palate to see if it is intact. Make sure to also palpate the palate for a submucosal cleft.
5. **Abdomen**. Palpate for masses and hepatosplenomegaly that might indicate intrauterine infection or other problems.
6. **Skin.** It is not uncommon to find bruising or a few petechiae after a difficult delivery; these should be few and localized to the face or other area of pressure. In addition, look for signs of congenital vascular malformation or infection. Examine the back for dimpling or tufting of hair over the sacrum that might indicate spina bifida.
7. **Extremities.** Be sure to check and count all fingers and toes. Extra digits are surprisingly common and are usually not associ-

ated with any particular syndrome. Examine the hips for developmental dysplasia by performing the Ortolani and Barlow maneuvers; read about these in a pediatric textbook.

8. **Neurologic examination.** Check for tone, ability to suck, and reflexes. The Moro reflex, which should be present at birth, can be elicited by placing the infant face up and gently lifting the head so that the weight of the body is supported. The head is suddenly released and allowed to fall back briefly but caught before contacting any surface. Generally, the infant flings out her arms and "is startled" before resuming her original position. It is useful to look for any asymmetry in the movements during the reflex, which would suggest weakness.

C. **Course in the nursery.** The goals of the newborn are fairly simple. He has to learn to feed, defecate, and urinate.

1. **Weight gain.** It is normal for the child to lose weight over the first 48 hours (expect it to be regained by 2 weeks) as he learns to coordinate feedings and waits for the mother's breast milk to become available. However, weight loss of more than 10% in the first 2 days should merit closer examination of the child's feeding. Most institutions routinely check a hematocrit and dextrose stick at 4 hours of life. After 24 hours, a federally mandated screen for treatable congenital disease is sent to the laboratory; the diseases included in the screen vary by state.
2. **Jaundice.** A newborn must be watched for jaundice as well. Although mild jaundice is very common after 48 hours of life (peaking at 3 to 5 days), jaundice noticeable before 24 hours of life is concerning and must be evaluated. The level of bilirubin roughly corresponds to the level of jaundice (increasing from head to toe). Risk factors for jaundice include Rh incompatibility with the mother (if she is Rh negative, she should have received Rh immune globulin during her pregnancy to prevent sensitization) and ABO incompatibility (if she is O and baby is A, B, or AB). In both cases, a test is usually sent that looks for active antibodies in the infant's blood (Coombs' test). Other common risk factors include a large cephalohematoma and poor feeding, which lead to dehydration.

HOT
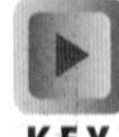
KEY

To remember the requirements for possible ABO incompatibility, use the mnemonic mOm/bABy.

VI **Outpatient Clinic**

A large portion of pediatric practice occurs in the context of the outpatient clinic. Your experience in the clinic will likely include some combination of urgent care, well child care, and subspecialty clinics. Some clinics combine urgent care visits into the continuity clinic, whereas others preserve the continuity clinic for well visits only. Overall, the principles discussed in Section II apply. Below are a few tips for urgent care and well child visits.

A. Urgent care. Generally, a high volume of mildly ill children need to be seen efficiently. It is critical to stay alert for the very ill ones. **Vital signs are critical and should be up front in your analysis and presentation.** As noted above, normal values vary with age (see Table 40-2).

1. Tachycardia is the first sign of hypovolemia in children, whether from dehydration, blood loss, or shock. Tachycardia can also result simply from fever, pain, or agitation.
2. Tachypnea is a very important sign of respiratory difficulty that should be looked for carefully in any child with respiratory complaints.
3. Blood pressure is not always recorded by nurses in triage, because it is difficult to obtain. However, it should be checked if relevant to the presenting illness.
4. The weight should always be checked for drug dosing and to get a sense of recent weight loss or gain.
5. Hydration status and a child's ability to feed, drink, and maintain hydration should be ascertained in **every** child, especially infants. On examination, look for tears and moist mucous membranes. Always consider an oral challenge trial (observed eating and drinking) as an observation option if you are concerned about a child.
6. Often, urgent care is where the underserved (especially recent immigrants or recently homeless patients) obtain their health care. Be sure to confirm immunization status, and consider administering vaccines to children whose immunizations are not up-to-date (see Figure 40-1).
7. It is important to ensure that all children have a primary provider. If they do not, they should obtain an appointment with a new provider before leaving clinic.
8. Never let parents leave without reviewing with them the indications for bringing the child back for further medical attention. For example, if the child is brought to the urgent care clinic with a cold, review the signs of respiratory distress. Remember that even if a child comes in with a "benign" diagnosis, the caregivers should leave with a new understanding of their child's condition; they should know how to assess their child and how to manage the illness in the future.
9. Always be on the alert for nonaccidental trauma such as bruises, burns, or fractures, especially when there are multiple injuries. Child abuse rates are surprisingly high, and incidents are often retrospectively missed by health care providers before finally being detected. Whenever a child comes in with a physical injury,

always ask yourself if the story makes sense. Does the injury fit the story? Was the child being properly supervised? If abuse or neglect is suspected, immediately consult a supervisor.

B. Well child visits

1. Start the visit by finding out if the patient or caregivers have any concerns or questions, and make sure to address them before the end of the visit.
2. The history covers the activities of daily living: eating and diet, elimination (bedwetting or constipation), sleeping, and activities and school. It helps to ask parents specifically about each activity, because it often reminds patients and caregivers about questions they have.

C. Routine screening involves measuring hearing, vision, weight, and height. (With the increase in childhood obesity, many clinics are calculating each patient's body mass index.) The practice of screening urinalysis and tests for anemia and lead vary with each clinic.

D. Sport physical examinations. In these cases, family history is very important. Ask about a family history of sudden deaths of unknown causes and early heart attacks. Ask patients if they have had exertional chest pain, fainting, or seizures. In addition, ask what sport and position the patient plans to play. For example, a linebacker in football is not an optimal position for a small-sized person and would be worrisome for serious injuries. Finally, complete a thorough musculoskeletal examination, looking especially for joint stability.

E. Anticipatory guidance is essential and is based on chronologic and developmental age. Television and video viewing has become epidemic in the United States, and many pediatricians ask how much television children watch. A maximum of 1 to 2 hours a day, with parental supervision, is recommended.

F. Immunizations (see Figure 40-1)

VII ADOLESCENTS

In general, adolescent medicine encompasses patients of 12 to 18 years of age. In adolescent medicine, remember that the teenager is your primary patient, although working with caregivers is also essential. Whether or not they express it, most parents of teenagers are concerned that their child is engaged in risky behaviors. In addition, it is important that you spend time alone with the patient, if possible.

A. General approach

1. Provide an overview of the visit early. After greeting the patient and family, start by giving an overview of the visit. By doing so, when you ask the caregivers to leave, they will not think it is something particular to their child. You might say, "What we usually do in our teen clinic is talk all together in the beginning. Then I will have you (the parent) leave so that ______ (the pa-

tient) and I can talk together and complete the physical examination. At the end, we will all discuss the plan together. What particular concerns do you have today?"

2. Establish confidentiality early. Most states have confidentiality laws that aim to protect healthcare providers and adolescents. Make sure you check with your supervisor and find out what the confidentiality policy is in the clinic. Before you start your interview with the teenager, review the confidentiality policy. "I will be asking you a lot of questions, and I want you to know that I will not be discussing this with anyone else without your permission. However, if you tell me that you are _____ or ______ (e.g., suicidal or homicidal), I have to inform others and involve them—in your best interest."
3. Ask sensitive questions first indirectly, then directly. "Do you any of your friends smoke cigarettes or marijuana? Do you feel pressure from your friends to smoke? How much do you smoke?"
4. Have the patient tell you the consequences of his actions. This approach is more effective than simply lecturing teenagers about why they should wear a seatbelt, use a condom, or quit smoking.

B. Questions specific to teenagers. Use the mnemonic **HEADSS** to help remember the areas unique to the adolescent medicine history (Table 40-3).

TABLE 40-3. Questions to Use When Taking the History in Adolescents: The HEADSS Mnemonic.

H: Home. Who lives with the patient? How are things at home?

E: Education/Employment. Where do you go to school? What kind of grades do you get? Do you receive any extra help? Do you work?

A: Activities. What do you do after school—sports, hobbies, extracurricular clubs? How much time do you spend watching TV or using video games or computers? Do you drive or ride in a car? Do you have a bicycle, a scooter, or motorbike? If so, do you use their seatbelt or helmet?

D: Drugs. Include sport enhancers.

S: Sexuality. Use gender-neutral terms. Are you attracted to females, males, or both? Have you had sex? (You may need to be specific. Have you ever had oral, anal, or vaginal sex?) How was the experience? Ask about the number of partners and contraception used.

S: Suicidality/Depression. Ask about depression symptoms such as sleep disturbance, changes in weight, or feelings of withdrawal. Eventually, ask about thoughts of/attempts at hurting themselves.

C. Unique aspects of the adolescent physical examination

1. Genital and breast examination. Check with your supervisor to find out whether he would like to be present for the genital examination. If your patient is of the opposite sex, offer to have a provider of the same sex perform the examination or to have a provider of the same sex present during the examination. Tanner staging (Figure 40-2) is a tool to measure the pubertal development of patients and is based on pubic hair growth, development of genitalia in boys, and development of breasts in girls.

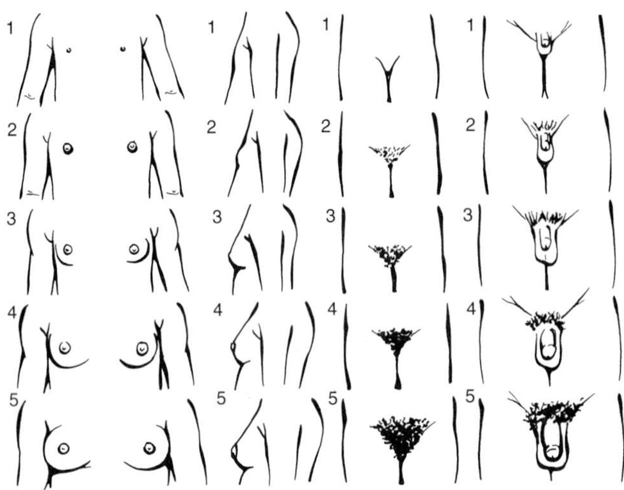

FIGURE 40-2. Tanner stages of development. **Female:** *Breast development*—Stage 1: preadolescent; no breast tissue. Stage 2: elevation of breast and nipple as small projections; areolar enlargement. Stage 3: enlargement of breast; no separation of areola and breast. Stage 4: areola and nipple project to form secondary mound above level of breast. Stage 5: only nipple projects; areola usually recedes to contour of breast; adult breast size. *Pubic hair development*—Stage 1: no pubic hair. Stage 2: sparse, long, downy hair along labia. Stage 3: darker, coarser, curlier hair. Stage 4: coarse and curly adult-type hair covering symphysis pubis. Stage 5: adult-type hair spread onto medial surface of thighs. **Male:** Stage 1: preadolescent; no pubic hair; prepubertal testes. Stage 2: testes larger; scrotum larger with reddened and coarser skin; sparse, long, downy hair. Stage 3: testes further enlarged; penis length enlarged; darker, coarser, curlier hair. Stage 4: darkening of scrotal skin; penis length and width increased, glans develops; coarse and curly pubic hair extending over symphysis pubis. Stage 5, testes and penis adult in size and shape; adult-type pubic hair that spreads to medial surface of thighs.

2. **Screening tests.** Most clinics have pregnancy, gonorrhea, and chlamydia urine tests. All females who have had sexual intercourse should have a Pap test. Check with your supervisor regarding routine testing for syphilis and HIV, because this differs from clinic to clinic.
3. **Scoliosis.** Check for scoliosis, which generally progresses during puberty.

41. Psychiatry

I Introduction

A. Psychiatric disorders affect clinical practice in every specialty of medicine. Psychiatric disorders may cause real physical disease, and underlying medical illness may induce psychiatric disease. Even if psychiatry is not your chosen career, this rotation is a great opportunity to augment your ability to deal with psychiatric issues in your chosen career.

B. Psychiatry has been the subject of many theories. Most departments have adopted the biopsychiatric model focusing on the mind–brain interaction; other departments still concentrate on the psychotherapy model. **Expect that some faculty members will have a completely different approach to the same disease** because they may subscribe to a different theory.

C. Psychiatric rotations may occur in inpatient psychiatric units (including specialized units for geriatric patients, adolescents, children, and "dual diagnosis" patients), consultation services, outpatient clinics, or psychiatric emergency departments and crisis centers.

II The Team

A. The team is similar to that on other rotations except that **resident and students have much greater autonomy.** Patients assigned to you will be *your* patients.

B. Attending rounds are likely to occur around a conference table instead of the bedside. The attending physician may not see each patient each day, because interval progress may not be expected on a day-to-day basis. This makes your observations particularly important; **your input may be all that the attending uses to make diagnostic and treatment decisions.**

C. **The team will be heavily augmented by non-physicians,** including nurses, social workers, psychologists, and recreational therapists. Most of the treatment decisions are made on the basis of thought and mood changes.

III What to Expect

A. The schedule of the typical day on an inpatient psychiatric service is shown in Table 41-1.

B. Pre-rounds may be nonexistent, because interval change in psychiatry takes place over days, not hours. Most management decisions are based on patient conversations held the previous day.

TABLE 41-1. Schedule for Typical Day on Inpatient Psychiatric Service.

Time	Activity
8:00 AM	Pre-rounds; community meeting (for patients and selected staff)
8:30 AM	Pre-rounds
9:00 AM	Attending rounds or morning report/rounds. NOTE: Patients may be scheduled for rounds today or according to another schedule.
10:30 AM	Activities such as meeting with patients or families, checking laboratory results, calling consults, meeting with social workers, contacting outpatient providers, and writing notes
12:00 PM	Noon case conference
1:00 PM	Talking with patients (may be referred to as "supervision"); meet to discuss cases with resident or attending physician

C. Before rounds, collect information about each patient by reviewing the chart, reviewing the medication administration record (MAR), and meeting briefly with the patient. Note the following in particular:
   1. Refusal to take any medication
   2. Number and amount of PRN medications given
   3. Quality and amount of sleep
   4. Occurrences of side effects
   5. Changes in vital signs
   6. Laboratory tests and current mental status examination (see below)
   7. Events that took place the previous evening (e.g., seclusion and restraint, altercation with peers, nature of family visit, consultations performed late in the day)

D. You will need to **exert greater initiative** on this rotation, because your time will be less structured than on other rotations. There are several ways to become an integral part of the psychiatric team.
   1. Demonstrate genuine interest in psychiatric diagnosis and treatment.
   2. Respectfully engage the patient, family, and all members of the team.
   3. Diligently obtain collateral history (e.g., from the family, primary care providers) and past medical history. The medical record is especially important because of the chronicity of mental illness. Insist on past medical histories, even from other hospitals.
   4. Exclude medical causes of psychiatric symptoms (see below).

E. Laboratory tests are less frequently used in psychiatry than in other medical disciplines, and IVs are almost never allowed. However, when laboratory samples are obtained, make the most of the late morning to check them and make adjustments. This is also the optimal time to call medical consults.

IV PSYCHIATRIC INTERVIEW

A. The clinical interview is vital in psychiatry, because laboratory and radiographic studies are less useful in making the diagnosis than on other services. Simple conversation with the patient can provide indirect evidence as to the health of the three key components of psychiatric function: **thought, mood, and cognition.**

B. The interview is best performed in a quiet and private setting (e.g., a designated interview room, a quiet corner of the common room). Find a quiet location where you will not be distracted.

C. Assess psychiatric functions in addition to thinking about what you are going to say next. To do this well, **you will have to learn how to listen much more intently than you do in normal conversation.** Look directly at the patient, and block everything from your mind. Here are some tips:

1. **Assess how the patient makes you feel.** These feelings may reflect the patient's psychological functioning. For example, depressed patients may generate feelings of depression, anxious patients may stir feelings of anxiety, and manic patients may make you feel energized and want to laugh.
2. **Assess the patient's language and sentence structure.** Pressured speech, tangential thoughts, and word salad (a mixture of words in no logical sequence) suggests that the patient has a thought disorder that does not give him enough time to cogently put thoughts into words. The inability to make eye contact with you suggests that he requires maximum concentration (i.e., not looking at you) to put thoughts into words.
3. **Listen for delusions and thoughts of reference.** Delusions are due to thought disorders: **a delusion is a fixed, false idiosyncratic belief. Hallucinations are seeing or hearing sensory input when none is present.** Be prepared for the patient to seek confirmation of delusions or hallucinations by asking you if you believe her. Saying that hallucinations are not real may invoke anger and frustration; confirming the delusion is a step back in therapy. Seek middle ground by telling the patient, "I believe that you believe it is real."
4. **Observe the patient's appearance, posture, dress, and ability to sit still.** Disorganized thought manifests in a disorganized life. Posture and activity give clues to agitation and depression. Shifting visual and physical focus is a clue to paranoia or delusions of persecution.

5. Use the **Mini-Mental State Examination** to assess cognition, memory and concentration.

D. **Expect the unexpected in the psychiatric interview.** Conversation is engagement, and, as in all forms of engagement, there are tacit rules of what is and is not acceptable. This keeps conversation safe. These rules have become a part of your subconscious; what you say and how you respond is within the context of these rules.

1. Psychiatric patients do not always obey these rules, and you must be consciously cognizant of what you say and how you say it. Do not assume that what is out of bounds in the regular world will be obeyed by the psychiatric patient.
2. Conversation with the psychiatric patient cannot be easy and relaxed. The psychiatrist in conducting an interview employs the same concentration the surgeon uses for a delicate surgery. You should feel tired at the end of the conversation; this is the degree of concentration required.

E. **Structuring the interview.** It is important to clarify the purpose of the interview at its outset and the degree to which the information will be shared with others (e.g., "I'm Mike Shlipak, a medical student working with your doctors. The purpose of our meeting is so that I can understand what was happening with you before you were brought to the hospital. I will discuss what we talk about with the rest of your team here in the hospital, but no one else.")

1. Begin the interview with open-ended questions (e.g., "What was happening at home that led your mother to call the ambulance?") and conclude with more closed-ended questions (e.g., "Have there ever been times in your life when you felt like life was not worth living?").
2. Begin with more focused questions if it is clear that the patient is unable to answer open-ended questions adequately (e.g., due to disorganized thought processes, poverty of thought content, lack of motivation related to depression).

F. **Setting limits and keeping the interview on track**

1. **Keep your personal life to yourself.** Many patients with chronic psychiatric disease have learned compensatory strategies to deflect discussion of their disease. One such strategy is to deflect the focus of conversation away from their disease and toward your life. If the patient asks about your life, respond with, "My goal is to help you, so my life is really unimportant here. I want to talk about you."
2. **Another compensatory strategy is to split the team by pitting one member of the team against another** (nurse versus physician; physician versus physician). This defense creates a sense of control for the patient, and diverts the team members' focus away from the patient and toward each other. **Splitting can**

wreak havoc on the team. Do not engage in discussions about other members of the healthcare team and do not side with the patient against other team members. When the conversation turns that direction, refocus the patient by saying, "I want to talk about you, not your nurse."

G. **Establishing and maintaining rapport.** Rapport facilitates patient cooperation and increases the probability that designed therapies will work. See Chapter 6 II for strategies in establishing rapport.

H. **Staying safe.** As a function of their disease, psychiatric patients may not have control over their emotions and impulses. It is important that you remain keenly aware of safety issues.

1. During the interview, **position yourself** so that you are closer to the open door than the patient; this will enable your escape if necessary. Do not block the door, however, because this may make the patient feel trapped.
2. If there is ever a question of your safety, ask security personnel to be present outside of the room while you conduct the interview.
3. Exercise particular caution if the patient has a history of assaultive or threatening behavior or is highly disorganized. In any situation in which you feel unsafe, terminate the interview prematurely by excusing yourself. You can then reassess the situation before resuming the interview under conditions in which you do feel safe. Do not be afraid of offending the patient by leaving the interview early; potentially violent patients are often afraid of their own aggressive impulses and so frequently feel safer with added security measures.

V MENTAL STATUS EXAMINATION

The mental status examination is an objective description of the patient's mental status; it is **the psychiatric correlate of the physical examination.** Be specific in your descriptions; use the **patient's own words** and include descriptions of **specific behaviors.** When a full mental status examination cannot be done, Folsom's Mini-Mental State Examination can also be used. Characteristics of the full mental status examination include the following:

A. **Appearance.** Aim to be sufficiently specific so that the patient could be easily identified on the basis of your description. For example, "Mr. Hude is a Caucasian man who looks significantly older than his 30 years. He wears his hair in waist-length dreadlocks and is dressed in a tie-dyed caftan. Multiple tattoos with women's names are evident on his forearms. He was malodorous and disheveled. His posture was stooped. His eye contact was intense."

B. **Psychomotor behavior.** Describe the patient's gait, level of psychomotor behavior (e.g., agitation or retardation), and extent to which behaviors are purposeful (e.g., a patient frenetically rearranging furniture in his room) or purposeless (e.g., a patient pacing back and forth while talking). In addition, note any involuntary or abnormal movements (e.g., tics, mannerisms, choreoathetoid movements, tremors).

C. **Speech.** Note articulation, volume, rate, and rhythm. Note this is just the verbal component of the conversation; the degree to which his words make sense are addressed in the assessment of thought (see below)

D. **Attitude.** The patient's attitude is the context for interpreting the remainder of the examination. Note whether the patient is cooperative, guarded, or hostile.

E. **Mood and affect. Mood refers to the patient's predominant internal emotional state,** and it is derived from the **patient's report.** For example, "Mr. Strand states 'I've been sick with fear for weeks. I can't shake the feeling.' " **Affect is the patient's external appearance;** it is evaluated by noting the patient's intonation, facial expressions, and body movements. It is also important to determine whether the patient's affect is congruent with the words that he says. For example, "Mr. Willis' affect was intense and fearful throughout the interview. This was consistent with his verbalizations."

F. **Thought process and content.** Thought process refers to the organization and expression of thoughts. There are two components: form and content.

1. **Normal thought form is goal-directed, logical, and coherent.** Examples of abnormal thought forms include "flight of ideas," perseveration, and tangential thought.
2. **Normal thought content is consistent with reality.** Abnormal content may include delusions (fixed, false, idiosyncratic beliefs), in which the content is paranoid, grandiose, erotomanic, obsessive, impoverished, or bizarre (violating the physical laws of the universe). Alternatively, thought content may include **thought broadcasting** (belief that others can hear one's thoughts) or **thought insertion** (belief that others are placing thoughts in one's mind).
3. Assessment of **suicidal and homicidal ideation** is a critical component of the mental status examination. If a patient discloses suicidal or homicidal ideation, you must assess whether he intends to act on this ideation and whether he has a plan. If you have any concerns about suicidal or homicidal potential, consult immediately with your supervising physician.
4. Perceptual disturbances. An **illusion** is an **erroneous impression resulting from an actual stimulus.** A **hallucination** is a **perception (auditory, visual, tactile, or olfactory) without**

external stimuli. Internal preoccupation or responding to internal stimuli (e.g., talking to oneself) may suggest their presence.

5. **Cognition.** Describe the patient's level of alertness. The Mini-Mental State Examination is an efficient instrument for assessing the components of cognition.
   a. **Orientation** to the four spheres: person, place, time, and situation (e.g., why he is here).
   b. **Attention** is the ability to focus on a task, such as repeating digits forward and backward.
   c. **Concentration** is the ability to maintain focus on an internal thought process, such as "serial 7s."
   d. **Memory. Short-term memory** is assessed by recounting items named 5 minutes earlier. **Recent past memory** is assessed by asking the patient to recall the events of days ago. **Remote memory** is assessed by asking the patient to recall childhood memories.
6. **Abstract thought** is assessed by asking the patient to note similarities and differences or proverb interpretation.
7. **Intelligence** may be assessed from the patient's vocabulary and fund of knowledge.
8. **Insight** is the awareness of one's problem and its meaning.
9. **Judgment** is assessed by noting the patient's ability to set realistic life goals and approach them in an appropriate way.
10. **Impulse control** is control over inappropriate verbal or physical impulses. This is assessed in the context of taking the history.

VI Psychiatric Diagnoses: The Five Axes

A. A full discussion of the treatment of psychiatric disease is beyond the scope of this book; however, it is worth noting how diagnoses in psychiatry are established.

B. Criteria for psychiatric diagnoses are listed in the *Diagnostic and Statistical Manual of Mental Disorders,* 4th ed. (DSM-IV). The DSM-IV does not provide lists of criteria necessary to make diagnoses, but rather provides guidelines that suggest diagnoses. The more criteria that are fulfilled, the more likely the patient has that disorder. The following five axes are intended to provide a biopsychosocial perspective.

C. Chapter 43 has a list of high-yield textbooks to guide you through the specifics of psychiatric diagnosis and management. It is useful to read the book *The Four Perspectives of Psychiatry* before starting the psychiatric rotation. It is a short book that will teach you the four perspectives of psychiatric diagnosis and treatment and the fundamental rule of psychiatric therapy—successful therapy matches the etiology of the disease (Table 41-2).

TABLE 41-2. The Four Perspectives and Their Treatment.

Perspective	Primary Treatment
Organic disease	Medications
Life story	Counseling/psychotherapy
Congenital/behavioral	Counseling/psychotherapy
Environmental	Counseling/psychotherapy

VII AXIS I: PRIMARY PSYCHIATRIC DISORDERS

Axis I includes depression, bipolar disease (manic-depressive disease), schizophrenia, adjustment disorders, anxiety disorders, and psychotic disorders.

A. **Depression.** Simple depression (unipolar depression) is usually successfully managed in an internal medicine or primary care clinic. The treatment is selective serotonin reuptake inhibitors (SSRIs). Depression with psychotic features or bipolar disease (manic depression), however, usually requires treatment in a psychiatry ward or clinic. Complicated depression rarely responds to psychotherapy alone, and neuroleptics are usually required.

B. **Bipolar disease** is also known as manic-depressive disease because patients fluctuate from periods of depression to periods of mania. Manic periods are characterized by delusions of grandeur, hypersexuality, and hyperspending. Treatment is usually lithium alone or in combination with SSRIs or neuroleptics.

C. **Schizophrenia.** Schizophrenia is diagnosed by symptoms of disordered thought, an age of onset <35, and family history.

1. **Positive symptoms** of schizophrenia are thoughts that are in addition to those a healthy person has; these are the predominate feature of early schizophrenia. Positive symptoms include audible thoughts, arguing or criticizing voices, interference with thought, thought broadcasting, delusional perception, and a perception that all drives, acts, and feelings are under someone else's control.
2. **Negative symptoms** are an absence of thoughts that a normal person has: flat affect, depression, and loss of motivation. Negative symptoms become more prominent as positive symptoms wane over time (i.e., in the late 40s to 60s).
3. **Treatment is with neuroleptics** that block dopamine receptors in the mesolimbus. These are very effective in reducing positive symptoms but less effective in treating negative symptoms. Excessive blockade over time can induce Parkinsonian symptoms (see Chapter 34).

D. Adjustment disorder is impairment of social function **within 3 months of exposure** to a stressful event. This is distinguished from posttraumatic stress disorder (PTSD) (see below) in that the disorder resolves after the life stressor is removed. Psychotherapy is particularly for adjustment disorder, because the therapist can empower the patient to avoid the stressor or develop coping mechanisms.

E. Anxiety disorders are divided into five categories (see below). For all anxiety disorders, exclude medical conditions that cause anxiety, such as thyroid disease, Cushing's disease, and carcinoid syndrome. Exclude also prednisone therapy, caffeine, withdrawal from alcohol, amphetamines, and cocaine. Anxiety disorders are usually treated with benzodiazepines in the short term and SSRIs such as buspirone and sertraline for long-term management. Psychotherapy can play an important adjunctive role, especially if the origin of the disease is from the life story perspective (see Table 41-2).

1. **Primary anxiety disorder** is due to endogenous anxiety; that is, the anxiety is unprovoked by a precipitating event. Attacks (i.e., panic attacks) are sudden and spontaneous, characterized by tachycardia, hyperventilation, and a sense of impending doom. Because patients cannot predict the attack, over time they develop anxiety of the anxiety attack itself.
2. **Posttraumatic stress disorder** (PTSD) is continued anxiety for up to 6 months after a stress (e.g., anxiety attacks following the Gulf War). Psychotherapy can be very useful, although anxiolytic or SSRI therapy is often required.
3. **General anxiety disorder** is the unrealistic worry about at least two life stressors for greater than 6 months.
4. **Phobias** are an irrational fear of a situation leading to pathologic avoidance of situations that result in impairment of the patient's life functions. Psychotherapy or desensitization therapy can be useful.
5. **Obsessive-compulsive disorder** (OCD) is recurrent thoughts, ideas, or feelings that the patient tries, but is unsuccessful in resisting.

F. Psychotic disorders not otherwise specified (NOS). This diagnosis refers to patients with psychosis (abnormal thought) but who do not meet the criteria for one of the diagnoses listed above. Neuroleptics are usually instituted.

G. Dementia. Dementia is a global decline in cognition (see Chapter 34).

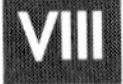

VIII Axis II Disorders: Personality Disorders

Personality disorders are **inflexible, maladaptive personality traits associated with functional impairment or distress.** Personality disorders have been grouped into three clusters: A, B, C (Table 6-1). It is important to recognize these disorders, because the approach to providing care to the patient can be very different from your standard approach (Table 6-2). Treatment is usually focused on psychotherapy.

IX Axis III: Medical Conditions Relevant to the Patient's Psychiatric Condition

Several important medical diseases can mimic psychiatric disease:

A. Hypothyroidism (dementia) or hyperthyroidism (acute thyrotoxicosis-induced psychosis)
B. Chronic subdural hematoma (dementia, altered sensorium)
C. Syphilis, either tertiary or secondary
D. Lupus cerebritis or primary central nervous system vasculitis
E. Obstructive sleep apnea
F. Vitamin deficiencies, especially B vitamins necessary for neuron function. Thiamine (vitamin B_1) deficiency causes Wernicke-Korsakoff disease; niacin (vitamin B_6) deficiency causes pellagra; and cobalamin (vitamin B_{12}) deficiency causes dementia.
G. Steroid-induced psychosis
H. Recreational drugs

X Axis IV: Social and Environmental Influences

A. Cocaine or drug intoxication (PCP, LSD, ecstasy, hallucinogenic mushrooms, cocaine, heroin), or excessive nicotine, caffeine, or stimulants can induce psychosis.
B. Alcohol withdrawal and benzodiazepine withdrawal. Both conditions can induce an acute psychosis characterized by disorientation and visual hallucinations, and a hyperadrenergic state that can induce stroke, seizures, or myocardial infarction.
C. In treating patients with substance abuse, you must first recognize the difference between introverts and extroverts.

1. **Introverts primarily focus on the future, not the present.** They have an ability to conceptualize the future and make changes in the present to alter the future. **Deferred gratification** and **risk avoidance** are features of the introvert. You are likely an introvert (otherwise, how could you defer so many of years of your life in medical training for the prospect of a great future career?).
2. **Extroverts are those who exclusively live in the present.** They have little conceptualization of the future, and their decisions are based on **maximizing pleasure for today.**
3. The problem with counseling substance drug abusers is that most physicians are introverts and most substance abusers are extroverts. Admonishing drug abusers to stop using heroin because of its long-term effects on the body is useless, because the heroin user does not conceptualize tomorrow; he is thinking about today.

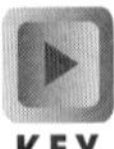

HOT KEY

To persuade the heroin user to quit, you must find an alternative reward or some pain that can be avoided now if he stops using the drug.

XI Axis V: Global Assessment of Functioning Score (1 to 100)

This axis assesses the patient's overall physical, social, and psychological function. A score of 1 indicates a serious danger of harm or inability to care for oneself, and a score of 100 indicates superior functioning.

XII Types of Psychiatric Treatment

A. **Somatic treatment** includes **medications** or **electroconvulsive therapy.**
   1. Medication may be aggressively titrated in acute care settings; it is critical that patients be carefully and regularly assessed for side effects and signs of toxicity.
   2. Interactions with other medications must be carefully considered. Prescription and over-the-counter medications, including herbal remedies, must be evaluated.

B. **Psychotherapeutic** treatment includes verbal interventions used to modify behavior and ameliorate emotional distress. Psychotherapy may involve individuals, couples, families, or groups.
   1. Psychodynamically oriented interventions focus on unconscious conflicts and defenses.
   2. Supportive interventions focus on strengthening current ego functions.
   3. Cognitive interventions focus on changing thoughts as a way of changing feelings and behavior.

C. **Milieu** interventions refer to the use of the inpatient psychiatric unit's very environment as a therapeutic intervention.
   1. The structure of the unit and interpersonal interactions with other patients and staff may enhance patients' feelings of security, by providing opportunities for enhancing self-esteem through competence.
   2. Milieu treatment may involve social interventions (e.g., helping the patient to mobilize supports), and therapeutic community systems and token economies are sometimes used.

XIII Psychiatric Note and Treatment Plan

The psychiatric admission note follows the same pattern discussed in Chapter 13 with the following additions:

A. **Reason for referral.** The "reason for referral" may be substituted for the chief complaint if the patient cannot verbalize the reason for his hospitalization.

B. In addition to describing the patient's symptoms, note any **precipitants** (e.g., changes in relationships) and any **sequelae** (e.g., loss of job, housing, or relationship as a result of behavior or symptoms).

C. The second paragraph should describe the conversation, with relevant data defined by those parts of the conversation (quotation marks) that give insight into the patient's inner thoughts, mood, and cognition. Note current treatment and compliance. Include the patient's understanding of the meaning of the symptoms (e.g., Are the symptoms a punishment? Do they mean that I am going crazy?).

D. **Past psychiatric history.** Include age of onset of symptoms, changes in presentation over time, previous inpatient and outpatient treatment (including number of admissions; longest admission; previous medications, including doses, duration, side effects, therapeutic effects, and compliance), and any history of suicidal, assaultive, or homicidal ideation or behavior.

E. Conclude with a **brief psychiatric review of systems.** Screen for depression, mania, psychosis, and anxiety disorders.

F. **Substance use history.** Ask about drug, alcohol, and tobacco use, and abuse of prescription medications. Ask about any treatment for substance use and duration of any abstinence.

G. **Family history.** Ask about relatives' psychiatric history, including past hospitalizations and suicides.

H. **Social history** is vital in psychiatry; homelessness in America is commentary on the care of the psychiatric population. Psychiatric disease alienates social support (family and friends), leaving many patients homeless; unless you address this, the homeless patient will return to the street. Know the patient's finances, housing, and access to community services (e.g., shelters, substance abuse clinics). Over the course of the hospitalization, it is also important to learn informa-

> "Mr. X is a 30-year-old Caucasian male with strong genetic loading for psychotic disorders. He was diagnosed with schizophrenia, paranoid type at age 18. Current symptoms include command auditory hallucinations to hurt himself and a paranoid delusion about being sought by the Mafia for execution. The symptoms began to reemerge 3 weeks ago when the patient discontinued his antipsychotic medication because of sexual side effects. Despite his current active symptoms, the patient has insight into the etiology of his decompensation and displayed good judgment in seeking medical help when he felt unsafe. Because of his symptoms, Mr. X recently lost his job as a taxi driver. His mother (with whom he resides) and his girlfriend remain highly supportive."

FIGURE 41-1. Patient presentation.

tion about the patient's childhood, interaction with parents, history of physical or sexual abuse, life crises, school performance, cultural and religious beliefs, and occupational history. All of this gives a context of the patient's life story and may be an important diagnostic clue to her current situation.

I. Mental status examination. In lieu of the full physical cxamination, substitute the patient's mental status examination (see V above). A biopsychosocial formulation should be a concise summary of the salient biologic, psychological, and social factors associated with the patient's presentation (Figure 41-1). If the Mini-Mental State Examination was performed, note the score obtained.

J. The assessment and plan follows the same formula discussed in Chapter 13. Be sure, however, to discuss each of the five axes. If there are no disorders present within an axis (e.g., no medical issues for Axis III), simply list "Axis III: none."

42. Working in the Outpatient Clinic

I Introduction

A. The outpatient clinic is one of the most important components of clinical medicine. The goal of inpatient care is to improve patients' health enough so that they can be treated in the outpatient clinic. The goal of outpatient care is to maintain health to prevent hospitalization. This is achieved by identifying and treating problems early, when small interventions can solve them, and by preventing problems before they occur (health maintenance).

B. Regardless of specialty, the vast majority of physicians spend most of their time in the clinic. There are three overriding goals for training in the clinic.

1. Becoming familiar with the line that separates the clinic patient from the hospitalized patient (i.e., knowing the severity of a disease that warrants hospitalization)
2. Managing time well
3. Preventing disease

II Key Elements of a Successful Clinic Experience

A. Make the paradigm shift. Outpatient medicine has a very different philosophy from inpatient medicine. Here, you do not have the luxury (or constraint) of addressing each complaint thoroughly. Your goal is to address the most important problem. If time remains after discussion of this problem (but only after this discussion has concluded), you can consider other topics. The philosophy of clinic is to treat the patient sequentially over several visits.

B. Greet the patient. Even when rushed and harried, take a few moments to look the patient in the eye, greet her (e.g., "Hello Mrs. Jones, it's good to see you today"), and ask her a general question about how she is doing (e.g., "How are things?" or "How have you been feeling?").

C. Set an agenda.

1. Ask the patient to list all of her concerns (e.g., "I'd like to find out if you have any problems or concerns today"). Make a list. The patient might say, "My back is hurting me." Note this as problem No. 1, but before asking about the back, say, "OK, what else?" The patient might say that she has been short of breath. Note this as problem No. 2, and ask again, "What else?" Continue until you have a complete list of problems, and then review the list with the

patient: "I note seven problems here, but today we have time to deal with only two or three; which ones are concern you the most?"

2. This technique allows you to focus on the most important problems from the patient's perspective, while keeping you aware of the full picture. It also prevents the end-of-the-visit comment, "Doctor, I forgot to tell you about my crushing chest pain," or "I think I may be depressed." These "hidden" concerns can ruin your time management if you do not elicit them up front. After you have established your list, spend time taking a history and performing a physical examination addressing the problems that are the focus of the visit.

D. After you have identified the problem, put your pen down and **listen attentively.** Maintain eye contact.

E. See Chapter 6 for how to deal with the talkative patient.

III Keeping Discussions with Patients on Target

A. **Provide reassurance that you are listening.** Rephrase each paragraph of patient data with a sentence. Then ask your next question. For example, after 5 minutes of the patient describing her bowel movements, start with "It sounds as if you are having difficulty with constipation, and this sometimes changes to diarrhea. Have you had abdominal pain?" This keeps the patient from circling back to talk about the bowel movements again.

B. **Use the physical examination like a test.** Only perform a physical examination maneuver if it will help you determine the etiology or severity of a problem you are addressing. Note that this is a departure from the Tier I examination philosophy in the inpatient arena, where a full Tier I examination is performed on all patients.

C. **Do not write as you talk.** You may note details on paper, but do not write the clinic note as the interview progresses. You are likely to waste more time asking questions twice to learn information you missed while your attention was on writing.

D. **Be efficient with your note writing.** Most computerized systems allow you to "cut and paste" past medical history and medications. Update these as necessary, and add only relevant new history, physical examination findings, and test results. Be sure to review and properly edit any "pasted" material.

E. **Formulate a management plan before a patient leaves.** This ensures that you have not forgotten to order tests or new treatments. Review the plan with the patient, and ask her to repeat it. Discuss an appropriate follow-up visit.

IV Managing Time Well

A. **Strive to be on time** and reduce waiting. Patients appreciate your concern for their time and will likely be more efficient with yours.

B. Listen well.

C. End the clinic visit successfully. Occasionally, patients do not want to end the clinic visit, usually because of fear that all of their problems have not been addressed. The remedy is reassurance. Restate the problems you have addressed, the plans you have made, and your optimism that these plans will work. "And if they don't, I will see you again soon and we will come up with a plan B." In addition, note when you will address any problems not discussed today.

D. Deal with paperwork at the end of the clinic day. Patients may bring many forms to clinic (e.g., disability forms, Medicare forms), which require time and are rarely an emergency. Collect the forms, and tell patients you will complete them at the end of the day. They can pick up the forms later, or the clinic staff can mail them.

E. As you progress into a clinic practice, **learn to schedule your most talkative patients late in the day.** Urgent care visits should come in the early part of the day; if they require hospitalization or consultation, both are easier to obtain at 1:00 PM than at 5:00 PM.

V DEALING WITH THE FAMILY IN CLINIC

A. Make it clear that this is the patient's time. If family is present, set the tone early: "Well, this is what I would like to do. I would like to hear Mr. Smith's thoughts about his health, and then I will get your (the family member's) input." This validates the family members but emphasizes your focus on your patient.

B. If the family tries to derail the discussion with a tangential comment, listen to the comment and then respond, "I see; very important. I would like to hear more about that in just a minute. Let me get Mr. Smith's story first, and then we can explore that further."

C. If the family is very persistent, skip to the physical examination and conduct the rest of the history at that time. "Well, if you will excuse us, I am going to do the physical examination now. I'll call you back in about 5 minutes." If the family refuses to leave, saying, "Can I stay for the examination?," reply, "Actually, it is my policy to always do the examination alone. I am better at focusing my examination techniques that way."

VI ENSURING GOOD CLINIC VISITS

You (or your consultant) cannot act until you have data on which to act.

A. Set aside time before clinic to review your patients. Ideally, make a note of items to discuss or highlight with each patient (e.g., Mr. Jones: discuss angina symptoms, review any symptoms as a result of starting the β-blocker at the last visit, discuss colon cancer screening).

B. If a laboratory value or study (e.g., HbA_{1c} for a patient with diabetes, creatinine level for a patient just started on an ACE inhibitor, stress test for a patient with suspected coronary disease) predicates your next decision, make sure that data have been acquired before the visit. Enlist the patient's help whenever possible: "Please make sure you go to the lab at least a few days before our next clinic visit. I need to know the results of these tests to decide what to do next."

C. Similarly, if you refer a patient to a specialty clinic, anticipate what he is likely to need. If you are sending your patient to an orthopedic clinic for evaluation for back surgery, make sure the patient has radiographs of the back performed before the visit.

VII Medications in the Clinic

Always assess compliance.

A. Normalize the question of compliance by saying the following:

1. "I know remembering to take medications is tough. How often would you say you have missed taking this medication in the last week?"
2. "This is a lot of pills. What's your system for remembering to take your medications?"

B. Ask the patient to bring all medications to clinic. Ask about vitamins, herbs, supplements, and OTC medicines as well. Review each one. Make sure the patient knows what each medicine is designed to do. Simple lists showing medicine dosage, times to take them, and reasons for use (e.g., blood pressure, diabetes, cholesterol) are very helpful.

VIII Writing Prescriptions

A. For prescriptions used chronically, **make the quantity for 90 days,** if possible (e.g., for a three-times-a-day dosing, the quantity is 270).

B. Make the number of refills enough to last the patient well beyond his next scheduled appointment.

C. Write OTC prescriptions on a prescription pad. This implicitly tells your patient that the medication (e.g., aspirin) is no less important just because it is OTC. Write OVER THE COUNTER on the prescription. Write the generic name of the medication instead of the trade name, and tell the patient to ask the pharmacist to help him find a generic brand that contains the active ingredient. This saves the patient money and contributes to compliance.

IX Health Care Maintenance

A. An essential part of the clinic philosophy is to detect problems that might occur or prevent problems before they occur. Health care maintenance is key to this philosophy.

B. Remind all patients who use tobacco, alcohol, or other drugs or do not exercise that you care whether they stop using these drugs or start exercising. Do this at every clinic visit, no matter how short. Even short reminders have been shown to be effective for helping some patients quit bad habits or start helpful ones.

PART VI

Self-Improvement Strategies: Maximizing Your Potential

43. Time Management

I **INTRODUCTION** There is much to do on the clinical wards. You must manage all of your patients in a limited amount of time. Remember that in addition to the patients you care for now, you will have patients to care for in the future. In addition to completing the ward work, you must also find time to read and develop. This chapter discusses the general features of time management.

II **PRIORITIZATION: IMPORTANCE VERSUS URGENCY** The key to time management is **prioritizing tasks based on their relative importance, *not* their urgency.** Look at Figure 43-1.

A. **Importance** is defined by you and is ultimately determined by your patient's needs. For example, performing a lumbar puncture on your patient is important; the nurses request to fill out the patient's admission form is urgent. Never sacrifice important tasks for urgent tasks.

B. **Urgency** is defined by other people. Most people believe that their task is the most vital, and they create a sense of urgency to accomplish these tasks first. This does not mean that these tasks are vital to **you,** your team, or your patients. Some of these tasks may be vital, but others may not be.

C. Using this approach, tasks can be classified into four groups: important and urgent, important but not urgent, urgent but not important, and neither urgent nor important. Tasks that are both urgent and important are done first, followed by those that are important but not urgent, and then followed by those that are urgent but not important. Tasks that are neither urgent nor important are done at the end of the day or the next day.

III **THE "BIG 7"** Make a list of the day's anticipated tasks. Number them from 1 to 7, with 1 having the highest priority. Do not

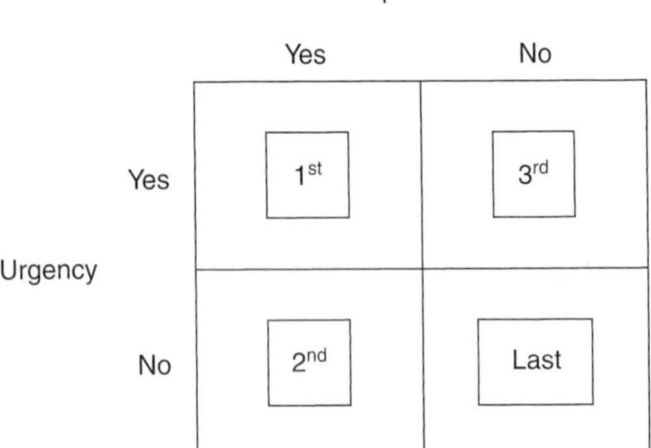

FIGURE 43-1. Prioritizing tasks.

perform any other tasks until the "Big 7" tasks are completed. After these seven tasks are accomplished, feel free to reprioritize with seven new tasks. Stick to this method for 2 weeks and you will have developed valuable discipline in time management.

IV Importance on the Wards

A. Submit your orders early (i.e., when everyone else is not submitting theirs) to make sure that your orders are addressed first.

B. Nurses make things happen on the wards, but they work in shifts. Time your orders so they fit in with the nurses' schedule.

C. Schedule radiologic studies and other procedures as early in the day as possible and beware of difficult weekend and holiday scheduling.

1. You want the results before going home so that you can act on them (e.g., discharge a patient). You are competing against all other physicians, so do this early. If you are ordering a test or procedure in the morning, take the time to call the physician who is performing the procedure to put your patient on the list. Merely writing the order places your order in line with all of the other orders written during the morning, and your patient has no priority. If necessary, ask for permission to break from rounds to make the call.
2. For laboratory tests and blood draws, know when the phlebotomy service goes on rounds. Place laboratory draws at least 1 hour before this time. Write laboratory orders the night before.

D. As a general rule, use the following list to **prioritize tasks** on the wards. Remember that some tasks have a long "wait" time.

1. **Radiologic tests and procedures**
2. **Consults** (see VI)

3. **Discharge** (see VII)
4. **Orders**
5. **Procedures**
6. **Family conferences**
7. **Progress notes**

V Specific Time Management Strategies on the Wards

A. **Begin the day efficiently.**
   1. Start the day earlier than necessary. The 15 minutes of sacrificed sleep is worth an hour of productivity. A great amount of energy is lost as you rush to work and worry about being late.
   2. Think through your day while going to work. This is your time to mentally assemble your "Big 7" list (see III).

B. **Prioritize tasks** (see IV).

C. **Know your intern's schedule.** Have your notes and orders ready for her when you know she will be available.

D. **Group similar tasks.** Develop a scut list of your own and one for the team. If your interns know you routinely have this list, you will be in a position to trade tasks (e.g., "I'll check the labs if you'll call the consultants").

E. **Always order procedure trays well ahead of time.** Allow plenty of extra time for procedures, because they often take longer than expected and you do not want to be hurried.

F. **Schedule patient/family conferences late in the day.** These can take a great deal of time, and you cannot afford to lose valuable morning time or cut family conferences short because of other commitments.

G. **Write progress notes last.** This is the best time to complete you notes, because you will have more data to communicate to your sign-out physician in your note.

H. **Keep a list of commonly called telephone numbers.** Even though you rotate every 1 or 2 months, you will likely remain in (or eventually return to) the same hospital.

I. **Use your pager wisely.**
   1. Page smartly. When you page another physician, you can enter the number you want him to call, then *, and then your own pager number. If he is busy and does not call you back for 10 minutes, he will have your pager number to page you to his phone. This keeps you from being tied to a phone waiting for a page to be returned. Do not page someone directly to a pager number; this is annoying.
   2. Do not be tied to your pager. Answer pages promptly when you can, but do not let paging fragment your day. Complete the task at hand, and then return the call.

J. Use on-call downtime to do time-consuming tasks. Do not put off tasks on call, believing that you will have more energy and time to do them on noncall days.

VI Obtaining Time-Efficient Consults

A. In most hospitals, consultants conduct rounds in the midafternoon. If you have a question, such as a simple knowledge question that does not require seeing the patient (e.g., should you use empiric vancomycin for penicillin-resistant pneumonia caused by *Streptococcus pneumoniae*?), catch the consultant during rounds and ask the question.

B. If it is late in the afternoon and you need a consult tomorrow, do not wait until then to make the request. Call the consultant and tell her you have a patient you would like her to see tomorrow morning. For consult services, mornings are slow, and your actions put your patient first on the list.

C. Try to call all consults before 12:00 noon.

D. If you have ordered a consult and you obtain new information about your patient, call the consultant with the new information before consult rounds.

VII Anticipating Discharge

A. Social workers, nurses, and patients' families need time to plan. The fewer patients you have in the hospital, the fewer the small distracting calls you will receive during the day; early discharge leads to exponential time savings.

B. If a patient is ready to be discharged today, do the discharge paperwork today. However, it is much easier to discharge a patient in the midmorning if you start the paperwork and alert the nurses (and thus the pharmacy) the day before. If the patient will be ready tomorrow, do the paperwork tonight. "Predischarging" patients allows discharge planning to begin a day early.

VIII Saving Time at Home

A. Try to simplify your home life so you can maximize your time for reading, sleep, and social activities.

B. Consider the following:

1. Automatic bill paying
2. Avoiding time drains such as:
    - **a.** Computer crashes. Back up frequently; get a computer that is stable.
    - **b.** Automobile trouble. Find a reliable car or other method of transportation.

c. Illness. Stay healthy. Avoid touching your nose or eyes with your fingers, because this is how most rhinoviruses and adenoviruses are spread. Eat well, and do not drink alcohol to excess. Exercise when you can.

d. Legal trouble. Do not speed. Things are different now; a $50 fine is $200 for you, because it will take 4 hours of valuable time to deal with the courts.

e. Unsolicited telemarketers. Block them using do-not-call lists.

44. Reading Strategies

I Introduction

INTRODUCTION Studying clinical medicine is about mastering the general aspects of diseases, comparing and contrasting these diseases to other disorders, and **visualizing yourself applying this knowledge on the wards.** The most common cause of difficulty with clinical medicine is not having a clear strategy when you read. This chapter describes the reading habits of the highly successful clinician.

II Make Reading a Habit

MAKE READING A HABIT The knowledge you will acquire in the near future is inconsequential compared to the knowledge you will acquire in your lifetime. **The goal is to become a habitual reader,** permitting a lifetime of learning.

III Pace Yourself

A. It is far better to read in small increments on a daily basis than to "binge" read. This will also maximize long-term retention, because only so much information from any given reading session can be retained long term. The brain can assimilate only so much. There is too much knowledge in clinical medicine to "cram" it all at the last minute; you will only become frustrated and discouraged.

B. Your goal should be increasing the amount of information in your long-term memory. To achieve this goal, **you should read something every day.** Volume does not matter; even one sentence is enough. Do not let a day go by without reading something. Soon this habit will become a part of your life. Read one sentence, then one paragraph, and then one article per day.

HOT
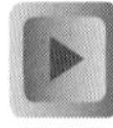
KEY

If you want to be well read, read something, however small, each day.

C. At each session, find satisfaction in what you read, read only until you are no longer satisfied, and then stop. "Binge" reading becomes like "binge" exercising; it becomes painful and you associate it with pain. If you make this negative association, you will find any excuse possible to avoid reading.

IV Read About a Disease in the Same Way You Would Watch a Movie

A. View each disease as its own movie, with its own cast of characters (symptoms), plot (progression, management), and conclusion (prognosis). Unless you become familiar with each of these, you cannot understand the movie.

B. When you start reading about a disease, do not stop or move to the next disease until you understand these three components.

V Build a Basic Foundation

Then add to that foundation. Try this method.

A. Start with a **"skeleton book."** These are books that have short chapters, requiring only about 5 minutes per chapter.

1. Skeleton books present **an overview of the most common diseases or symptoms,** giving you the essential facts. This will give you an outline of the disease of interest and a list of its symptoms.
2. Skeleton books also **provide perspective,** enabling you to compare and contrast a disease's symptoms and signs to those of similar diseases.
3. The added bonus is that if you are short of time, you will have learned **80% of what you need to know** about the disease. The remaining 20% can come later if you have time (via "flesh books").
4. Another reason a "skeleton" knowledge is so important is that the wards do not operate on the basic-to-complex sequence. For example, on one day you may admit a patient with lupus; on another a patient with endocarditis; and on still another, a patient with hypercalcemia. If you spend all your time mastering the details of lupus, you will lose the opportunity to learn from the next two patient encounters. **Your goal is to establish a basic knowledge of each common disease in medicine as soon as you can.** This will provide a scaffold on which you can hang the details of each disease as you encounter them on the wards. The sooner you construct this "skeleton," the more you will gain from the wards.
5. "Skeleton" books should be **portable** (i.e., pocket books), and you should carry them on the wards. See Chapter 45 III for a list of good "skeleton" books.

B. **"Flesh books."** After you have mastered the broad strokes of a disease, move to a flesh book if time allows. These books add "meat to the skeleton" by **providing details about diagnosis and management.** The common feature of flesh books is that they provide everything a physician needs to diagnose and manage a disease, but are usually without the pathophysiology and epidemiologic information contained in most "skin" books.

C. "Skin books." Skin books provide all details known about a disease, and thus serve as a **great reference** for preparing reports and presentations. Avoid these books in your daily reading; the time expended learning all of the details of one disease will come at the expense of learning about basic principles of other diseases.

D. Avoid fragmentation. Like a computer, the mind loses efficiency and wastes memory when it jumps around from one topic to another. Try to stay focused on one topic, completing the "skeleton" knowledge of one disease, before moving on to another.

VI Compare and Contrast

A. Use a book's table of contents to keep you moving from one topic to another. Because the table of contents is organized by similar diseases, this juxtaposes diseases with similar presentations (e.g., lupus versus rheumatoid arthritis), allowing you to compare and contrast diseases as you read. Before you proceed to another topic, make sure you can tell yourself the following:

1. Essentials of diagnosis (i.e., symptoms, examination findings, laboratory or radiographic studies)
2. Underlying physiology and how this explains the symptoms and signs
3. Management and how this relates to the physiology of the disease
4. Prognosis
5. People affected (i.e., race, gender, age)

B. Start with a symptom, list the diagnoses that could cause this symptom, and then read about one of these diagnoses. When you are finished, read about another diagnosis that could cause this symptom. This keeps the diseases in an order that makes sense in clinical practice. **Remember that comparing and contrasting is as important as knowing about the characteristics of each disease.**

VII Read the Right Books

A. Do not confuse activity with productivity. People usually fail the boards because they read the wrong things, not because they do not read. Read about common diseases (e.g., diabetes) instead of fascinating diseases (e.g., pheochromocytoma). **Your reading should parallel the incidence of disease.**

B. Avoid relying solely on question books and other "quick fixes." These books do not provide a solid and long-lasting understanding of the important concepts and skills.

C. Chapter 45 presents a list of books that provide **both understanding and knowledge.**

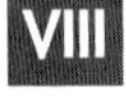

Read at the Proper Level If you do not understand large portions of an article, it is above your level of understanding. Use the following guidelines as a rule of thumb:

A. **Medical students** will get the greatest yield per unit of time by reading textbook chapters.
B. **Interns** should advance to reading review articles.
C. **Residents** should advance to reading original research articles.
D. **Attending physicians** should advance to reading original research articles and research that is soon to be published.

IX **READ WITH A PURPOSE** Reading is less fun when you feel you must do it. You will be tempted to read about medicine while on a surgical rotation, or surgery when you are on an internal medical rotation. Avoid this temptation.

A. **Use your patients' conditions to give your reading a purpose.** Your retention will be maximized by linking what you read to the patients for whom you provide care.
   1. After you are finished reading about a disease that affects a particular patient, write her name and presenting complaint in the margin. Your memory functions better with names and faces than it will with details about the disease. A year from now, when you look back at the chapter you just read, the patient's name and chief complaint will help you remember all of the knowledge you once had about this disease. This will also mark your progress and help you determine what you need to read in your spare time.
   2. When you have some downtime and can read about other diseases, flip through your flesh book and read chapters that do not have patient names in the margins. This method also forces you to read about the most common diseases (i.e., the ones you most often see on the wards) and keeps track of what you have and have not seen.

B. Reading surgery while on your surgical rotation will also allow you to make the most of your resident's expertise to determine what is and what is not important for that disease. Questions not answered by your reading can be directed to your resident.

X **VISUALIZE YOURSELF USING THE ACQUIRED INFORMATION** There will be times when you must read something that you do not enjoy. In these situations, visualize a scenario in which this information will be useful for one of your current patients. If you find yourself reading detailed information that you cannot visualize yourself using, you are reading the wrong material.

XI **WHAT TO DO WHEN YOU GET "STUCK."** There will be times when you get stuck mentally and cannot concentrate on what you are reading. Instead of reading the same paragraph over and over again, do something constructive. Find some small noncognitive task that is easily accomplished. Wash your car, clean the house, or organize some files. The simple act of starting and completing a task puts your mind back on track. Then begin reading again.

XII Find a Suitable Time and Place

Find a Suitable Time and Place Everyone has an optimal time for reading. If you are a morning person, rearrange your day so you go to bed early and read early in the morning before going to work. If you are a night owl, read later in the evening. Some people need absolute quiet. Other people study better in a coffee house. Find the place where you study best.

XIII Take Naps

Take Naps Once again, do not confuse activity with productivity. If you read while you are tired, you will read the same paragraph over and over again. It is better to spend 1 hour of study time napping and to have 3 productive study hours than it is to waste 4 hours reading the same page because you cannot concentrate.

XIV Develop a Strategy to Combat Loss of Knowledge and Skill

A. Everything fades over time, even knowledge. Knowledge you mastered 6 months ago has now faded; a percentage of the knowledge you acquire now will be gone in 6 months. This is known as "skills decline."

B. Four actions to slow skills decline.

1. **Acknowledge** that this is a natural phenomenon.
2. Expect that you will lose a percentage of what you know. Do not be discouraged about how much knowledge you have lost; **focus on the information you have retained.**
3. Learn new knowledge **methodically.** Methods of learning new information, in order of **worst to best,** are:
    a. **Pure memorization.** Memorized facts fade in a month.
    b. **Short-term learning.** Study properly to place information into your long-term memory. Do not read a chapter and then quiz yourself. This activates short-term memory storage. Instead, read a chapter and then visualize yourself using the information.
    c. **Mnemonics.** Mnemonics are useful as a bridge to organizing data until you have a good mastery of the physiology that underlies the disease. Mnemonics are useful for short lists. Beware of esoteric mnemonics that do not relate to the disease in question. The mnemonic PANCREATITIS relating to the disease pancreatitis is a good mnemonic, but CAMP MIST GUNCLOTH relating to altered mental status is not a good mnemonic. In addition, mnemonics with letters such as "M"

for "metabolic disease" or "O" for "other diseases" only introduce more confusion and may not contribute to understanding.

d. **Long-term memory.** Remember that memory is tightly joined with emotion. Make sure that your vision of yourself using the information is emotional. Envision a trauma room scenario or a grand rounds quiz session. Practice under mental stress, and the knowledge will be accessible when you are subject to the real-world stress of the wards.

e. **Physiologic-based methods.** Physiologic principles are applicable to many diseases and allow for long-term comprehension. See Appendix A for 10 key physiologic principles that are a good start in establishing your own methods for approaching disease.

4. **Make note of lessons that "speak" to you.**

   a. You will hear many lectures on the same topic. Some of these talks make sense of the topic. When a talk (or a book chapter or a journal article) makes sense to you, record your notes somewhere where you can find them at a later time. You may use cards, small blank books, a PDA, or a computer.

   b. A sample method follows:

      (1) **Buy a blank book.** Number the pages (every other page is sufficient). Assign a general topic to every 10 pages (e.g., cardiology, endocrinology, rheumatology).

      (2) Carry several 3 × 5 cards or a pocket notebook with you on the wards. When you hear something that makes particular sense to you, **write it down.**

      (3) When you get home, neatly **transcribe** the features of the talk or article that made sense to you. Do not be compulsive about including every detail about the topic. Focus on the broad outline.

      (4) Do the same for articles or chapters that you read. Do not note every detail, but instead **focus on the broad outline of the topic** and the details that make sense of the topic.

      (5) As you transcribe the information, focus on the method for approaching the problem. **Visualize yourself using the method to take care of a patient.**

      (6) As you gather other small pearls and nuggets related to a topic in your book, record them in the margins of the appropriate section. It is not necessary to have a perfect table of contents—**do not let perfect become the enemy of the good.** As long as you can flip through your book and find "thyroid disease," you are fine. The goal is to be able to read in 2 minutes what it took you 2 hours to read the first time around.

      (7) The art of this method is in *not* being compulsive. **Record only the main points** and only those that make sense to you.

45. Building a Home Library

I Why Build a Personal Library?

A. There should be no wasted time looking for a book when you need it, and there should be no wasted opportunities when you are struck with the desire to read.

B. ***Your* library should be a reflection of what speaks to *you.*** Your library will mark the passage of time: each book will represent a part of your life and the patients that were in that segment. It is at once a reminder of the richness that medicine has brought to your life and a motivation to understand your patients better.

II General Components of the Home Library

A great home library contains **four elements:**

A. Understanding disease: the science of medicine
B. Personal improvement and colorful speech
C. Understanding your patients: novels, plays, and poetry
D. Discovering mentors: great people in medicine

III Understanding Disease: The Science of Medicine

A. "Skeleton" books. These books present an overview of the most common diseases or symptoms. See Chapter 44 V A for a description of "skeleton," "flesh," and "skin books." Examples of books to consider are in Table 45-1.

B. "Flesh books." These books add "meat to the skeleton" in the form of **details about diagnosis and management.** These books should remain on your shelf or, if you are on call, in your locker (or bag). **If you are going into a particular specialty, read the corresponding "flesh" book from cover-to-cover.** If not, use these books as references. Table 45-2 has a list of high-yield flesh books.

C. "Skin books." These books are primarily used as **references** or a detailed source for presentations. Their density precludes them from daily reading, because it usually takes hours to read about each disease. **Buy only the book that corresponds to the specialty you choose;** cost prohibits buying them all. During other rotations, make use of your school's library. (Table 45-3).

IV Books for Personal Improvement and Colorful Speech

Success in clinical medicine requires multiple skills in addition to medical knowledge. Unfortunately, very little time is devoted to these skills in a standard medical school curriculum.

TABLE 45-1. Skeleton Books.

Book	Author
Internal Medicine	
Practical Guide to Care of the Medical Patient	F. Ferri
Saint-Frances Guide to Inpatient Medicine	S. Saint
NMS Medicine	A. Meyers
Surgery	
Mont Reid Surgical Handbook	S. Berry
NMS Surgery	B. Jarrell
Pediatrics	
Harriet Lane Handbook	C. Nechyba
Saint-Frances Guide to Pediatrics	D. Migita
NMS Pediatrics	P. Dworkin
Obstetrics and Gynecology	
Handbook of Gynecology and Obstetrics	J. Brown
NMS Gynecology and Obstetrics	W. Beck
Psychiatry	
Saint-Frances Guide to Psychiatry	M. McCarthy
NMS Psychiatry	J. Scully
Neurology	
Neurology: House Officer Series	H. Weiner

TABLE 45-2. Flesh Books.

Book	Author
Internal Medicine	
Current Medical Diagnosis and Treatment	L. Tierney
DeGowin's Diagnostic Examination	R. LeBlond
Surgery	
Essentials of General Surgery	P. Lawrence
Pediatrics	
Current Pediatric Diagnosis and Treatment	W. Hay
Obstetrics and Gynecology	
Current Obstetric and Gynecologic Diagnosis and Treatment	A. DeCherney
Neurology	
Clinical Neurology	D. Greenberg
Psychiatry	
DSM-IV	American Psychiatric Association
Intensive Care	
The ICU Book	P. Marino

TABLE 45-3. Skin Books.

Book	Author
Internal Medicine	
Harrison's Principles of Internal Medicine	D. Kasper
Cecil's Textbook of Medicine	L. Goldman
ACP Medicine	D.C. Dale
Rapid Interpretation of EKGs	D. Dubin
Marriott's Practical Electrocardiography	G. Wagner
Clinical Physiology of Acid-Base and Electrolyte Disorders	B. Rose
Surgery	
General Surgery	W. Ritchie
Principles of Surgery	S. Schwartz
Campbell's Operative Orthopaedics	S. Canale
Cope's Early Diagnosis of the Acute Abdomen	W. Silen
Practical Orthopedics	L. Mercier
Anatomy: A Regional Atlas of the Human Body	C. Clemente
Netter's Atlas of Anatomy	F. Netter
Pediatrics	
Nelson's Textbook of Pediatrics	R. Behrman
Obstetrics and Gynecology	
Williams Obstetrics	G. Cunningham
Danforth's Obstetrics and Gynecology	D. Danforth
Neurology	
Adams and Victor's Principles of Neurology	M. Victor
The Diagnosis of Stupor and Coma	F. Plumb
Psychiatry	
The Perspectives of Psychiatry	P. McHugh
Intensive Care	
The ICU Book	P. Marino
Emergency Medicine	
Emergency Procedures and Techniques	R. Simon
Dermatology	
Color Atlas and Synopsis of Clinical Dermatology	T. Fitzpatrick
Radiology	
Felson's Principles of Chest Roentgenology	L. Goodman
Fundamentals of Radiology	S. Squire
Physical Examination	
Sapira's Art and Science of Bedside Diagnosis	J. Orient
DeGowin's Diagnostic Examination	R. DeGowin
The CIBA Collection	F. Netter
Reading the Medical Literature	
Primer of Biostatistics	S. Glanz
Evidence-Based Medicine	D. Friedland
User's Guide to the Medical Literature	G. Guyatt

TABLE 45-4. Personal Improvement and Colorful Speech.

Book	Author
Teaching	
The Physician as Teacher	N. Whitman
Time Management	
Seven Habits of Highly Effective People	S. Covey
Time Management (Barron's Business Success Guide)	R. Hochheiser
The One Minute Manager	K. Blanchard
Interpersonal Skills	
How to Win Friends and Influence People	D. Carnegie
Communication	
The Articulate Executive	G. Toogood
The Gentle Art of Verbal Self-Defense	S. Elgin
How to Say It: Choice Words, Phrase, Sentences & Paragraphs for Every Situation	R. Maggio
The Elements of Style	W. Strunk
Designing Clinical Research	S. Hulley
Attitude and Motivation	
Aequanimitas and Way of Life	W. Osler
William Osler	C. Bryan
On Heroes, Hero Worship, and the Heroic in History	T. Carlyle
Selected Poems	W.C. Williams
Career Crisis	
Arrowsmith	S. Lewis
Finances	
Get a Financial Life: Personal Finance in Your Twenties and Thirties	B. Kobliner
Adding Color to Your Presentations	
Zebra Cards: An Aid to Obscure Diagnosis	J. Sotos
Classic Description of Disease	R. Major
Dictionary of Medical Eponyms	R. Edwards
Medical Meanings: A Glossary of Word Origins	W. Haubrich
The Medical Detectives	B. Roueché

For this reason, it is important that you acquire these skills by reading some of the books listed in Table 45-4.

UNDERSTANDING YOUR PATIENTS: NOVELS, PLAYS, AND POETRY The better you understand your patient, the more successful your rapport and the more applicable your management strategies will be. The problem is that it is difficult to truly

TABLE 45-5. Novels to Give Insight in Your Patients' Lives.

Book	Author
Substance Abuse	
The Lost Weekend	C. Jackson
Clockers	R. Price
Trainspotting	I. Welsh
Depression	
The Bell Jar	S. Plath
'Night Mother	M. Norman
Schizophrenia and Mental Illness	
Preparing for a Brief Descent into Hell	G. Lessing
A Beautiful Mind	S. Nasa
Zen and the Art of Motorcycle Maintenance	R. Pirsig
One Flew over the Cuckoo's Nest	K. Kesey
The Thantos Syndrome and The Second Coming	W. Percy
Chronic Diseases	
Death of Ivan Illyich	L. Tolstoy
The Problem of Pain	C.S. Lewis
How We Die	S. Nuland
Personal Triumph	
The Long Walk: The True Story of a Trek to Freedom	S. Rawicz
Night and Dawn	E. Wiesel
A Mass for the Dead	W. Gibson
A Day in The Life of Ivan Densiovich	A. Solheitzen
Homelessness	
Ironweed	W. Kennedy
Neurological Disorders	
The Man Who Mistook His Wife for a Hat	O. Sacks
The Doctor is Sick	A. Burgess
Life at the Bedside	
The English Patient	M. Ondaatjee
Love in the Time of Cholera	G. Marquez
Franny and Zooey	J.D. Salinger
Doctors, Their Power and Their Roles	
The Cider House Rules	J. Irving
Peyton Place	G. Metallious
The Plague	A. Camus
Books about Human Character	
Lord of the Flies	W. Golding
Lake Wobegon Days	G. Keillor
Winesburg Ohio	S. Anderson
Billy Budd	H. Melville

(Continued)

TABLE 45-5. Continued

Book	Author
A Separate Peace	J. Knowles
The Day of the Locust	N. West
Siddhartha and The Wall	H. Hess
Jude the Obscure	T. Hardy
Native Son	R. Wright
Crime and Punishment	F. Dostoyevsky
The Great Gatsby	F.S. Fitzgerald
The Fountainhead	A. Rand
The Catcher in the Rye	J.D. Salinger
The Wings of the Dove	H. James
The Magic Mountain	T. Mann
Cancer Ward	Solzhenitsyn
Fauste	Goethe
Conan Doyle's Tales of Medical Humanism and Values	A. Rodin
Catch-22	J. Heller
Slaughterhouse Five	K. Vonnegut
A Clockwork Orange	A. Burgess
Art in Medicine	
Medicine and the Artist	C. Zigrosser
Medicine: A Treasury of Art and Literature	Carmichael

understand your patient without having lived his life. Although it is no substitute for living a patient's life, the novel can give you insight into the lives of your patients. Table 45-5 has a list of novels (lives) commonly encountered in clinical medicine.

VI Great People: Bibliography and History

This shelf should include (Table 45-6):

A. **History books about your medical school, your hospital, and their famous physicians.** You are a part of something much grander than yourself; these books will show you the proud tradition that you now carry.

B. **Important times and physicians in medicine**

C. **Important philosophical books** (without requiring a degree in philosophy)

VII Journals

A. **Appropriate journal articles.** Reading the right articles may be tricky, because the journals you should read at the beginning of your

TABLE 45-6. Some Important History and Philosophy Books.

Book	Author
Books About Your Medical School, Your Hospital, and Their Famous Physicians	
Ask the local medical librarian for choices	
Important Times and Physicians in Medicine	
Guns, Germs and Steel	J. Diamond
Man and Microbes	A. Karlen
Mass Listeria	T. Dalrymple
Great Feuds in Medicine	H. Hellman
People's History of the United States	H. Zinn
Important Philosophical Books	
Six Great Ideas and Ten Philosophical Mistakes	M. Adler
Human, All Too Human	F. Nietzsche
The Blind Watchmaker and The Selfish Gene	R. Dawkins

career are not the journals you should read later. For now, focus on journals that explain difficult concepts and provide good general overviews of disease. Later, switch to journals with original articles that focus on the specifics of diagnosis and management of disease.

B. **Explanatory journals.** If you inform the publisher that you are a medical student, most are free.
   1. ***Mayo Clinic Proceedings*** (free for medical students). Focus on the concise review for physicians and the resident report section.
   2. ***Journal of the American Medical Association*** (JAMA). If you are a member of the American Medical Student Association (AMSA), this is free. Focus on the review articles.
   3. ***American Family Physician*** (free for medical students). This journal provides simple, high-yield reviews of common topics.
   4. ***Resident and Staff Physician.*** Free for medical students.

VIII File Cabinets

A. **Organization.** Label files by the table of contents of your favorite flesh book. Copy the table of contents and tape it to your file cabinet. This will save you time in filing new articles and even more time in finding articles you want to reference.

B. **Journal articles**
   1. **Do not file every journal article given to you.** The result will be stacks of articles you have never read; this will only remind you of how much you have not read, which will kill your motivation.

2. Instead, **file only those articles you find meaningful.** They should be articles that make sense to *you;* that is, articles you think will be worth referencing again in the future.
3. If you have a journal subscription, save the journals. At the end of the year, consider paying to have them bound into a book. Your school librarian has the address of the local bookbinder. This will remove all of the unwanted clutter (e.g., advertisements), making a three-foot stack into one book. Bind only the journals you are likely to reference in the future.

C. **Teaching files.** When you come across a great case, copy the admission note, OR report, ECGs, radiographs, and pathology pictures and file them. The day will soon come when you will be teaching students, and then you will want this material.

Appendix A. The Ten Equations

If you can master 10 simple equations, you can understand the physiology behind most diseases. As clinical problems present, use one or a combination of these equations to generate your differential diagnosis.

What's the big picture? At its simplest, medicine is about ensuring that the brain and vital tissues receive oxygen (Equations 1 to 7) and are able to eliminate waste (CO_2) from the body (Equation 8). Equations 9 and 10 address how the body manages fluid within compartments.

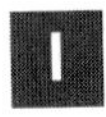

EQUATION 1. GETTING OXYGEN TO THE ALVEOL

The patient does not have enough oxygen.

$$PaO_2 = (760 - 47) \times FiO_2 - PaCO_2(1.25)$$

If the brain is not getting enough oxygen, the first step is to determine if the alveoli are getting enough oxygen.

A. The driving force of oxygen into the alveoli is barometric pressure (760 mm Hg). This is why it is harder to breathe at high altitudes, where atmospheric pressure is less.

B. Because the total pressure of a gas is the sum of all of the pressures of all of the gases in the mixture, you have to subtract the partial pressure of water vapor (47) in the alveoli. This is why it is harder to breath in a steam room than in a dry room.

C. Air is a combination of gases; only 21% of room air is oxygen. We are only concerned about the partial pressure of oxygen, so multiply the total pressure by 21%.

D. This is the amount of oxygen that could be in the alveoli. But oxygen shares the alveoli with CO_2: the more CO_2 there is in the alveoli, the less oxygen there is in the alveoli. CO_2 is freely permeable from the blood to the alveoli (even across water and fibrosis in the interstitial space); thus, we can estimate the pressure of CO_2 in the alveoli by measuring the CO_2 in the blood (arterial blood gas) and multiplying by 1.25. (Note that this is the same as dividing by 0.8, or the respiratory quotient.)

E. Importance: Equation 1 allows you to calculate how much oxygen pressure is in the alveoli (PaO_2). If you know the pressure of oxygen in the blood (via an arterial blood gas [PaO_2]), you can calculate the **A**lveolar to **a**rterial gradient (**A-a** gradient). This is important: **If the A-a gradient is high, the hypoxia is not a function of not having enough oxygen in the alveoli, it is a problem with something between the alveoli and the blood.** Equation 2 will help you with this second problem.

HOT 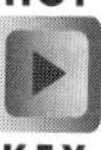 KEY

At room air $(760 - 47) \times 21\% = 150$. Always obtain blood gas values on room air, because this allows you to accurately assess the A-a gradient. Although every liter of supplemental O_2 increases the oxygen concentration by 3% (e.g., 4 L of oxygen by nasal cannula = 21% + 12% = 33%), you can never be sure just how much of this supplemental O_2 is being inspired.

II EQUATION 2. GETTING OXYGEN FROM THE ALVEOL TO THE BLOOD

What is impairing the flow of oxygen from the alveoli to the blood? Fick's law of diffusion of a gas across a membrane will give you the answer. Build your differential based on these categories.

$$\text{Diffusion} = \frac{\text{Pressure gradient} \times \text{Area}}{\text{Wall thickness}}$$

A. The A-a gradient is an example of a pressure gradient, described by the above equation. If the arterial oxygen is low and the A-a gradient is high, the only two remaining explanations are:

B. A decrease in **alveolar surface area.** Pneumonia, emphysema, alveolar hemorrhage, and aspiration all cause hypoxia by reducing the alveolar surface area.

C. An increase in the **interstitial wall thickness.** If the interstitium is thicker, less oxygen can pass from the alveoli to the blood. Pulmonary edema, ARDS, and interstitial lung disease (fibrosis) are causes of increased interstitial wall thickness. Use Equation 10 (see below) to understand why high pulmonary venous pressure from a failing heart or an increased permeability of sepsis (ARDS) causes more fluid to be pushed into the interstitium, increasing interstitial wall thickness.

D. Importance: Instead of memorizing the causes of hypoxia, use Equations 1 and 2 to generate your differential diagnosis and a method for solving the problem.

HOT 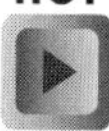 KEY

Hypoxia is not the same as dyspnea. When the patient says he is short of breath, he is saying he is dyspneic, which can be due to either low oxygen or high CO_2. Obtain an ABG and refer to Figure 10-4 to determine the cause.

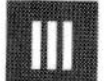 III EQUATION 3: DELIVERY OF OXYGEN

The oxygen in the blood is normal, it is just not being delivered to the brain.

$$DO_2 = \text{Cardiac output} \times (\text{Hgb} \times \text{Sat}\%)$$

A. Think of oxygen delivery to the brain as like a fruit delivery company trying to get fruit to its retail grocery stores. If the stores do not have enough fruit, it is due to:

1. Inadequate cardiac output (see Equation 4). The delivery trucks can't drive fast enough.
2. Inadequate hemoglobin. There are not enough trucks to deliver the fruit. This is why anemia causes weakness.
3. Inadequate oxygen saturation of the hemoglobin. Equations 1 and 2 explain the causes of inadequate oxygen in the blood. There are enough trucks and the trucks are driving fast enough; there is just not enough fruit per truck to satisfy the demands of the grocery stores.

EQUATION 4: CAUSES OF INADEQUATE CARDIAC OUTPUT Why are my trucks going so slow?

Cardiac output = Stroke volume × Heart rate

If the cardiac output is inadequate, it is due to one of the following:

A. Stroke volume. The amount of blood pushed forward with each pump is inadequate (see Equation 5).

B. The heart rate is inadequate.

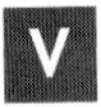

EQUATION 5: CAUSES OF INADEQUATE STROKE VOLUME

Stroke volume = Preload × Contractility

A. Preload. If there is no blood in the ventricle when it contracts, nothing will be pushed forward. The more volume there is, the greater is the volume that will be pushed forward with each stroke. Remember Starling's law: the greater the volume in the ventricle, the greater is the myocardial stretch, the greater is the ventricular recoil, and the greater is the contractile force. Causes of poor preload are dehydration, hemorrhage, third-spacing, and obstruction of blood flow into the left ventricle (diastolic heart failure from a stiff ventricle, pericardial disease, mitral stenosis).

B. Contractility. The stronger the contraction, the greater is the volume that will be pushed forward. A healthy heart pumps hard. Causes of poor contractility include ischemia, toxins (e.g., anthracyclines, cocaine), viral infections, and diseases that infiltrate the heart wall (e.g., amyloid).

C. Importance: When the brain does not get enough oxygen, the patient passes out (syncope). Solving syncope is easy: measure the hemoglobin and oxygen saturation (see Equation 3). If these are OK, there is a problem with cardiac output. Assess the pulse. If this is OK, there is a problem with stroke volume. Use your examination to assess the contractility and exclude valve obstruction to flow (see

Chapter 33). If these are OK there is a problem with preload. Give the patient IV fluids.

VI EQUATION 6: OHM'S LAW Why is my patient hypotensive?

Mean arterial pressure = Cardiac output × Systemic vascular resistance

This is Ohm's law: the pressure across a circuit (in this case, the arterial-venous circuit) is equal to the current times the resistance (P = IR). The mean arterial pressure determines the perfusion to the vital organs. It is composed of one-third of the systolic blood pressure and two-thirds of the diastolic blood pressure because the cardiac cycle is one-third systole and two-thirds diastole (at high heart rates, diastolic time is reduced: MAP = $^1/_3$ SBP + $^2/_3$ DBP). When a patient is hypotensive, use Equation 6 and the following method to discern the cause:

A. Feel the big toe. The hypotension is due to either inadequate cardiac output or inadequate systemic vascular resistance.
   1. If the toe is warm, a low SVR is usually the cause. The arterioles will have inappropriately dilated, allowing blood flow to go to the extremities, increasing skin warmth. Causes include sepsis, anaphylaxis, neurogenic shock, and hypothyroidism.
   2. If the toe is cool, a poor cardiac output is usually to blame. The body has compensated by constricting these vessels (increasing SVR) and reducing blood flow to the extremities.

B. If the big toe is cool, check the pulse (use Equations 4 and 5). If the heart rate is normal or high, heart rate is excluded as the cause of the hypotension.

C. With SVR and HR excluded, the only two possibilities are preload and contractility. Use your examination to assess preload (see Chapter 25: JVP, S_3, crackles) and contractility (see Chapter 31: PMI, S_1, S_3).

VII EQUATION VII. BALANCING OXYGEN DEMAND WITH OXYGEN SUPPLY How much is enough?

Metabolic needs of the tissues = CO × (Arterial content of O_2 − Venous content of O_2)

When the metabolic needs of the tissues increase (e.g., during exercise), the body compensates by increasing oxygen delivery. When oxygen demand exceeds supply, the body must compensate or tissues will die. How does the body compensate?

A. Increasing cardiac output. During exercise, the tissues need more oxygen. The heart rate increases to increase the supply (Equation 4).

B. Increasing oxygen extraction. The tissues extract more oxygen from the hemoglobin as the demand increases or as the cardiac output to the tissues decreases. It does this by recruiting more capillary beds and by shifting the oxygen dissociation curve so that more oxygen is removed from the hemoglobin. With more oxygen removed from the hemoglobin, the venous oxygen concentration will be less.

C. This is a trivial point until the body reaches the point at which it can no longer compensate for the discrepancy between oxygen demand and supply. At this point, cells die and so may the patient (see Figure 23-1).

1. If the delivery of oxygen decreases from point A to point B, nothing happens to the patient because he can compensate for the decline by extracting more oxygen from the blood.
2. If DO_2 further declines to point C, there is still no damage done: further compensation matches oxygen demand to oxygen supply.
3. Point C is where you come in. "C" is for **C**ritical point (as in **c**ritical **c**are). The patient cannot compensate for himself anymore: he needs your help to rematch supply to demand. If you do not help him, the patient will continue to point **D. D** is for **d**eath.

D. How do you prevent death? Either:

1. Increase oxygen delivery. Equation 3:
   - **a.** Increase saturation (Equations 1 and 2)
   - **b.** Increase hemoglobin. Transfuse blood.
   - **c.** Increase the cardiac output. (Equations 4 and 5)

E. This cadre of interventions—ventilators, transfusion, vasopressors, and antibiotics—are the key components of critical care medicine.

VIII EQUATION 8: MINUTE VENTILATION

After O_2 has made it to the cells and combines with glucose to create energy, how do I get rid of the CO_2?

$$\mathbf{PaCO_2 = CO_2\ produced - Minute\ ventilation}$$

(note that Minute ventilation = Respiratory rate × Tidal volume × [1 − deadspace%])

Like a bathtub that is too full, too much CO_2 is due to either too much being produced (too much faucet) or not enough being removed (too little drain). The drain is minute ventilation: the number of ventilations per minute. If your patient has too much CO_2 in her blood, follow this approach:

A. Is too much being produced? In the hospitalized patient, seizure is the only common cause. Treat the seizure, if present.

B. Assess the respiratory rate. If it is too low, correct the cause: naloxone for opiate overdose and mechanical ventilation for all other causes.

C. Assess the tidal volume. Remember that a percentage of tidal volume is dead-space ventilation, which is volume that remains in the mouth/

pharynx/trachea or goes to alveoli that are not perfused (normal is <30%).

1. Assess the rate and the depth of the patient's ventilation.
2. If the breaths are normal, the high CO_2 level is likely due to deadspace ventilation (which indicates an area of the lung where there is ventilation without perfusion). The most common cause of increased deadspace is emphysema, where air trapping increases alveolar pressure and reduces blood flow to the emphysematous parts of the lung.

IX Equation 9: Wall Tension

How does the body handle fluid in all of its chambers?

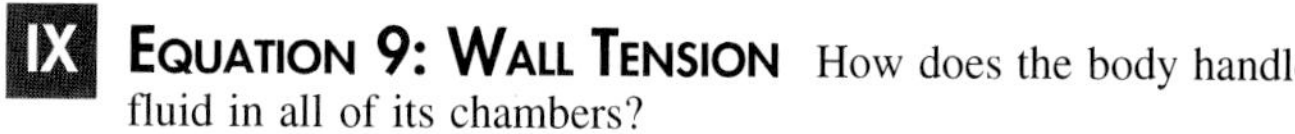

$$\textbf{Wall tension} = \frac{\textbf{Pressure} \times \textbf{radius}}{\textbf{Wall thickness}}$$

A. Wall tension is proportional to popping. A balloon pops under three conditions: when the pressure inside the balloon is high, when the radius is large, and when the balloon wall is thin. Chambers in the body pop under the same conditions. The body compensates by thickening the wall of the chamber. If pressure increases in a chamber, the wall of the chamber will thicken to decrease the wall tension, thereby reducing the risk of popping.

B. Example 1: Which is more urgent? A small bowel obstruction or a large bowel obstruction? The answer of course is the one that is going to pop the first. The small bowel has a thicker wall (relative to the bowel diameter) and a smaller radius than the large bowel. The large bowel will pop first. Medically manage the small bowel obstruction if you can; always obtain urgent surgical consultation on the large bowel obstruction.

C. Example 2: How does diabetes cause kidney disease, and how can I prevent it? Diabetes sugar-coats proteins making them bigger, stickier, and without their negative charge. These glycosylated end-products plug up the efferent arterioles of the kidney. This increases pressure in the glomerulus. The glomerulus will pop (increased wall tension) unless the mesangial cells hypertrophy (wall thickness) to offload the wall tension (crescentic glomerular sclerosis). The thickened glomerulus can no longer filter the blood, which leads to renal failure. ACE inhibitors preferentially dilate the efferent arteriole, decreasing the pressure at the glomerulus, thereby decreasing the impetus for thickening of the glomerular wall.

D. Example 3: Hypertension is the silent killer. How does it kill?

1. Stroke. Increased pressure = increased wall tension in the cerebral vessels—the vessels pop.
2. Heart disease. The increased arterial pressure increases the pressure in the left ventricle. The ventricle hypertrophies (increasing

wall thickness) to avoid popping as a result of the higher wall tension. The problem is solved, except there are now more muscle cells to feed, which increases the risk of myocardial infarction and may lead to poor relaxation of the heart (diastolic dysfunction).

3. Renal failure. Increased pressure at the glomerulus increases wall tension at the glomerulus. The glomerulus must hypertrophy to compensate for the wall tension or pop. It hypertrophies, and this decreases glomerular filtration, which leads to renal failure.

E. Example 4: When should I operate on an aortic aneurysm? The greater the radius of the aneurysm, the greater is the wall tension and the greater is the risk of popping. Operate when the aneurysm is >5 cm in radius. How do you medically manage until that time? Decrease the blood pressure to decrease the wall tension.

X EQUATION 10: FLUID MANAGEMENT

How do I approach fluid where fluid should not be?

$$\text{Fluid flow} = K[(P_{in} - P_{out}) - (\text{Oncotic } P_{in} - \text{Oncotic } P_{out})]$$

(where K = permeability constant and P = pressure)

There are many varieties of this problem: ascites, peripheral edema, pleural effusions, pericardial effusions, pulmonary edema, swollen joints; but they all have this in common. When faced with fluid where fluid should not be, use this equation to organize your thoughts. Increased fluid flow across a membrane is due to:

A. Increased pressure in the capillaries. Use the following method: start at the aortic root and work backward to the effusion. Any valve incompetence or stenosis will increase back-pressure; any failure of the pump or obstruction of the venous return to the heart will increase the venous pressure.

B. Decreased oncotic pressure in the veins. Think of the causes of low albumin (see Chapter 35).

C. Increased permeability. Common causes include inflammation (sprained ankle, infected joint, ARDS, hypothyroidism), anaphylaxis, or sepsis.

XI CONCLUSION

The field of medicine is too vast to memorize it all. Even if you could memorize every disease pattern, each patient is a different host and each disease looks different in different patients. Instead of memorizing facts, use the 10 equations to organize your thoughts and guide your therapy.

Appendix B. Common Procedures

Procedures are an essential part of taking care of a patient. This section provides an overview of the most common procedures a clinician is likely to perform as a student or house officer. Table B-1 describes some essential steps that apply to the majority of the procedures described in this section.

 Thoracentesis

A. **Definition:** removal of pleural fluid

B. **Indications**

1. **Diagnostic:** to determine the etiology of a pleural effusion
2. **Therapeutic:** to relieve dyspnea due to a pleural effusion

C. **Contraindications:** none

D. **Complications:** pneumothorax, hemothorax

E. **Before the procedure**

1. Obtain decubitus chest radiographs to confirm that fluid is free-flowing (i.e., forms a layer along the lateral chest wall) and is not loculated.
2. Consider ultrasound localization of the pleural fluid.

F. **Patient positioning:** seated at the edge of the bed, with arms resting on a bedside table

G. **Locating the point of entry**

1. Identify the highest point of the effusion by percussion and move one or two interspaces below.
2. Mark the skin at the superior aspect of the inferior rib of the interspace. Use a pen or the indentation of a needle hub.
3. Alternatively, mark the location of the pleural effusion with ultrasound guidance.

H. **Technique**

1. Clean the entry point with povidone-iodine solution.
2. Feel the lower rib of the interspace (i.e., inferior to the mark).
3. Anesthetize the skin at the mark with 1% lidocaine, using a 25-gauge needle.
4. Anesthetize the subcutaneous tissue and the periosteum of the rib (superior aspect), using a 22-gauge needle. Note that the planned trajectory is above the rib, avoiding the neurovascular bundle that courses *below* the rib.
5. Advance the needle over the rib, first withdrawing and then injecting anesthetic if there is no return of fluid. Appearance of pleural fluid in the syringe signifies entry into the pleural space (i.e., between the visceral and parietal pleura).

TABLE B-1. Essential Steps to Consider While Performing Procedures.

Before the Procedure

Obtain informed consent from the patient.

Inform the nurse of the procedure and enlist his or her assistance.

Prepare all equipment. An extra set of equipment is often helpful.

Remove your pager, stethoscope, and "lab" coat.

Comfortably position yourself and the patient.

Always wash your hands and observe universal precautions.

Wear a mask for all procedures.

After the Procedure

Dispose of all sharps in the sharps container.

Carry important or hard-to-obtain specimens to the laboratory yourself.

Write a procedure note, which should include the names of the operators (including supervisors); the procedure name and indication; a one-line description of the technique; complications and blood loss; and follow-up (e.g., chest radiograph pending, specimens sent to laboratory). Peripheral intravenous lines and arterial blood gas sampling generally do not require a procedure note.

6. Remove the needle, noting the site of insertion and trajectory.
7. Insert a 14- or 16-gauge catheter-over-needle apparatus along the same (anesthetized) path, carefully advancing over the rib.
8. Use the nondominant hand to stabilize the needle. Use the dominant hand to apply negative pressure to the syringe as you slowly advance.
9. With the return of pleural fluid into the syringe, stop advancing and withdraw 30 to 60 ml of fluid (for diagnostic studies) (Figure B-1.)
10. If therapeutic drainage is anticipated, advance the catheter-over-needle apparatus slightly further inward.
11. While maintaining the position of the syringe and needle with the dominant hand, use the nondominant hand to advance the catheter into the pleural space; then pull the needle out.
12. Quickly attach the end of the catheter to the extension tubing, which is then connected to vacuum drainage bottles. Alternatively, the catheter-over-needle apparatus can be attached to a three-way stopcock, initially opening to the syringe and then switching over to preattached extension tubing connected to vacuum drainage bottles (Figure B-2.)
13. Once all fluid is removed, remove the catheter and quickly apply a bandage.
14. Consider obtaining a chest radiograph, which is recommended to rule out a pneumothorax but is not always necessary if thora-

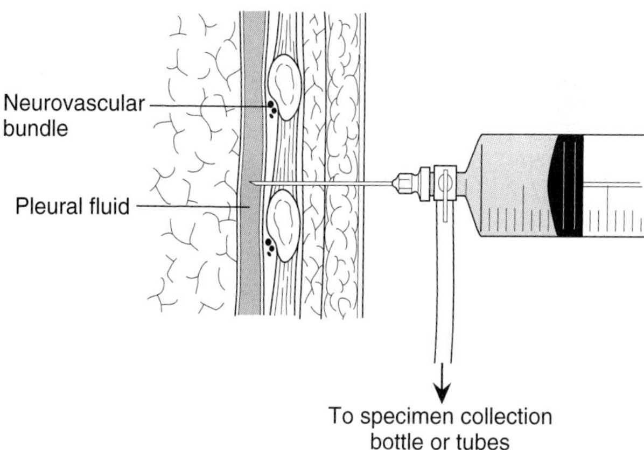

FIGURE B-1.

centesis has proceeded smoothly (i.e., without excessive pain or shortness of breath during fluid removal).

I. Fluid analysis

II Paracentesis

A. Definition: removal of peritoneal fluid

B. Indications

1. **Diagnostic:** to determine the cause of ascites, to diagnose or exclude peritonitis
2. **Therapeutic:** to relieve abdominal pain or dyspnea due to ascites

C. Contraindications: surgical scar or hernia at the site of needle entry. Note that **coagulopathy is not a contraindication.**

D. Complications

1. Bowel perforation, persistent leakage of peritoneal fluid, abdominal wall hematoma
2. Hypotension (after large-volume paracentesis)

E. Before the procedure

1. Have the patient empty her bladder; alternatively, insert a Foley catheter. (This step avoids the very rare complication of puncture of the bladder.)

F. Patient positioning: semi-recumbent

G. Locating the point of entry

1. Choose one of the following entry sites (the preferred site is not universally agreed on):

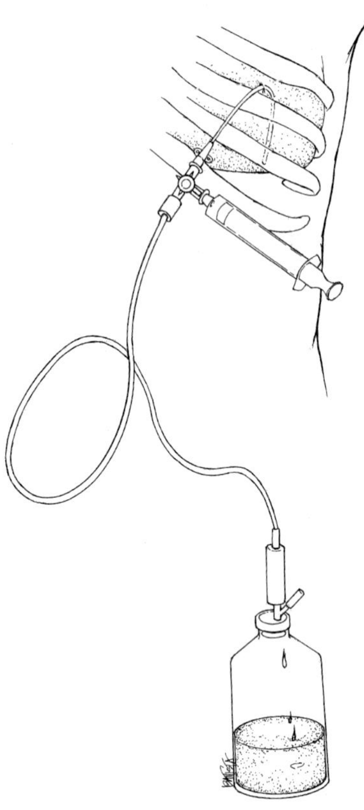

FIGURE B-2.

- **a.** At the midline, 2 to 3 cm below the umbilicus
- **b.** In either of the lower quadrants, lateral to the rectus abdominus muscle and below the level of the umbilicus (i.e., at the anterior superior iliac spine)

2. Localize the fluid by percussion or by ultrasound.

3. Mark the skin with a pen or the indentation of a needle hub.

H. Technique

1. Clean the entry site with povidone-iodine and apply the sterile drape.
2. Anesthetize the skin at the mark with 1% lidocaine, using a 25-gauge needle.
3. Inject additional anesthetic into the subcutaneous tissue and anterior abdominal wall.

4. Keep the needle perpendicular to the skin and aspirate before each advancement, both to avoid entry into a vessel and to detect peritoneal fluid (typically straw-colored).
5. With the return of peritoneal fluid, withdraw the needle, noting the site of insertion and trajectory.
6. Choose the needle for the next puncture.
   a. For **diagnostic paracentesis:** 22-gauge 1.5-inch needle attached to a 30-ml or 60-ml syringe
   b. For **therapeutic paracentesis:** 16-gauge catheter-over-needle apparatus (or 15-gauge multihole blunt needle with removable trocar) with an attached syringe
7. For large-volume (therapeutic) paracentesis, a "Z" technique is recommended. Before insertion, pull the skin 1 inch to the side and then insert the needle. (When the procedure is completed and the needle is withdrawn, the intact skin will slide back over the hole created in the abdominal wall, preventing a persistent track that can leak.)
8. Slowly advance the needle along the same track. Aspirate after each small advancement. If there is no fluid (or blood), release negative pressure on the syringe and advance further.
9. Withdraw 30 to 60 ml of peritoneal fluid into the syringe (for diagnostic studies).
10. After diagnostic paracentesis, withdraw the needle and apply a bandage.
11. For therapeutic paracentesis, use the nondominant hand to stabilize the catheter position and use the dominant hand to slowly pull back and remove the syringe and attached needle.
12. Quickly attach tubing to the end of the catheter.
13. Insert the needle attached at the other end of tubing into vacuum drainage bottles.
14. Drain up to 6 L of peritoneal fluid.
15. If fluid return decreases unexpectedly, gently manipulate the position of catheter, turn the patient, or both.
16. Once all fluid is removed, remove the catheter and apply a bandage.

I. Fluid analysis

III Lumbar Puncture

A. Definition: removal of cerebrospinal fluid (CSF)

B. Indications: diagnosis of various neurologic diseases (e.g., meningitis, subarachnoid hemorrhage, tertiary syphilis)

C. Contraindications

1. Infection at the site of lumbar puncture
2. Increased ICP secondary to a mass lesion
3. Coagulopathy or platelets <50,000/ml

D. Complications: postprocedure headache, local hematoma (rare), infection (rare), tonsillar herniation (rare)

E. Before the procedure

1. Rule out elevated ICP with funduscopic and neurologic examinations.
2. If papilledema or a focal neurologic deficit is present, obtain a CT scan of the brain to rule out a mass lesion.

F. Patient positioning

1. Lateral decubitus position, with the neck, back, hips, and knees all maximally flexed, putting the patient into the "fetal position."
2. Alternatively, the patient can be seated, leaning over a bedstand. With this technique, however, opening pressure measurements are not accurate.

G. Locating the point of entry

1. Find the intersection of a line formed by the spinous processes and a line formed between the superior iliac crests; this marks the L3-L4 interspace (Figure B-3).
2. Feel between the spinous processes for the site of entry, and mark the skin here with a pen or the indentation of a needle hub.

H. Technique

1. Clean the area with povidone-iodine solution (this is often provided in the lumbar puncture tray) and then apply the sterile drape.
2. Anesthetize the skin at the mark with 1% lidocaine, using a 25-gauge needle.
3. Anesthetize the subcutaneous tissues with 1% lidocaine, using a 22-gauge needle, injecting in the intended track of the lumbar

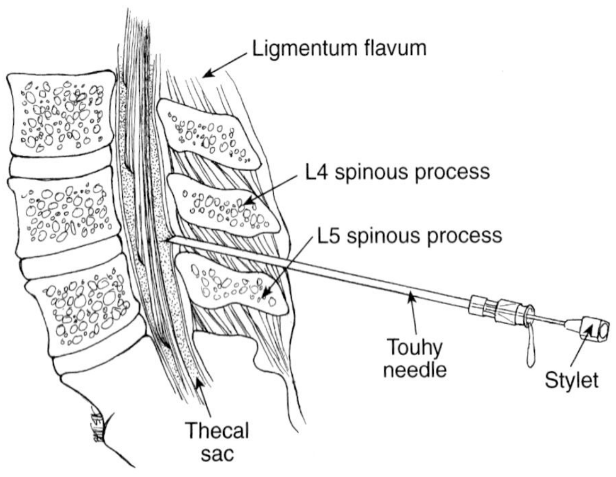

FIGURE B-3.

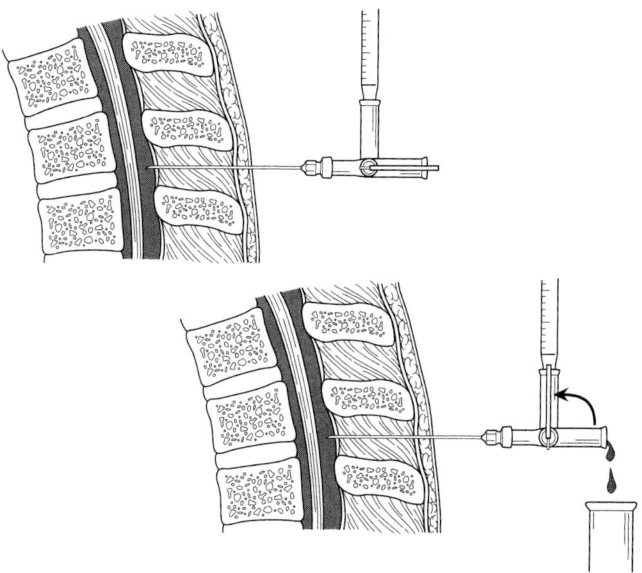

FIGURE B-4.

puncture (i.e., slightly toward the head and parallel to the midline).

4. Introduce the spinal needle (with the bevel upward, facing the ceiling) in the interspace along the same track.
5. Slowly advance the needle, frequently stopping to remove the stylet and check for the return of CSF.
6. If there is no CSF, replace the stylet and advance the needle slightly, then check again; a "pop" or giving-way is felt as the needle penetrates the dura.
7. With the return of fluid, attach the pressure manometer and measure the opening pressure. The patient must be relaxed and in the lateral decubitus position in order to obtain an accurate measurement.
8. Collect 2 to 3 ml in each of the four collecting tubes (Figure B-4, bottom).
9. Replace the stylet in the needle and withdraw the needle.
10. Apply a bandage over the entry site.

I. Fluid analysis

IV ARTHROCENTESIS

A. Definition: removal of synovial fluid from a joint

B. Indications

1. **Diagnostic:** to determine the etiology of a joint effusion or arthritis
2. **Therapeutic:** to drain large, hemorrhagic, or purulent effusions or inject medication into a joint

C. **Contraindications**
   1. Infection overlying the arthrocentesis site
   2. Prosthetic joint (procedure should be performed by an orthopedic surgeon)

D. **Complications:** septic joint (very rare), bleeding at injection site or into joint (very rare)

E. **Patient positioning (knee):** supine with the knee slightly flexed; place a roll under the knee

F. **Locating the point of entry (knee)**
   1. Confirm the presence of an effusion (ballottable patella, lateral or medial fluid bulge around the patella).
   2. The needle will be injected midway between the top (rostral) and bottom (caudal) of the patella, just under the inferior aspect of the patella (Figure B-5).

G. **Technique (knee)**
   1. *Optional:* Use sterile gloves instead of standard gloves.
   2. Clean the entry point with povidone-iodine solution.
   3. *Optional:* Anesthetize the entry site with 1% lidocaine.

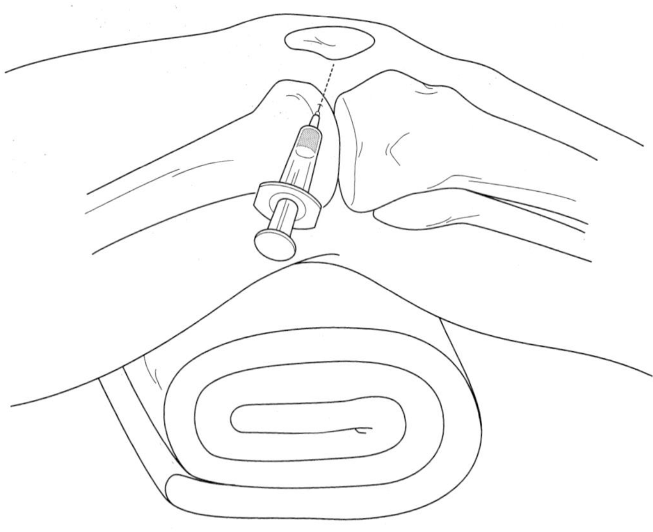

FIGURE B-5.

4. Advance a 1.5-inch, 18-gauge needle (attached to a 30- to 60-ml syringe) rapidly through the entry point, directed at the center of the joint.
5. Apply negative pressure on the syringe as you advance the needle.
6. Once synovial fluid enters the syringe, do not advance any further.
7. Stabilize the position of the needle with the nondominant hand and continue to withdraw fluid by applying negative pressure on the syringe with the dominant hand.
8. To attach another syringe to either withdraw more fluid or inject a medication, secure the position of the needle with a sterile hemostat.
   a. Remove the first syringe, and carefully attach a second syringe to the needle.
   b. Inject or withdraw.
9. Withdraw the needle and apply a bandage

H. Fluid analysis

V Central Line Placement (Femoral Line)

Note that femoral vein cannulation is the easiest central venous procedure to learn and perform. More often, internal jugular and subclavian vein cannulation are preferred; however, these procedures have a higher risk with different anatomic considerations and are not outlined here.

A. Definition: catheterization of the central venous circulation via the femoral vein

B. Indications

1. Administration of multiple intravenous medications or medications that require central venous delivery
2. Frequent blood draws
3. Inability to place a peripheral intravenous catheter

C. Contraindications

1. Overlying skin infection
2. Inability to leave a leg in the extended position

D. Complications

1. Arterial puncture with or without local hematoma
2. Retroperitoneal hemorrhage
3. Infection and thrombosis of the line

E. Patient positioning: recumbent

F. Locating the point of entry

1. Palpate the femoral pulse
2. Locate the point of entry into the femoral vein, 2 to 3 cm below the inguinal ligament and 1 cm medial to the femoral arterial pulsation (Figure B-6).
3. Alternatively may use bedside ultrasonographic localization of femoral artery and vein.

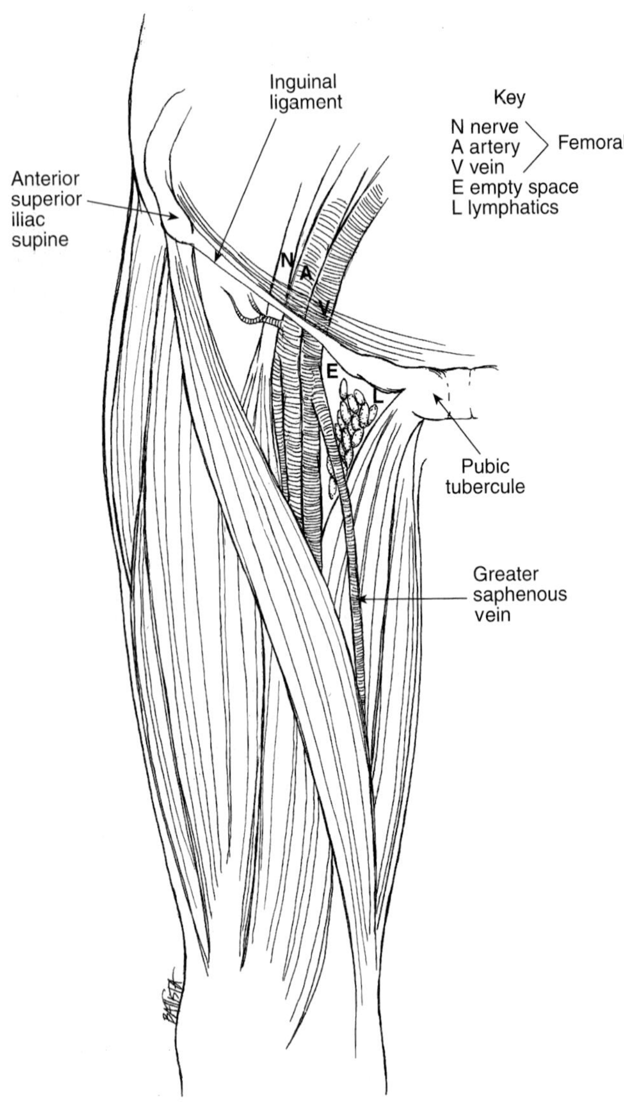
Inguinal
ligament
Key
N nerve
A artery
V vein
Femoral
E empty space
L lymphatics
Anterior
superior
iliac
supine
N
A
V
E
L
Pubic
tubercule
Greater
saphenous
vein

FIGURE B-6.

G. Technique

1. Sterilize the entry site and a wide field with chlorhexidine gluconate solution.
2. Anesthetize the overlying skin with 1% lidocaine using a 25-gauge needle.
3. Anesthetize the underlying subcutaneous tissue with 1% lidocaine using a 20-gauge needle.
4. With the nondominant hand palpating the femoral artery, use the dominant hand to insert a 18-gauge needle on a syringe at a 45-degree angle aiming cephalad and slightly medially (Figure B-7).
5. While applying negative pressure to the syringe, slowly advance the needle forward until blood enters the syringe.
6. If there is no blood return, slowly withdraw the needle, watching for a flash of blood that may occur if the vein was completely punctured on the first pass.
7. When good blood flow is achieved, maintain the position of the needle with the nondominant hand, which is braced on the patient's skin.
8. Lower the angle of the needle and aspirate to confirm good flow (i.e., that the needle remains in the vessel).

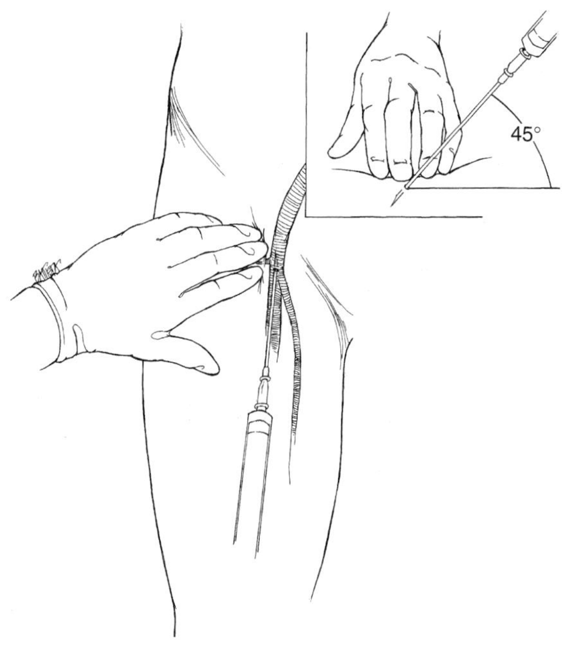

FIGURE B-7.

9. With the position of the needle secured with the nondominant hand, remove the syringe from the needle with the dominant hand.
10. Assess the flow of blood (via the needle), which should be dark and steady but not bright red or pulsatile (which would suggest femoral artery puncture).
11. Feed the guidewire through the needle. Be sure to have control of the guidewire at all times.
12. Remove the needle over the guidewire.
13. Make an incision in the skin at the entry of the guidewire. The scalpel should penetrate both the skin and the subcutaneous tissue.
14. Pass the dilator over the guidewire, dilating down to the subcutaneous tissue.
15. With the dominant hand, pass the triple-lumen catheter (distal port uncapped) over the guidewire.
16. When the end of the catheter nearly reaches the skin, advance the guidewire **backward,** until it just exits the distal port.
17. Grab this end of the guidewire, and then advance the entire catheter over the guidewire into the vein.
18. Remove the guidewire.
19. Aspirate blood from each port and flush with saline.
20. Sew the catheter into place and apply a sterile dressing.

VI Arterial Line Placement

A. **Definition:** introduction of catheter into the (radial) artery
B. **Indications**
   1. Continuous monitoring of heart rate and blood pressure
   2. Frequent arterial blood gas measurement
C. **Contraindication:** digital ischemia
D. **Complications**
   1. Hematoma at the insertion site
   2. Arterial pseudoaneurysm
   3. Thrombosis or infection of the arterial line
   4. Hand or digit ischemia or infarction
E. **Technique**
   1. Place a roll under the dorsal surface of the wrist, leaving it in dorsiflexion (i.e., hyperextended) (Figure B-8).
   2. Secure the fingers and forearm to an armboard.
   3. Localize the radial artery pulsation proximal to the wrist crease.
   4. Sterilize the entry site with povidone-iodine or chlorhexidine gluconate solution.
   5. *Optional:* Anesthetize the skin at the entry site with 1% lidocaine.
   6. Advance a 20-gauge catheter-over-needle apparatus at a 45-degree angle while gently palpating the radial artery proximal to the site of insertion (too much pressure will occlude the pulse).

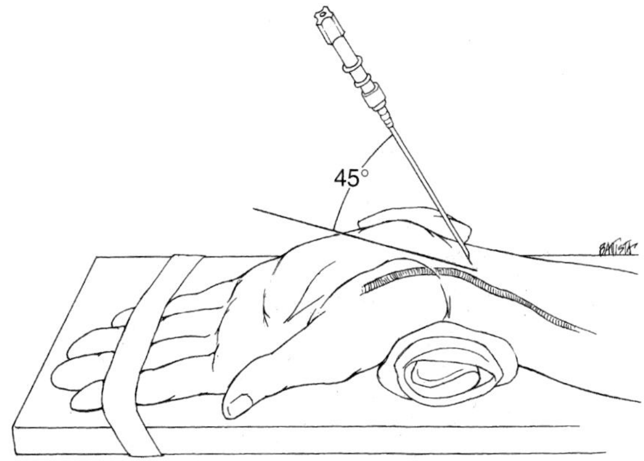

FIGURE B-8.

7. Stop when bright red blood appears in the hub of the needle; this signifies entry of the **needle** into the artery.
8. Slowly lower the entire apparatus, making a more acute angle with the skin.
9. Advance the entire apparatus approximately 2 mm; this places **the catheter,** as well as the needle, into the lumen of the artery.
10. While resting the dominant hand against the skin to stabilize the position of the needle (i.e., do not pull back on the needle), slowly advance the catheter with the nondominant hand until the hub is at the skin (Figure B-9).
11. With compression applied proximal to the catheter insertion site, remove the needle with the dominant hand.
12. Release compression; the return of pulsatile bright blood signifies the presence of successful arterial cannulation.
13. If there is no blood return, then the catheter is not within the artery lumen.
    a. Remove the catheter and apply pressure for 5 minutes.
    b. Repeat the process at a more proximal entry site.
14. Attach the catheter to the flush system and sensors, and check for an adequate arterial waveform on the monitor.
15. Secure the catheter with a suture and/or sterile dressing and remove the arm board.

VII Arterial Blood Gas

A. Definition: sampling of (radial) arterial blood

B. Indications

1. Measurement of pH

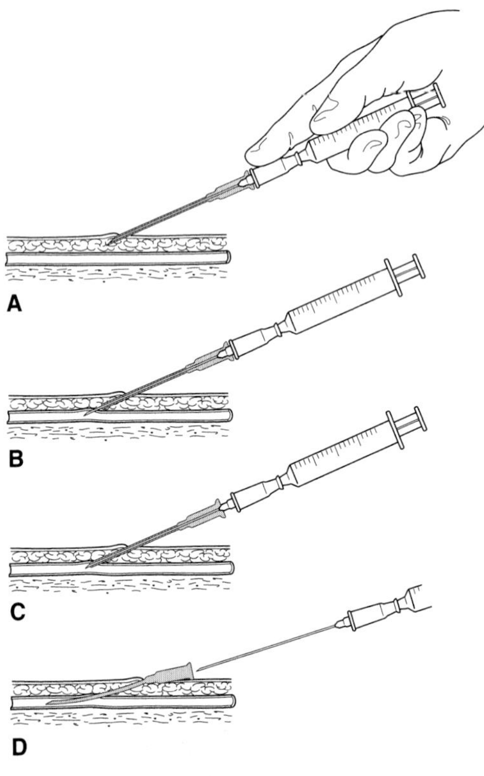

FIGURE B-9.

2. Measurement of partial pressures of oxygen and carbon dioxide (Po_2, Pco_2)
3. Assessment of methemoglobinemia and carboxyhemoglobinemia

C. **Contraindications:** none

D. **Complications:** insertion point hematoma, arterial thrombosis

E. **Patient positioning:** patient seated or recumbent with the wrist in a slightly hyperextended position

F. **Locating the point of entry:** Palpate the radial artery at the proximal wrist crease.

G. **Technique:**
1. Clean the overlying skin with an alcohol swab.
2. *Optional:* Anesthetize the skin with 1% lidocaine, using a 25-gauge needle.
3. Flush the blood gas needle and syringe with heparin, and leave 1 ml of air in the syringe.

4. With your nondominant hand lightly palpating the artery, enter the artery at a 45-egree angle. The return of briskly flowing bright red blood signifies arterial puncture.
5. Keep the needle in the same position, collecting 2 to 3 ml of blood.
6. Remove the needle, and quickly apply pressure.
7. Cover the puncture site with a bandage.
8. Remove the needle from the syringe.
9. Place a cap on the syringe.
10. Ensure that the specimen remains anaerobic by advancing the blood in the syringe up to the point of the cap.
11. Transport the sample immediately to the laboratory.

VIII Peripheral Intravenous Line

A. **Definition:** introduction of a catheter into a peripheral vein
B. **Indication:** administration of intravenous medications or fluids
C. **Contraindication:** infection overlying the insertion site
D. **Complications:** infection, bleeding, or hematoma
E. **Technique**
1. Locate the vein with inspection and palpation, preferably in the upper extremity at a point of vein bifurcation.
2. Apply a tourniquet proximal to insertion point, allowing the vein to engorge.
3. Clean the overlying skin at the puncture site with alcohol or chlorhexidine gluconate solution.
4. Apply slight pressure distal to the insertion site, securing the vein position.
5. Insert a 20-gauge catheter-over-needle apparatus into the vein at an acute angle (as flat as possible), with the bevel facing upward.
6. Stop when blood enters the flashback chamber.
7. Advance the apparatus 1 mm further into the vessel.
8. Maintain the position of the needle with the dominant hand.
9. Slowly advance the catheter into the lumen of the vessel with the nondominant hand.
10. Remove the tourniquet.
11. Withdraw the needle.
12. Quickly apply pressure to the vein proximal to the catheter, interrupting the return of blood.
13. Attach tubing and fluids to the catheter.
14. Apply a sterile dressing.

Appendix C. Commonly Used Abbreviations

3-0 silk (say three-oh silk) size and type of suture. Sizes in the format #-0 mean that the larger the number, the smaller is the suture. Rarely, you will encounter 0, 00, or even 000 suture. These are large sutures; the more 0s, the larger the suture.
4 × 4 pads 4-inch by 4-inch gauze pad
11-blade: type of scalpel blade. Numbers correspond to specific blade shapes.
A-a alveolar-to-arterial (gradient)
ABG arterial blood gas
ABI ankle-brachial index
Abx antibiotic
AC ssist-control (mode)
ACL anterior cruciate ligament
ALT alanine aminotransferase
ALS amyotrophic lateral sclerosis
AMA against medical advice
AMS altered mental status
ANA antinuclear antibody (test)
ARDS acute respiratory distress syndrome
ASD atrial septal defect
AST aspartate aminotransferase
A&P assessment and plan
BE base excess
bid twice daily
BM bowel movement
BMP basic metabolic panel (same as Chem 7) Na, K, Cl, HCO_3, BUN, Cr, glucose, and often Ca
BNP brain natriuretic peptide
BP blood pressure
BSOO bilateral salpingooopherectomy (that is both tubes and both ovaries)
BTP breakthrough pain. Pain med order to preempt pain with medication
BUN blood urea nitrogen
CBC complete blood count
C/C/E clubbing/cyanosis/edema
CHF congestive heart failure
CMP complete metabolic panel (same as Chem 10) same as BMP plus Ca, Mg, and P

CN I to XII cranial nerve I to XII
CNS central nervous system
c/o complains of
COPD chronic obstructive pulmonary disease
CP chest pain
CPR cardiopulmonary resuscitation
CREST calcinosis, Raynaud phenomenon, esophageal dysfunction, sclerodactyly, telangiectasia
C/S cesarean section
CSF cerebrospinal fluid
CT computed tomography
CTA clear to auscultation
CVP central venous pressure
CXR plain chest radiograph
D_5 5% dextrose solution
$D_{5 1/2}$NS c 20 meq KCL fluid order for D_5 water that contains 77 mEq of sodium and 20 mEq of potassium
DBP diastolic blood pressure
DIP distal interphalangeal (as in DIP joint)
DNI do not intubate
DNR do not resuscitate
DO_2 oxygen delivery
DVT deep venous thrombosis
EBL estimated blood loss
ECG electrocardiogram (also EKG)
EEG electroencephalogram
ELISA enzyme-linked immunosorbent assay
EOMI extraocular muscles intact
EtOH ethanol (recreationally or professionally)
ETT endotracheal tube
Ex lap exploratory laparotomy
f/c fevers/chills
F/E/N fluids/electrolytes/nutrition
FEV_1 forced expiratory volume in 1 second
FIO_2 fraction of inspired oxygen
Fr French (common catheter measurement, the bigger the number the bigger the diameter)
FVC forced vital capacity
ga gauge (sizing used for needles, the larger the gauge, the smaller the needle bore)
GABA γ-aminobutyric acid
GCS Glasgow Coma Scale
GETA general endotracheal anesthesia
GSW gunshot wound
HD hospital day
HIV human immunodeficiency virus
HMO health maintenance organization

HPI history of present illness
HR heart rate
IBW ideal body weight
ICF intracellular fluid
ICU intensive care unit
IHSS idiopathic hypertropic subaortic stenosis
INR International Normalized Ratio
I/O intake/output
IS incentive spirometry
IV intravenous
IVF intravenous fluids
JP drain Jackson-Pratt drain
JVP jugular venous pulsations
LAD lymphadenopathy
Lap Chole laparoscopic cholecystectomy
LCL lateral collateral ligament
L&D labor and delivery
LLQ left lower quadrant
LMP last menstrual period
LPN licensed practical nurse
LR lactated Ringer's solution
LUQ left upper quadrant
MAP mean arterial pressure
MAR medication administration record
MCL medial collateral ligament
MCP metacarpophalangeal (as in MCP joint)
mm Hg millimeters of mercury
MRI magnetic resonance imaging
MVC motor vehicle collision (or MVA: motor vehicle accident)
NABS normal active bowel sounds
NAD no apparent distress
NG nasogastric tube
NKDA no known drug allergies
NOS not otherwise specified
NP nurse practitioner
NPH normal pressure hydrocephalus
NPO nothing by mouth
NS normal saline
NSAID nonsteroidal antiinflammatory drug
NSR normal sinus rhythm
N/V nausea and vomiting
OB/GYN obstetrics and gynecology
OCD obsessive-compulsive disorder
OD oculus dextra
OR operating room
OS oculus sinister
OT occupational therapy

OTC over-the-counter
OU oculi unitas
PA physician's assistant
PaCO_2 partial pressure of arterial carbon dioxide
PACU postanesthesia care unit
PAO_2 partial pressure of alveolar oxygen
PaO_2 partial pressure of arterial oxygen, arterial oxygen tension
Pap Papanicoloau (test)
PCL posterior cruciate ligament
PCO_2 partial pressure of carbon dioxide
PDA personal digital assistant
PEEP positive end-expiratory pressure
PERRLA pupils equal, round, and reactive to light and accommodation
PIP proximal interphalangeal (as in PIP joint)
PMI point of maximal impulse
PO by mouth
PO_2 partial pressure of oxygen
POD postoperative day
PPD purified protein derivative (test)
PPO preferred provider organization
PRBC packed red blood cells
PRN as required
PRT pit recovery time
PS pressure support (mode)
PT physical therapy
PTSD posttraumatic stress disorder
PT/PTT prothrombin time/activated partial thromboplastin time
q every
RBC red blood cells
RLQ right lower quadrant
RN registered nurse
RPR rapid plasma reagin (test)
RR respiratory rate
RRR regular rate and rhythm
RTC return to clinic
RUQ right upper quadrant
SaO_2 oxygen saturation
SBP systolic blood pressure
SICA surgical intermediate care area (i.e., surgical stepdown unit)
SICU surgical intensive care unit
SIMV synchronized intermittent mechanical ventilation
SLE systemic lupus erythematosus
S/ND/NT soft/nondistended/nontender (as in S/ND/NT abdomen)
SOAP abbreviation for standard note format: subjective, objective, assessment, and plan
SOB shortness of breath

s/p status post (after)
SSRI selective serotonin reuptake inhibitors
SV stroke volume
SVR systemic vascular resistance
TAH total abdominal hysterectomy
TED antiembolism stocking
TIA transient ischemic attack
TM tympanic membrane
TPN total parenteral nutrition
T/S type and screen for blood products
TV tidal volume
U/A urinalysis
UOP urine output
U/S ultrasound
V/Q ventilation-perfusion
VS vital signs
WBC white blood cells
WNL within normal limits

Appendix D.

Name				#

History

PMH:

Meds:
1.
2.
3.
4.
5.
6.
7.
8.
9.
10.
11.
12.
13.

All:________ ETOH: ______/d Tob _____pk/yrs Drugs ______________

Physical Exam

Problems/Assessment

1)__________	2)__________	3)__________	4)__________	5)__________
* * * * *				

Day 1	Day 2	Day 3
Day 4	Day 5	Day 6

Date							
BP							
Pulse							
T max							
RR							
Sat %							
Weight							
HCT							
WBC							
PLT							
PT/INR							
PTT							
Na+							
K+							
Cl–							
HCO3–							
BUN							
Creat							
Gluc							
Trop							
AST							
ALT							
Alk. P							
T. bili							
UA							
Cultures							

Echo: ____ EF%

Cath: ____ LAD
____ RCA
____ Circ

CT:

Index

Page numbers set in *italics* denote figures; those followed by a t denote tables